Clinical Research Methods

in Speech-Language Pathology and Audiology

Second Edition

Clinical Research Methods

in Speech-Language Pathology and Audiology

Second Edition

David L. Irwin, PhD, CCC-SLP
Mary Pannbacker, PhD, CCC-SLP
Norman J. Lass, PhD

PLURAL
PUBLISHING
INC.

SAN DIEGO
OXFORD
MELBOURNE

MW

PLURAL PUBLISHING
INC.

5521 Ruffin Road
San Diego, CA 92123

e-mail: info@pluralpublishing.com
Web site: http://www.pluralpublishing.com

49 Bath Street
Abingdon, Oxfordshire OX14 1EA
United Kingdom

Typeset in 10½/13 Garamond by Flanagan's Publishing Services, Inc.
Printed in the United States of America by McNaughton & Gunn, Inc.

Library of Congress Cataloging-in-Publication Data

Irwin, David (David L.)
  Clinical research methods in speech-language pathology and audiology / David
Irwin, Mary Pannbacker, Norman J. Lass.—2nd ed.
       p. ; cm.
  Includes bibliographical references and index.
  ISBN-13: 978-1-59756-508-0 (alk. paper)
  ISBN-10: 1-59756-508-3 (alk. paper)
  I. Pannbacker, Mary H. II. Lass, Norman J. III. Title.
  [DNLM: 1. Biomedical Research—methods. 2. Audiology—methods. 3. Research
Design. 4. Speech-Language Pathology—methods. W 20.5]

  616.85'50072—dc23
                                                          2012042891

3/17/14

Contents

List of Tables

10 Multimethod Research

11 Reporting and Disseminating Research

12 Evaluating Tests and Treatments

13 **Evidence-Based Practice: Application of Research to Clinical Practice**

List of Figures

11 Reporting and Disseminating Research

12 Evaluating Tests and Treatments

13 Evidence-Based Practice: Application of Research to Clinical Practice

Preface

This book is intended for speech-language pathology and audiology students as well as practicing professionals who wish to learn more about conducting clinical research and its application to the professions. In line with the first edition of this text, more speech-language pathologists and audiologists are being asked to conduct more research due to increased interest in evidence-based practice and demands for accountability.

Revisions to the Second Edition

As with the first edition of this text, many of the chapters include a general orientation to research design and statistical analysis, followed by specific discussion of various types of research methods and conclude with a chapter focusing on the acquisition of research grants. Furthermore, the utilization of the discussion questions at the end of each chapter function as a guide to focus learning and prompt further inquiry for the reader.

Major changes for the second edition include the following: (1) the impact of HIPAA on research; (2) the use of social media for research; (3) a chronology of ethical misconduct with human subjects; (4) an update with the ASHA 2010 Code of Ethics focusing on research; and (5) new references for print and online information related to grants.

Acknowledgments/ Use of Royalties

The authors of this book thank the publishers who granted with a waiver or reduction in the fees to republish material in this book. Gratitude is extended for the late Dr. S. Singh who was instrumental in the idea for the overblending research and clinical activities. The second author of this book would like to extend sincere appreciation to David Duggar and Janice Morgan for their assistance with the preparation of this text. The third author would like to extend sincere appreciation to Georgia McClure for her assistance with this text. Royalties paid to the authors for this text will be donated to universities for the advancement of student scholarships. Royalty payments will be made to the University of Louisiana at Monroe Foundation, the Louisiana State University Health Sciences Foundation, and the West Virginia University Foundation.

David L. Irwin, PhD, CCC-SLP
Mary Pannbacker, PhD, CCC-SLP
Norman J. Lass, PhD

1

Introduction to Research

Upon completion of this chapter the reader will be able to:

- Discuss the importance of research to clinical practice
- Describe the historical evolution of research in the professions
- Briefly describe the sources of knowledge used in the professions
- Describe descriptive research including strengths and weaknesses
- Describe exploratory research including strengths and weaknesses
- Describe experimental research including strengths and weaknesses
- Describe survey research including strengths and weaknesses.

Introduction

The vitality and endurance of a profession are dependent on the quantity and quality of its ongoing research programs. The curricula of speech-language pathology and audiology programs traditionally have reserved the study of research methods and responsibilities for advanced graduate training. By that time, students may have developed an attitude of apprehension about research. Sometimes, these attitudes develop into sheer terror. Some academic advisors in programs having a thesis option rather than a requirement have difficulty persuading entering graduate students to consider pursuing a thesis project. By the time the students become informed and confident about doing research, they are so far along in their graduate programs that doing a thesis would delay graduation.

The purpose of this text is to remove the mystery surrounding research by teaching basic principles and providing practice in gathering and summarizing data. It is hoped that this information will be conveyed to students early in their training in an effort to increase the number of research projects conducted by speech-language pathology and audiology students. Once students have developed research skills under the direction of productive faculty, they are more likely to continue the practice as they move into varied professional settings.

Importance of Research in Communication Disorders

There are a number of reasons for doing research in communication sciences and disorders. Short-term or survival objectives for doing research include doing projects to complete one's education or to improve one's job security in an academic setting where tenure and promotion depend on research productivity.

More important reasons for doing research include contributing to the professional pool of knowledge about treatment of clients presenting a variety of communication disorders and maintaining quality clinical services while realizing a sense of professionalism by active involvement in learning through discovery. For the person who enjoys receiving professional recognition along with opportunity to be creative, satisfy curiosities, and engages in problem solving with a team of colleagues having similar interests, research provides numerous secondary rewards (Pannbacker & Middleton, 1991–1992).

A profession's image is readily enhanced by the integration of research along with the provision of clinical services. This has become more important with an increased emphasis on the use of *evidence-based practice*. Such practice increases professionalism, accountability to clients and other professionals, and the social relevance of the health services delivered in an economy with increased costs and decreased resources. *Clinical research* may readily integrate into the assessment, planning, intervention, and evaluation phases of clinical management (Portney & Watkins, 2009). Findley and DeLisa (1990) stress the importance of integrating clinical and research activities for the following reasons. The best clinicians and strongest research are providing clinical services and conducting research. Furthermore, staff training and awareness about new procedures and technology followed by improved client care are direct results. Both lead to the establishment of a rewarding, stimulating professional environment that contributes to improved staff recruitment and retention.

There is also an ethical reason for accepting the challenge of doing research. The speech-language pathologist or audiologist is frequently asked by clients or their relatives, "Does this treatment really work?" or "Is this hearing aid going to make a difference?" These questions are very difficult to answer ethically and truthfully without controlled research to substantiate an affirmative response. Ferketic (1993) stated, "We can't ignore the challenge to promote efficacy research. There are many questions to be answered. We all have something to offer and we need to work together to answer the questions. It's an opportunity to strengthen our professional credibility and viability" (p. 12). Collaboration between researchers and clinicians has been identified as a priority by the American Speech-Language-Hearing Foundation (ASHF) (http://www.ashfoundation.org) and the National Institute on Deafness and Other Communication Disorders (http://www.nidcd.nih.gov). According to Rao (2011), there is a resource for SLPs and AUDs about assessing and treating specific communication disorders (http://www.asha.org/members/ebp/compendium).

Distinguishing two terms at this point is important. In research, *efficacy* is the benefit of an intervention plan as compared to a control or standard program. This type of research lets us examine theory and draw generalizations to large populations. *Effectiveness* in research is defined as the benefits and use of the procedure under "real world" conditions. Effectiveness involves the expectation that when researchers apply treatments, they do so without being able to control

all circumstances (Portney & Watkins, 2000). Understanding the distinction and also the relationship between these two terms helps researchers ask answerable questions that meet the rigor of scientific methods and produce usable results.

Historical Evolution of Research in Communication Disorders

During the academic year, 1968 to 1969, Dr. Elaine Pagel Paden began to write a history of the American Speech-Language-Hearing Association (ASHA). In 1970, Paden authored a book which covered the years from 1925 to 1958. This is a summary of the early efforts by the membership to compile completed projects and continue research in speech disorders.

A small group interested in speech disorders met, beginning in 1919, at the annual meeting of the National Association of Teachers of Speech (NATS) and continuing until 1925. Lee Edward Travis reported a study in which he described the effects on phonatory pitch of stutterers and nonstutterers following the firing of a blank pistol at close range without warning. The teachers of public address (public speaking) in attendance were outraged at such inhumane treatment of subjects under investigation. Following this incident, it was decided that a separate organization for individuals interested in researching speech disorders should be established.

In December of 1925, the American Academy of Speech Correction was organized by 11 individuals, 5 men and 6 women. Conducting research about speech disorders was one of the three minimal requirements for membership. From the very beginning, the group emphasized the importance of a working, productive organization. The projects initially assigned to the membership were all research in nature. They included establishing the classifications and terminology for the field, summarizing thesis projects in progress, developing bibliographies on topics in speech correction, and investigating topics including stuttering, foreign accent problems, and phonetic description of "careless speech."

Realizing the need for a vehicle for publishing studies in speech correction, the group initially mimeographed 28 studies and made them available for $3.00 each. Having made money on the project, the group continued the practice. The *Journal of Speech Disorders* was established in 1935. The University of Illinois library has in its collection the early issues of this journal.

In the first issue of the new journal, published in 1936, three articles appeared covering the topics of foreign dialect, cleft palate, and stuttering. Also a bibliography covering speech, voice, and hearing disorders was included. Gradually, the journal became less devoted to news items and increasingly dedicated to quality scholarly content. The camaraderie and friendships established among the young energetic contributors with similar professional interests remained.

Eventually the *Journal of Speech Disorders* was renamed the *Journal of Speech and Hearing Disorders*. The majority of articles that appeared in the journal for the first 20 years covered topics on stuttering followed by articles on general topics and therapy and "audiometry." Also, between 1936 and 1949, the articles were more clinically oriented. In 1950, the journal's focus shifted to articles with a research orientation until 1957 when the reverse trend began.

With the explosion of submitted research, the *Journal of Speech and Hearing Research* (JSHR) began publication in 1958. This journal adopted a research orientation whereas the *Journal of Speech and Hearing Disorders* (JSHD) published research with clinical application. Because individuals working in school settings were interested in clinical applications and felt that neither journal served their needs, another ASHA journal, *Language, Speech, and Hearing Services in Schools* (LSHSS), began publication in 1970.

In an effort to increase the relevance of the ASHA journal program to all members, in 1990, the *Journal of Speech and Hearing Disorders* was divided into two separate publications and its title was discontinued. Two new journals were initiated. The *American Journal of Audiology: A Journal of Clinical Practice* and the *American Journal of Speech-Language Pathology: A Journal of Clinical Practice* were first published in the fall of 1991. With these changes, both audiologists and speech-language pathologists have subject-specific periodicals in which to publish clinical and experimental research. Supporting research by the ASHA will continue to evolve as the needs of the professions change. In 2004, ASHA took action to develop the Advisory Committee on Evidence-Based Practice (ACEBP). This committee has been charged to address several issues relative to EBP in communication disorders. According to Mullen (2005), ASHA has also established the National Center for Evidence-Based Practice in Communication Disorders (N-CEP). Mullen (2005) stated that ASHA "members will be introduced to the basic principles of

EBP and provided with the necessary support tools to assist them with integrating quality evidence into their practice" (p. 1). Duchan (2006) has developed a website that documents the history of speech-language pathology during the 19th and 20th centuries. The historical review contains numerous references and efforts of various fields on the evolution of research in speech-language pathology. These fields include phonetic studies, brain studies, technology, testing, and child study.

The American Academy of Audiology (AAA) was founded in January 1988 when a group of audiology leaders met. The purpose of the study group was to establish an independent freestanding national organization run by and for audiologists. The AAA published the first edition of the *Journal of the American Academy of Audiology* (JAAA) in 1990 (http://www.audiology.org).

Sources of Knowledge

Information used by clinicians and other types of researchers can come from a variety of sources. As consumers of research, we may accept some findings based on tradition, authority, trial and error, and logical reasoning (deductive and inductive). For a summary of these sources, one should consult Portney and Watkins (2009). Each of these sources of knowledge may be limited by a lack of empirical research principles, an unsystematic use of variables, lack of control for critical variables, or stifling of new knowledge and thought.

Research is conducted to answer questions, and it is an increasingly important component in speech-language pathology and audiology because both basic and clinical questions remain unanswered. In an effort to determine cause-and-effect relationships, researchers conscientiously apply scientific methodology to carefully control variables. Kerlinger (1973) defined the *scientific approach* as a systematic, empirical, controlled, and critical examination of hypothetical propositions about the association among natural phenomena. Portney and Watkins (2000) assert that the element of control is "the most important characteristic that sets the scientific method apart from the other sources of knowledge" (p. 11). It is important for any researcher to attempt to control factors that are directly related to the variables in question.

Lieske (1986) described the systematic study of a problem or question as a cyclical process beginning with an unanswered question followed by a clear statement of the problem, development of appropriate hypotheses, data collection, and finally interpretation of the information gathered in an effort to accept or reject hypotheses.

Portney and Watkins (2009) caution researchers that the scientific method may have limitations when applied to human behavior. Because humans are unique and capacities vary widely, there will always be some uncertainty regarding the interpretation and generalization of data. It is almost impossible to control for all variables in clinical research. This does not mean that clinicians should allow for less control, but rather that they should recognize that other variables may be happening that could influence results.

Types of Research

Classification of research into specific categories is not easy because there are a number of different research strategies. There is also a lack of agreement about these categories as well as overlap among the various types of research so that specific research projects may fit more than one classification (Schiavetti, Metz, & Orlikoff, 2011). Portney and Watkins (2009) view research on a continuum and describe the major categories: descriptive, exploratory, and experimental. Figure 1–1 shows how these types of research may be viewed along a continuum and that some share properties with all three categories (e.g., survey research) whereas others are specific to a particular category (e.g., randomized controlled trials).

Figure 1–1. A continuum of research. Adapted with permission from *Foundations of Clinical Research* (2nd ed.), by L. G. Portney and M. P. Watkins, 2000, p. 13, Upper Saddle River, NJ: Pearson Education. Copyright 2000 Pearson Education, Inc.

Descriptive Research

Descriptive research is designed to systemically describe situations or events as they naturally occur, in other words, the status of phenomena of interest as they currently exist (Polit & Beck, 2010). It is a type of research in which the distributions of selected dependent variables is observed and recorded (Hegde, 2003). Descriptive research is used to study group differences, developmental trends, and relationships among variables (Schiavetti, Metz, & Orlikoff, 2011). Sometimes this type of research is called normative or developmental research (Hegde, 2003). Developmental research that focuses on changes over time may be cross-sectional, longitudinal, or semilongitudinal (Maxwell & Satake, 2006; Portney & Watkins, 2009; Schiavetti, Metz, & Orlikoff, 2011; Shearer, 1982). Not all research is developmental in the maturational sense; it may be designed, for example, to study the course of progress for a pathology.

Cross-Sectional Research

Cross-sectional research involves selecting subjects from various age groups and observing differences between the behavior and characteristics of the group. This approach has several advantages: (1) it is less costly and less time consuming than longitudinal research and (2) it is relatively immune to subject attrition. The greatest disadvantage is the possibility that results could be attributable to biased selection of the cross-sectional groups. A variety of terms are used to describe cross-sectional research: disease, frequency, survey, and prevalence study (Rosenfeld, 1991).

Longitudinal Research

Many consider longitudinal research stronger than cross-sectional research because the same group of subjects is followed over time. This approach has the disadvantages of being expensive, time consuming, and vulnerable to subject attrition. Because of these problems, only a small number of subjects can be studied. Synonyms for longitudinal research include cohort study, follow-up study, incidence study, and perspective study (Rosenfeld, 1991).

Semilongitudinal Research

The semilongitudinal approach is a compromise designed to maximize the strengths and minimize the weaknesses of the cross-sectional and longitudinal approaches. This involves dividing the total age span to be studied into several overlapping age spans, selecting subjects whose ages are at the lower edge of each new age span, and following them until they reach the upper age of the span (Schiavetti, Metz,& Orlikoff, 2011; Shearer, 1982).

Historical Research

Historical research, sometimes referred to as archival or library research, is a type of research aimed at establishing facts and relationship about past events (Bordens & Abbott, 1988; Portney & Watkins, 2000). It may summarize a specific topic, sometimes in a type of review article entitled "State of the Art" or "Tutorial." Tutorial papers have been published about a variety of topics in communication disorders: facilitated communication (Duchan, 1993); and hearing loss, speech, and hearing aids (Van Tassell,

1993). Such papers are often written at the request of a journal editor who wants to present a summary from the viewpoint of a recognized scholar (Shearer, 1982).

Shearer (1982) pointed out that "nearly every example of published research contains a miniature library study as part of the introductory section that refers to related research. More extensive reviews of the literature commonly comprise the second chapter of theses and dissertations" (p. 17).

The following characteristics of historical research were identified by Isaac and Michael (1987):

1. Historical research depends on data observed by others rather than the investigator.
2. Historical research must be rigorous, systematic, and exhaustive. Much "research" claiming to be historical is an undisciplined collection of inappropriate, unreliable, or biased information.
3. Historical research depends on two kinds of data: primary sources where the author was a direct observer of the recorded event, and secondary sources where the author reports the observation of others and is one or more times removed from the original event.
4. Two basic forms of criticism weight the value of the data: external criticism, which asks, "Is the document or relic authentic?" and internal criticism, which asks, "If authentic, are the data accurate and relevant?" This critical evaluation of the data is what makes true historical research so vigorous—in many ways more demanding than experimental methods (p. 45).

Case Study Research

Case study research is an intensive study of the background, current status, or environmental interactions of an individual, group, institution, or community (Isaac & Michael, 1987). Most case studies are descriptive studies that examine relationships among different variables or trends over time (Maxwell & Satake, 2006; Polit & Beck, 2010.)

The primary strength of case study research is that it may be the only method available for studying some phenomena when few subjects are available or when financial restrictions preclude the use of other types of study (Schiavetti, Metz, & Orlikoff, 2002). In some instances, case studies should be considered pilot studies because they need to be combined with appropriate follow-up studies using larger numbers of subjects having the same phenomena and focusing on specific hypotheses (Isaac & Michael, 1987). Table 1–1 presents several case studies that been done in communication disorders.

On the other hand, case studies also have weaknesses. Because of their narrow focus on a few subjects, case studies are limited in their generalizability. Also case studies are vulnerable to subjective bias. This may happen because the subjects were selected because of dramatic or atypical attributes.

Secondary Analysis

Secondary analysis involves research that uses previously gathered data (Polit & Beck, 2010). It may involve examining unanalyzed variables, testing unexplored relationships, focusing on a specific subsample, or changing the unit of analysis.

Table 1–1. Examples of Case Studies in Communication Disorders

Author(s)	Topic
Apel & Masterson (2001)	Effects of an intensive group intervention focusing on spelling and oral reading.
Bauch, Olsen, Lynn, Radin, & Dale (1999)	Hearing sensitivity and acoustic reflexes following a nail gun accident
Friel-Patti, DesBarres, & Thibodeau (2001)	Outcome of the Fast ForWord program with children presenting language-learning disabilities
Guitar, Schaefer, Donahue-Kilburg, & Bond (1992)	Change in parent speech variables and in child's stuttering
Kent, Sufit, Rosenbek, Kent, Weismer, Martin, et al. (1991)	Speech intelligibility, pulmonary function, and voice functions for a woman with amyotrophic lateral sclerosis (ALS).
McGann & Paslawski (1991)	Communication devices with two patients with locked-in syndrome (LIS)
Ray (2002)	Phonological disorder of 5-year-old bilingual child
Williams (2000)	Different models of intervention for 10 children with moderate-to-profound phonological impairments
Wilson, Onslow, & Lincoln (2004)	Use of Lindcombe Program for Early Stuttering with 5 children using low-tech telehealth
Windsor, Doyle, & Siegel (1994)	Study of a woman with autism from age 10 to acquisition of spoken language to age 26.

Because secondary analysis uses existing data, it has the advantage of reducing time and cost. It has the disadvantage of little or no control over data collection (Hearst & Hulley, 1988). There is also the possibility the data are inaccurate.

Evaluation Research

Evaluation research involves collection and analysis of information related to the effects of a program, policy, or procedure (Hegde, 2003; Polit & Beck, 2010). Four types of evaluation research have been described in the literature: process or implementation evaluation, outcome and impact evaluation, cost-benefit analysis, and comprehensive evaluation. This type of research can be used to ensure compliance with quality assurance policies and third-party payors such as Medicare and Medicaid.

Process or implementation evaluation is designed to answer questions about the function of a program or policy (Polit & Beck, 2010). Typically, this type of research involves intensive examination of a program and often involves collection of both qualitative and quantities data gathered through interviews with clients and staff, observation of the program in operation, and analysis of records related to the program.

A process or implementation evaluation may focus on improving a new or ongoing program. Such an evaluation is sometimes referred to as a formative evaluation. In other instances, the evaluation may be designed primarily so that the program can be replicated by others (Polit & Hungler, 1999).

Outcome and impact evaluation is concerned with the effectiveness of a program. In other words, the purpose is to determine whether a program should be discontinued, replaced, modified, continued, or replicated. The evaluation may be referred to as a summative evaluation. An outcomes evaluation is fairly descriptive but does not utilize a vigorous experimental design (Polit & Beck, 2010). Such an evaluation documents the extent to which the goals of the program are achieved, the extent to which the goals of the program are achieved, and the extent to which positive outcomes result.

Impact evaluation is designed to identify the impact(s) of an intervention, in other words, the impact(s) that can be attributed to the intervention rather than to other factors. Polit and Hungler (1999) believe that impact evaluation usually involves "an experimental or quasi-experimental design, because the aim of such evaluations is to attribute a casual influence to the specific intervention" (p. 200). Hegde (1994) agrees to an extent because he feels that "in some ways, an impact evaluation resembles experimental research. However, in practice, appropriate experimental methods are not used in impact evaluation" (p. 101).

Evaluations that determine whether the benefits of the program outweigh the cost are referred to as cost-benefit analyses. Such analyses are often done in conjunction with impact evaluations (Polit & Beck 2010).

Evaluation research combines process and outcome-impact evaluations which were previously described. Hegde (2003) believes that comprehensive evaluation is the only truly useful type of evaluation research because the usefulness of process or impact evaluation is limited. A comprehensive model of evaluation, which includes multiple types of evaluation, was described by Isaac and Michael (1987) and is presented in Figure 1–2. The greatest problem with evaluation research is that it can be threatening to individuals. Even though the focus of evaluation research is on a program, procedure, or policy, people develop and implement the entity. Some people think they or their work are being evaluated. It can also be difficult to determine goals of the program (Polit & Beck, 2010). Often, the objectives of a program are multiple and diffuse.

Exploratory Research

An exploratory researcher examines how one event or events relate to other factors. Correlational research is used to determine possible relationships among factors (Portney & Watkins, 2009). Examples of correlational research include studying the role of home literacy practices and children's language and emergent literacy skills (Roberts, Jurgens, & Burchinal, 2005), frequency processing in listeners with hearing impairment (Healy, Kannabiran, & Bacon, 2005); and frequency discrimination and literacy skills for children with mild to moderate sensorineural hearing loss (Halliday & Bishop, 2005).

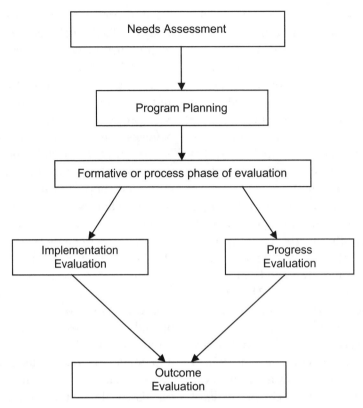

Figure 1–2. Comprehensive model of evaluation from needs assessment to outcome evaluation. From *Handbook in Research and Evaluation* (3rd ed.), by S. Issac and W. B. Michael, 1995, p 11, San Diego, CA: Edits Publishing. Copyright 1995 Edits Publishers. Reproduced with permission.

Correlational Research

Portney & Watkins (2000) state "predictive research studies are designed to predict a behavior or response based on the observed relationship between that behavior and other variables" (p. 278). For example, predictive studies can be used to study the scores achieved on standardized tests (e.g., Graduate Record Examination) and performance in a graduate program. Predictive research is being used more often in outcomes for making clinical decisions. For example, Daniels, McAdam, Brailey, and Foundas (1997) studied whether risk factors detected in the clinical examination approximated the videofluoroscopic swallow study in the identification of dysphagia severity. They studied six clinical features: dysphonia, dysarthria, abnormal volitional cough, abnormal gag reflex, cough after an oropharyngeal evaluation, and a clinical swallowing examination.

Case-Control Studies

Case-control studies are done when individuals are selected whether they have a particular disorder or not. Cases have the disorder or disease being studied and controls are chosen because they do not have the disorder or disease (Portney & Watkins, 2009). The researcher may utilize a variety of techniques including interviews, questionnaires, or chart review to determine why an individual may or may not have a disorder/disease based on exposure factors. A study by Tallal, Hirsch, Realpe-Bonilla, Miller, Brzustowicz, Bartlett, et al. (2001) conducted a case-control study in which the current language related ability of all biological, primary relatives (mother, father, siblings) or probands with specific language impairment and compared them to matched controls.

Portney and Watkins (2000) suggest that "one advantage of case-control design is that samples are relatively easy to gather. Therefore, case-control studies are useful for studying disorders that are relatively rare, because they start by finding cases in a systematic manner" (p. 325). Case-control studies are typically done for diseases or disorders that have a long latency period.

Cohort Studies

A cohort study is where the "researcher selects a group of subjects who do not yet have the outcome of interest and follows them to see if they develop the disorder" (Portney & Watkins, 2000, p. 328). Cohort studies allow the researcher to follow the temporal sequence of factors that may have impacted the development of a disorder. Grievink, Peters, van Bon, and Schilder (1993) examined the relationship between early otitis media with effusion (OME) and later language ability in a group of children systematically documented with bilateral OME. The children in this study received tympanometry every 3 months, between the ages of 2 and 4, and at age 7, three groups participated in language-testing.

Cohort studies can be either prospective or retrospective. If a researcher determines that subjects have already been exposed to risk factors, then the study would be retrospective. If the researcher contacts the subjects before they develop the disorder, but after exposure to risk factors, then it would be prospective (Portney & Watkins, 2000).

Experimental Research

In experimental research, the independent variable is controlled to measure its effect on the dependent variables (Shearer, 1982). In other words, experimental research is used to examine possible cause-and-effect relationships by exposing one or more experimental groups to one or more conditions and comparing the results to one or more control groups (Isaac & Michael, 1987). This type of research has also been referred to as the cause-and-effect method, the pretest-posttest control group design, and the laboratory method (Leedy, 1989). The distinguishing feature of experimental research is the experiment and control of the main variables; other types of research do not involve an experiment (Hegde, 2003; Shearer, 1982). Experimental research is considered by many to be the best or most powerful research design, but it is not the only acceptable type of research (Hegde, 2003; Ottenbacher, 1990; Portney & Watkins, 2009). Shearer (1982) points out that the most appropriate type "of research is the one that best fits the problem and the situations available" (p. 10).

The three characteristics of experimental research described by Polit and Hungler (1999) were: (1) "manipulation —the experimenter does something to at least some of the subjects in the study; (2) control—the experimenter introduces one or more control over the experimental situation, including the use of a control group and (3) randomization—the experimenter assigns subjects to a control or experimental group on a random basis" (p. 152).

Isaac and Michael (1987) have outlined the steps in experimental research (Table 1–2). This outline is useful in understanding experimental research and knowing the procedures that a researcher might utilize.

Hegde (2003) stated, "the strengths of experimental research are the strengths of science itself" (p. 170). It is the most appropriate method for testing hypotheses of cause-and-effect relationships between variables. Experimental research offers greater corroboration than any other type of research in that if the independent variable is manipulated in a certain way, then certain consequences in the dependent variable may be expected to ensue.

Experimental research has several weaknesses. First, there are many situations in which experimental research cannot be conducted because of ethical or practical considerations (Polit & Beck,

Table 1–2. Seven Steps in Experimental Research

1. Survey the literature relating to the problem.
2. Identify and define the problem.
3. Formulate a problem hypothesis, deducing the consequences and defining basic terms and variables.
4. Construct an experimental plan.
a. Identify all nonexperimental variables that might contaminate the experiment, and determine how to control them.
b. Select a research design.
c. Select a sample of subjects to represent a given population, assign subjects to groups, and assign experimental treatment to groups.
d. Select or construct and validate instruments to measure the outcome of the experiment.
e. Outline procedures for collecting the data, and possible conduct a pilot or "trial run" test to perfect the instruments or design.
f. State the statistical or null hypothesis.
5. Conduct the experiments.
6. Reduce the raw data in a manner that will produce the best appraisal of the effect which is presumed to exist.
7. Apply an appropriate test of significance to determine the confidence one can place on the results of the study.

Source: From *Understanding Educational Research* (Rev. ed.), by D. B. Van Dalen and W. J. Meyer, 1966, New York, NY: McGraw-Hill. Copyright 1966 by McGraw-Hill. Reproduced with permission of The McGraw-Hill Companies.

2010; Portney & Watkins, 2009). Another problem with experimental research is the Hawthorne effect. This refers to the effect on the dependent variable caused by changes in subjects' behavior because they know they are participating in a study (Huck, Cormier, & Bounds, 1974; Portney & Watkins, 2000). Despite problems inherent in research, Hegde (2003) believes none of the "weaknesses of experimental research seem to be valid" (p. 169).

Randomized Controlled Trial

The basic structure of an experiment involves the pretest-posttest design (Portney & Watkins, 2009). Some researchers (Portney & Watkins, 2009) regard the "gold standard" for clinical research to include the randomized controlled trial (RCT). This involves the experimental group receiving the variable of interest and the control group not receiving any form of treatment. Measuring the differences between the two groups, with all other factors being equal or constant, are due to the impact of the experimental variable. In RCT, the assignment of subjects to groups is randomized. An example for the use of RCT by speech-language pathologists includes Roy, Weinrich, Gray, Tanner, Stemple, and Sapienza (2003) who studied three treatments for teachers with voice disorders. Cohen, Hodson, O'Hare, Boyle, Durrani, McCartney, et al. (2005) used RCT when studying 77 children between the ages 6 to 10 and the effects of computer-based intervention through acoustically modified speech (i.e., Fast ForWord; Scientific Learning Corporation, 1998). Portney and Watkins (2009) assert that this design is strong in internal validity and selection bias can be controlled through random assignment of subjects.

Quasiexperimental

Variations of "true" experimental research are considered quasiexperimental because they have the same degree of experimental control or inferential confidence (Ottenbacher, 1990). This type of research is sometimes referred to as pseudoexperimental or pre-experimental (Huck, Cormier, & Bounds (1974). Quasiexperimental research, like experimental research, involves manipulation of an independent variable but does not have a comparison group or randomization (Polit & Beck, 2010). The two characteristics of quasiexperimental research identified by Isaac & Michael (1987) are: "(1) quasiexperimental typically involves applied setting where it is not possible to control all the relevant variables but only some of them; and (2) the distinction between true and quasiexperimental research is tenuous, particularly where human subjects are involved" (p. 54).

Sequential Clinical Trials

The use of sequential clinical trials (SCTs) addresses two concerns often seen with experimental designs. First, SCT does not require a fixed sample size before the study can begin. Subjects can be added to the study as they become available or develop a disease. Second, SCT allows for the analysis of data to occur when the subject has completed the trial. Other forms of experimental research require the collection of the data from the entire sample before data analysis begins (Portney & Watkins, 2009). The use of SCTs has application to the field of speech-language pathology and audiology because it allows for the comparison of a "new" treatment to an "old" treatment. This may address the ethical concerns of true experimental designs being used in clinical research.

Single-Subject Designs

Single-subject designs focus on the behavior of one or a few subjects. These designs are also referred to as applied behavioral analysis designs or behavioral analysis, idiographic designs, single-subject experimental designs, single-case designs, intrasubject replication designs, small N-approach, and within-subjects designs.

It is misleading to consider any design that uses one or a few subjects as a single-subject design. Designs that use single subjects also can be classified as case studies or single-subject designs (Warren, 1986). Single-subject designs are experimental designs that attempt to establish cause-and-effect relationships (Hegde, 2003).

Meta-Analysis

Meta-analysis is similar to secondary analysis because it also uses previously gathered data. In meta-analysis, statistical techniques are used to compare results across previous studies (Bordens & Abbott, 1988; Cooper, 1993). Meta-analysis by speech-language pathologists and audiologists has included various topics such as clinical outcomes in the treatment of aphasia (Robey, 1998), the efficacy of treatment for children with developmental speech and language delay/disorder (Law, Garrett, & Nye, 2004) and otitis media and language development (Casby, 2001).

Meta-analysis provides a method for integrating and synthesizing research studies and theory development. It involves: (1) identification of relevant variables, (2) location of relevant research to review, and (3) conducting the metaanalysis (i.e., comparing or combining results across studies) (Bordens & Abbott, 1988). Cooper (1993) identified several problems in meta-analysis including publication bias, missing information, reliability, independent effect sizes, correlated moderators, and interpreting effect sizes.

Survey Research

Survey research can be used with descriptive, exploratory, and experimental research. Survey research, which is often called sample survey, is designed to provide a detailed inspection of the prevalence of conditions, practices, or attitudes in a given environment by asking people about them rather than observing them directly. Surveys can be classified by the method by which data are obtained: controlled observation, mail questionnaire, panel, personal interview questionnaires, and telephone interviews (Kerlinger, 1973). The most powerful type of survey data is collected through personal interview (Polit & Beck, 2010). This method has the advantage of encouraging subject cooperation, which results in good response rates and a better quality of data (Polit & Beck, 2010). Table 1–3 gives several other advantages. Personal interviews, however, have limitations: they are rather costly and considerable time is required to conduct the interviews. A variety of formats is used for questionnaires: fill in the blank, multiple choice, true/false, and selecting a number to indicate strength of agreement or disagreement with a specific term (Johnson, 1991). There are a variety of methods which can be used to distribute surveys including the Internet (e.g., http://www.survey

Table 1–3. Comparison of Personal Interviews and Questionnaires

Advantages of Personal Interviews	Advantages of Questionnaires
Clarity: Clarify questions; avoid problems of illiteracy.	Economy: Self-administration reduces staff time.
Complexity: Obtain more complex answers and observations about respondent's appearance and behavior.	Standardization: Written instruction reduces biases from difference in administration or from interactions with interviewer.
Completeness: Minimize omission and inappropriate responses.	Anonymity: Privacy encourages candid, honest answers to sensitive questions.
Control: Order sequence of questions.	

Sources: From "Planning the Measurements in a Questionnaire," by S. R. Cummings, W. Strull, M. C., Nevitt, and S. B. Hulley. In S. P. Hulley and S. R. Cummings (Eds.), *Designing Clinical Research*, 1988, p. 43, Baltimore, MD: Williams & Wilkins, with permission. Copyright 1988 Williams and Wilkins. Reprinted with permission.

monkey.com), Facebook (http://www.facebook.com), direct E-mail, "snail" mail, and telephone. The most important component of any survey, regardless of how it is distributed, is the response rate. High response rates are important for at least three reasons: (1) they increase sample size and statistical power, (2) they tend to produce a more representative sample, and (3) they reduce wasted time and materials (Dodd, Bosell, & Litwin, 1988). A response rate of 50% is considered adequate, a response rate of at least 60% is considered good, and a response rate of 70% or more is very good (Babbie, 1973). Shewan (1986) suggests pretesting questionnaires so that potential problems can be identified prior to disseminating them. Answers to the following questions are requested:

1. How long did it take you to complete the questionnaire?
2. Did you understand the instructions? What, if anything, was unclear?
3. Did you ever feel forced to make a choice that didn't fit your particular situation? If so, on which question(s) and why?
4. Were the questions reasonable and appropriate? How, in your judgment, could the questions be improved?

A cover letter should accompany all questionnaires (electronic or paper) briefly explaining the purpose of the survey, conveying researcher's thanks and appreciation for the reply, that the survey has been approved by the appropriate committee or advisor, and offering to provide a summary of the results. Contact information for the researcher should be listed such as telephone number, E-mail, and fax number. A self-addressed envelope should be enclosed for paper questionnaires. There are several resources for conducting surveys (Dillman, 1978; Groves, 1989; Portney & Watkins, 2009).

Surveys have been used to study a variety of topics in speech-language pathology and audiology. Garcia, Chambers, and Molander (2005) surveyed the practice patterns of speech-language pathologists in their use of thickened liquids. Zipoli and Kennedy (2005) utilized a questionnaire to examine attitudes of 240 speech-language pathologists toward and use of research and evidence-based practice. Hoffman, Yorkston, Shumway-Cook, Ciol, Dudgeon, and Chan (2005) utilized the results from a Medicare Current Beneficiary Survey to determine how many respondents over 65 years of age were categorized by level of communication disability.

The use of surveys makes it possible to obtain a great deal of information from a large population (Kerlinger, 1973). They are also economical because of the amount and quality of information they yield. Surveys, however, have a number of weaknesses. First, survey research tends to be relatively superficial; in other words, it does not usually penetrate much below the surface (Kerlinger, 1973; Portney & Watkins, 2000). Second, survey research does not permit cause-andeffect conclusions because of a lack of experimental manipulations (Hegde, 2003; Portney & Watkins, 2000). A third weakness is that surveys tend to be demanding of time and other resources and tend to focus on "soft" (i.e., opinions) dependent variables (Hegde, 2003).

Summary

This chapter has provided an introduction to the research process, historical overview of how it evolved during the early years of the professions, reviewing various sources of knowledge when making clinical decisions, and an overview of the scientific method and various types of research. It is important for all readers to understand that this chapter is not complete and exhaustive of all aspects related to research. In subsequent chapters, more information is discussed in greater detail. Although many research projects ask very important and viable questions, it is important to remember: The best research project is one that is done and properly disseminated. Subsequent chapters are designed to guide students through this process so that they can complete a research project that adheres to standards and answers important questions for the professions of speech-language pathology and audiology.

DISCUSSION QUESTIONS

1. What might be personal, professional, and ethical reasons to conduct research?
2. Differentiate between efficacy and effectiveness. What is used in speech-language pathology and audiology?
3. How did research evolve in the speech-language pathology and audiology professions?
4. What are some sources of knowledge? What might be some problems with these sources?

5. Describe the scientific method. Why is the issue of experimental control difficult for some studies in clinical practice?

6. What are three major types of research? How can these be viewed along a continuum?

7. What is developmental research?

8. Compare cross-sectional, longitudinal, and semilongitudinal research.

9. What are some problems with doing historical research? How might these problems be controlled or resolved?

10. Under what circumstances do researchers tend to use case studies?

11. What are some types of evaluation research? Why might this research be difficult to conduct?

12. Give some examples of exploratory research in speech-language pathology and audiology?

13. What has ASHA done to collect more data using EBP?

14. Compare case-control and cohort studies.

15. What is the distinguishing aspect of experimental research according to Portney and Watkins (2000)?

16. What is considered the "gold standard" for experimental research? Why?

17. Why might sequential clinical trials be valuable to a researcher involved in clinical practice for speech-language pathology or audiology?

18. What are some advantages and weaknesses of meta-analysis?

19. Surveys can be in various formats. Describe the pros and cons of each format.

20. What is considered an "adequate," "good," and "very good" response rate to a survey?

21. Describe why a questionnaire should be tested with some subjects prior to dissemination.

22. What are some weaknesses associated with surveys?

References

Apel, K., & Masterson, J. J. (2001). Theory-guided spelling assessment and intervention: A case study. *Language, Speech, and Hearing Services in the Schools, 32*(3), 182–195.

Babbie, E. R. (1973). *Survey research methods.* Belmont, CA: Wadsworth.

Bauch, C. D., Olsen, W. O., Lynn, S. G., Reading, C. C., & Dale, A. J. (1999). Penetrating injury to the brainstem after a nail gun accident: A case study. *American Journal of Audiology, 8*(1), 57–64.

Bordens, K. S., & Abbott, B. B. (1988). *Research designs and methods.* Mountain View, CA: Mayfield.

Casby, M. W. (2001). Otitis media and language development: A meta-analysis. *American Journal of Speech-Language Pathology, 10*(1), 65–80.

Cohen, W., Hodson, A., O'Hare, A., Boyle, J., Durrant, T., McCartney, E., Mattey, M., & Naftalin, L. (2005). Effects of computer-based intervention throughout acoustically modified speech (Fast ForWord) in severe mixed receptive expressive language impairment: Outcomes from a randomized controlled trial. *Journal of*

Speech, Language, and Hearing Research, *48*(3), 715–729.

Cooper, H. (1993). Children and hospitalization: Putting the new reviews in methodological context. *Developmental and Behavioral Pediatrics, 14*(1), 45–49.

Cummings, S. R., Strull, W., Nevitt, M. C., & Hulley, S. P., (1988). In S. P. Hulley & S. R. Cummings (Eds.), *Designing clinical research* (p. 43). Baltimore, MD: Williams & Wilkins.

Daniels, S. K., McAdam, C. P., Brailey, K., & Foundas A. L. (1997). Clinical assessment of swallowing and prediction of dysphagia severity. *American Journal of Speech-Language Pathology, 6*(4), 17–24.

Dillman, D. (1978). *Mail and telephone surveys: The total design method.* New York, NY: John Wiley.

Dodd, D. K., Boswell, D. L., & Litwin, W. J. (1988). Survey response rate as a function of number of signatures, signatures ink color, and postscript on covering letter. *Psychological Reports, 63,* 538.

Duchan, J. F. (1993). Issues raised by facilitated communication for theorizing research on autism. *Journal of Speech and Hearing Research, 36*(6), 1108–1119.

Duchan, J. F. (2006). *Judith Duchan's short history of speech pathology.* Retrieved from http://www.acsu.buffalo.edu/~duchan/new_history/hist19c/science.html

Ferketic, M. (1993). Professional practices perspective on efficacy. *Asha, 35*(1), 12.

Findley, T. W., & DeLisa, J. A. (1990). Research in physical medicine and rehabilitation XI: Research training: Setting the stage for lifelong learning. *American Journal of Physical Medicine and Rehabilitation, 68*(5), 240–251.

Friel-Patti, S., DesBarres, K., & Thibodeau, L. (2001). Case studies of children using Fast For Word. *American Journal of Speech-Language Pathology, 10*(3), 203–215.

Garcia, J. M., Chambers IV, E., & Molander, M. (2005). Thickened liquids: Practice patterns of speech-language pathologists. *American Journal of Speech-Language Pathology, 14*(1), 4–13.

Grievink, E. H., Peters, S. A., van Bon, W. H., & Schilder, A. G. (1993). The effects of early bilateral otitis media with effusion on language ability: A prospective cohort study. *Journal of Speech and Hearing Research, 36*(5), 1004–1012.

Groves, R. M. (1989). *Survey errors and survey costs.* New York, NY: John Wiley.

Guitar, B., Schaefer, H. K., Donahue-Kilburg, G., & Bond, L. (1992). Parent verbal interactions and speech rate: A case study. *Journal of Speech and Hearing Research, 35*(4), 742–754.

Halliday, L. F., & Bishop, D. V. M. (2005). Frequency discrimination and literacy skills in children with mild to moderate sensorineural hearing loss. *Journal of Speech, Language, and Hearing Research, 48*(5), 1187–1203.

Healey, E. W., Kannabiran, A., & Bacon, S. P. (2005). An across-frequency processing deficit in listeners with hearing impairment is supported by acoustical correlation. *Journal of Speech, Language, and Hearing Research, 48*(5), 1236–1242.

Hearst, N., & Hulley, S. B. (1988). Using secondary data. In S. B. Hulley & S. R. Cummings (Eds.), *Designing clinical research* (pp. 53–62). Baltimore, MD: Williams & Wilkins.

Hegde, M. N. (1994). *Clinical research in communicative disorders.* Austin, TX: Pro-Ed.

Hegde, M. N. (2003). *Clinical research in communicative disorders* (4th ed.). Austin, TX: Pro-Ed.

Hoffman, J. M., Yorkston, K. M., Shumway-Cook, A., Ciol, M., Dudgeon, B. J., & Chan, L. (2005). Effect of a communication disability on satisfaction with health care: A survey of Medicare Beneficiaries. *American Journal of Speech-Language Pathology, 14*(3), 221–228.

Huck, S. W., Cormier, W. H., & Bounds, W. G. (1974). *Reading statistics and research.* New York, NY: Harper Collins.

Isaac, S., & Michael, W. B. (1987). *Handbook in research and evaluation.* San Diego, CA: Edits Publishers.

Kent, R. D., Sufit, R. L., Rosenbek, J. G., Kent, J. F., Weisner, G., Martin, R. E., & Brooks, B.

R. (1991). Speech deterioration in myotrophic lateral sclerosis: A case study. *Journal of Speech and Hearing Research, 34*(6), 1269–1275.

Kerlinger, F. N. (1973). *Foundations of behavioral research.* New York, NY: Holt, Rinehart & Winston.

Law, J., Garrett, Z., & Nye, C. (2004). The efficacy of treatment for children with developmental speech and language delay/disorder: A meta-analysis. *Journal of Speech, Language, and Hearing Research, 47,* 924–943.

Leedy, P. D. (1989). *Practical research.* New York, NY: Macmillian.

Lieske, A. M. (1986). *Clinical nursing research: A guide to undertaking and using research in nursing practice.* Rockville, MD: Aspen.

Maxwell, D. L., & Satake, E. (2006). *Research and statistical methods in communication sciences and disorders.* Clifton Park, NY: Thomson-Delmar Learning.

McGann, W. M., & Paslawski, T. M. (1991). Incomplete locked-in syndrome: Two cases with successful communication outcomes. *American Journal of Speech-Language Pathology, 1*(1), 32–37.

Mullen, R. (2005). Evidence-based practice planning addresses members needs, skills. *ASHA Leader,* pp. 1, 21.

Ottenbacher, K. J. (1990). Clinically relevant designs for rehabilitation research: The idiographic model. *American Journal of Physical Medicine and Rehabilitation, 69*(12), 286–292.

Paden, E. (1970). *A history of the American Speech and Hearing Association 1925–1958.* Washington, DC: American Speech-Language Hearing Association.

Pannbacker, M. H., & Middleton, G. F. (1991–1992). Common myths about research. *Journal of the National Student Speech-Language-Hearing Association, 19,* 128–137.

Polit, D. F., & Beck, (2010). *Essentials of nursing research.* Philadelphia, PA: Lippincott, Williams, and Wilkins.

Polit, D. F., & Hungler, B. P. (1991). *Nursing research: Principles and methods.* Philadelphia, PA: Lippincott.

Polit, D. F., & Hungler, B. P. (1999). *Nursing research: Principles and methods* (6th ed.). New York, NY: Lippincott.

Portney, L. G., & Watkins, M. P. (2000). *Foundations of clinical research: Applications to clinical practice* (2nd ed.). Upper Saddle River, NJ: Prentice-Hall Health.

Portney, L. G., & Watkins, M. P. (2009). *Foundations of clinical research: Applications to clinical practice* (3rd ed.). Upper Saddle River, NJ: Pearson.

Rao, P. R. (2011). Evidence-based practice: The coin of realism in CSD. *ASHA Leader,* p. 7.

Ray, J. (2002). Treating phonological disorders in a multilingual child: A case study. *American Journal of Speech-Language Pathology, 11*(3), 305–315.

Roberts, J., Jurgen, J., & Burchinal, M. The role of home literacy practices in preschool children's language and emergent literacy skills. *Journal of Speech, Language, and Hearing Research, 48*(2), 345–359.

Robey, R. (1998). A meta-analysis of clinical outcomes in the treatment of aphasia. *Journal of Speech, Language, and Hearing Research, 41*(1), 172–187.

Rosenfeld, R. (1991). Clinical research in otolaryngology journals. *Archives of Otolaryngology-Head and Neck Surgery, 117,* 164–170.

Roy, N., Weinrich, B., Gray, S. D., Tanner, K., Stemple, J. C., & Sapienza, C. (2003). Three treatments for teachers with voice disorders: A randomized clinical trial. *Journal of Speech, Language, and Hearing Research, 46*(3), 670–688.

Schiavetti, N., Metz, D. E., & Orlikoff, R. R. (2011). *Evaluating research in communicative disorders.* Boston, MA: Allyn & Bacon.

Scientific Learning Corporation. (1998). Fast ForWord—Language. [Computer software]. Berkeley, CA: Author.

Shearer, W. S. (1982). *Research procedures in speech, language and hearing.* Baltimore, MD: Williams & Wilkins.

Shewan, C. M. (1986, November). *The survey: An important data collection tool.*

Miniseminar presented at the annual meeting of the American Speech-Language-Hearing Association, Detroit, MI.

Survey Monkey. Retrieved March 21, 2006 from http://www.surveymonkey.com/

Tallal, P., Hirsch, L. S., Realpe-Bonilla, T., Miller, S., Brzustowicz, L. M., Bartlett, C., & Flax, J. F.. (2001). Familial aggregation in specific language impairment. *Journal of Speech, Language, and Hearing Research, 44*(5), 1172–1182.

Van Dalen, D. B., & Meyer, W. J. (1966). *Understanding educational research.* New York, NY: McGraw-Hill.

Van Tassell, D. J. (1993). Hearing loss, speech, and hearing aids. *Journal of Speech and Hearing Research, 36*(2), 228–244.

Ventry, I., & Schiavetti, N. (1986). *Evaluating research in speech pathology and audiology.* New York, NY: Macmillan.

Warren, R. L. (1986). Research design: considerations for the clinician. In R. Chapey (Ed.), *Language intervention strategies in adult aphasia* (pp. 66–79). Baltimore, MD: Williams & Wilkins.

Williams, A. L. (2000). Multiple oppositions: Case studies of variables in phonological intervention. *American Journal of Speech-Language Pathology, 9*(4), 289–299.

Wilson, L., Onslow, M., & Lincoln. (2004). Telehealth adaptation of the Lidcombe Program of early stuttering intervention: Five case studies. *American Journal of Speech-Language Pathology, 13*(1), 81–93.

Windsor, J., Doyle, S. S., & Siegel, G. M. (1994). Language acquisition after mutism: A longitudinal case study of autism. *Journal of Speech and Hearing Research, 37*(1), 96–105.

Zipoli, R. P., & Kennedy, M. (2005). Evidencesbased practice among speech-language pathologists: Attitudes, utilization, and barriers. *American Journal of Speech-Language Pathology, 14*(3), 208–220.

2

Ethics of Research in Speech-Language Pathology and Audiology

LEARNING OBJECTIVES

Upon completion of this chapter the reader will be able to:

- Explain the need for ethical research
- Trace historical background of ethics in research
- Define responsible conduct of research and research misconduct
- Apply ethical principles to research
- Identify and avoid research misconduct
- Compare the AAA and ASHA Codes of Ethics related to research
- Identify content and methods for teaching ethics
- Explain current and future issues related to research ethics.

Research requires knowledge about scientific methods as well as the responsible conduct of research. The proliferation of research in speech-language pathology and audiology has increased interest in research ethics. Research requires careful consideration of ethical issues.. The American Academy of Audiology (AAA and American Speech-Language-Hearing Association (ASHA) provide information about the responsible conduct of research. Both the AAA (2011) and ASHA (2010) Codes of Ethics have guidelines, principles, and rules related to research in ethics. The Codes of Ethics for these organizations are in Appendixes 2–A and 2–B. This chapter discusses the major ethical issues related to research.

Need For Ethical Guidelines

Research has not always been conducted ethically. Also, there has been inadequate training in the responsible conduct of research. Currently, ethical issues related to research have high visibility because of past ethical transgressions such as lack of informed consent, unfavorable risk-benefit ratio, and use of vulnerable populations such as children, students, and prisoners. Furthermore, ethical standards have changed over time. Previously, specific protection of human subjects did not exist and ethical standards were considerably more lax than today. Last, ethical considerations have not always been given adequate attention. In the following section, the historical reasons for the development of ethical guidelines are considered.

Historical Background

There is a long history of research misconduct. Meline (2006) described ethical abuse as early as the first century BC There has been considerable interest in research ethics since the Nazi medical experiments of the 1930s and 1940s. The Nazi research used prisoner of war and "racial enemies" in studies to test the limits of human endurance and human response to disease and untested drugs. The studies were unethical because "participants" were exposed to permanent physical harm, even death, and not given an opportunity to refuse participation (Polit & Beck, 2010).

There have been numerous reports about unethical research involving humans in the United States. This research has involved surgical experiments, exposure to pathogens, disease, radiation, chemicals, drugs, and psychological experiments. A historical summary of this research is in Table 2–1. There is limited information about the long-term adverse effects of this research; there is limited information about unethical research in speech-language pathology and audiology except for the Tudor study in 1939.

It was not until the 1970s and beyond that researchers in the United States considered inform consent and the risks and benefits of research (Horner & Minifie, 2011). Limited attention has been given to the use of animals in research (Horner & Minifie, 2011). Relevant issues included the emergence of human treatment of animals; animals welfare versus animal rights, and evolving regulations and guidelines for animal research. It is noteworthy that the ASHA Code of Ethics did not include protection of animals until 2003.

Table 2–1. Chronologic Listing of Unethical Research in the United States 1840–1972

Year(s)	Investigators/Site	Subjects
Surgical Experimentation:		
1840s	Dr. J. Marion Sims	Surgical experiments on enslaved African women without anesthesia; operated on one woman 30 times
1874	Dr. Robert Barthlow Good Samaritan Hospital	Treated Irish women servant for cancer; cut open head and inserted needle electrodes into exposed brain
1896	Dr. Arthur Wentworth Boston Children's Hospital	Performed spinal taps on 29 children without parental consent
1913–1951	Dr. Leo Stanley San Quentin Prison	Experiments on 100s of prisoners; many involved testicular implants
Pathogens, Disease, and Biological Agents:		
1880s	California physician Hawaii Hospital for Lepers	Injected 12 young girls under 12 with syphilis
1895	Dr. Henry Heiman	Infected two mentally disables boys, 4 and 16, with gonorrhea
1900	U.S. Army doctor Philippines	Infected 5 prisoners with bubonic plague; induced beriberi in 29 prisoners
1906	Professor Richard Strong Harvard University	Infected 24 Filipino prisoners with cholera; all became sick and 13 died
1908	3 Researchers St. Vincent Hospital, Philadelphia	Infected dozens of children with TB causing permanent blindness or painful lesions and inflammation of eyes
1909	C. Knowles	Infected 2 children at orphanage
1911	Dr. Hideyo Noguchi Rockerfeller Institute for Medical Research	Injected 146 patients, some children, with syphilis
1932–1972	U.S. Public Health Service Tuskegee, AL	400 improvised black males with untreated syphilis

Table 2–1. *continued*

Year(s)	Investigators/Site	Subjects
1941	Dr. Francis and Jonas Salk University of Michigan	Infected patients at several hospitals with influenza virus
1941	Dr. William C. Black	Inoculated 12-month-old with herpes
1943–1970	Statesville Penitentiary Joilet, IL University of Chicago Medical School U.S. Army and State Department	Effects of malaria on 441 prisoners
1944–1946	Dr. Alf Alving University of Chicago Medical School	Infected psychiatric patients with malaria
1946	Guatemala U.S. Public Health Service National Institute of Health Pan American Health Sanitary Bureau	Used prostitutes to infect prisoners, psychiatric patients, and Guatemalans with syphilis and other sexually transmitted diseases
1950	U.S. Navy	Sprayed large quantities of bacteria over San Francisco, CA; numerous pneumonia-like illnesses; killed at least one.
1950	Dr. Joey Stokes University of Pennsylvania	Infected 200 female prisoners with viral hepatitis
1952–1972	Willowbrook State School Staten Island, NY	Mentally disabled children infected with viral hepatitis
1952	Chester M. Southam Sloan-Kettering Institute	Injected live cancer cells into prisoners at the Ohio State Prison, half were black, other half were not
1955	CIA	Released whooping cough bacteria from boats outside Tampa Bay, FL, caused epidemic: killed at least 12
1956–1957	U.S. Army	Released millions of infected mosquitoes on Savannah, GA, and Avon Park, FL; hundreds affected

continues

Table 2–1. *continued*

Year(s)	Investigators/Site	Subjects
1962	Chester M. Southam Jewish Chronic Disease Hospital Brooklyn, NY	22 elderly patients injected with live cancer cells
1966	U.S. Army	Released *Bacillus globigis* into subways of New York and Chicago

Source: From *Children As Research Subjects*, by M. A. Grodin and L. H. Glantz, 1994, New York, NY: Oxford University Press; *Acres of Skin*, by A. M. Hornblum, 1998, New York, NY: Routledge Press; *Sentenced to Science*, by A. M. Hornblum, 2007, University Park, PA: Pennsylvania State University; *Lesser Harms*, by S. A. Halpern, 2004, Chicago, IL: University of Chicago Press; *Medical Apartheid*, by H. A. Washington, 2006, New York, NY: Random House; *Unethical Human Experiments in the United States,* by Wikipedia (n.d.), Retrieved from http://en.wikipedia.org/wiki

There has been little discussion of ethical misconduct in speech-langue pathology and audiology except for the Tudor study which was conducted in 1939 at the University of Iowa. Twenty-two normally fluent children were taught to stutter (Annett, 2001; Dyer, 2001; Yairi & Amrose, 2001). These children were orphans at the Soldiers and Sailors Orphan's Home in Davenport, Iowa. The study was a master's thesis conducted by a graduate student, Mary Tudor, and directed by Wendell Johnson. Ambrose and Yairi (2002) reviewed the Tudor study and concluded that there were " . . . fundamental flaws in its design and execution" (p. 201). They also indicated that their assessment of related ethical issues " . . . should be viewed within the common standards of the period that there is no evidence of intent to harm, and that the objective in increasing diffluent speech should not be confused with instilling chronic stuttering in normally fluent children" (p. 201). Obviously, such

a study would not be permitted under current ethical standards. Ambrose and Yairi (2002) believe that " . . . in spite of the controversy regarding the Tudor thesis, there is no question that Johnson's contribution to the study of stuttering remains very significant in many positive ways" (p. 201). Conversely, Silverman (1988a) reviewed the study and stated that, "The implications of the findings seem clear—asking a child to monitor his speech fluency and attempt to be more fluent can lead to increased disfluency and possibly stuttering" (p. 231). Goldfarb (2006) edited a comprehensive review of the Tudor study and current ethical issues in clinical research. Johnson stated that the Tudor study ethics compare favorably not only tip the standards of its own time in 1939 but to those of 2000 as well.

It is also important to know about the history of the responsible conduct of research. Horne and Minifie (2011a) provided a detailed chronology of the major documents relevant to the responsible conduct of research pertaining to human and animal experimentation.

Research Misconduct

Research misconduct is relatively rare in speech-language pathology and audiology although it has increased over the past several years. Horner and Minifie (2011) noted that " . . . the actual prevalence of misconduct is unknown." Data from the Office of Research Integrity (2007, 2010) indicates an increase in research misconduct among public health service researchers. Possible increase in research misconduct may be related to a number of factors such as greater attention to responsible conduct of research, awareness and knowledge of research misconduct, and publish or perish culture. It is possible that junior employees may bear the burden for sanctions for scientific misconduct.

Research misconduct in any form threatens to undermine not only the progress and public support for science but it also has the potential to cause harm to those who receive the erroneous treatment. Those involved in research must specifically address these issues (Society for Clinical Trials, 2003).

Research misconduct involves fabrication, falsification, or plagiarism in proposing, performing, reviewing, or in reporting research. It does not include honest error or differences of opinion. *Fabrication* is making up data or results and recording or reporting data for experiments that were never con-ducted. Falsification of data is probably rare (Knapp & Van de Creek, 2006). It involves manipulating research materials, equipment, processes, or altering data or results, such that the research is not accurately represented in the research record. The research record includes, but is not limited to, research proposals, laboratory records; progress reports abstracts, theses, dissertations, oral presentations, and journals. *Plagiarism* is the use of another person's ideas, procedures, results, or words without giving appropriate credit. It has been further defined as stealing someone else's work and using it for personal gain. Plagiarism can relate to the theft of ideas as well as text (Association of American Medical Colleges, 1994). In recent years, plagiarism has become more problematic because of the proliferation of documents available on the Internet (Knapp & Van de Creek, 2005). Furthermore, some sources offer to sell papers on specific topics or prepare them for a fee.

Self-plagiarism is duplicate submission or publication. Duplicate/previous submission means that the manuscript is simultaneously being considered for publication elsewhere. It is essentially publication of the same content by the same author(s) (Bennett & Taylor, 2003; JAMA, 2006).

Research misconduct is a significant failure to adhere to prevailing, professional standards, and is considered a violation of the AAA (2011) and ASHA (2010) Codes of Ethics. Seriousness of research misconduct ranges from obvious to subtle. Several forms about research misconduct have been identified (ASHA, 2008; Bailar, 1995; Sales & Lavin, 2001). Examples of research misconduct are listed in Table 2–2.

Table 2–2. Examples of Research Misconduct

Arbitrary or biased selection of data	Inadequate supervision
Bias in manuscript	Incompetent supervision
Censorship	Lazy writing
Coercion	Misrepresentation
Conflict of interest	Multiple authors
Cyber-cheating	Multiple relationships
Data recycling	Negligent data collection or analysis
Deception	Not fully informing IRB of participant
Duplicate publication	Not maintaining complete records
Dual relationships	Not protecting participants' confidentially
Exploitive supervision	Public bias
Failure to comply with guidelines for handling research misconduct	Role conflicts
	Software piracy
False representation of manuscript	Supervision abandonment
Forging of academic documents	Tardy reviews
Fragmented publication	Unauthorized use of confidential information
Ghost authorship	
Honorary authorship	Undisclosed repetition of study
Improprieties of authorship	Violating research protocol
Inadequate maintenance of records	Wrongful manipulation of data or results

Reporting research misconduct is the responsibility of every speech-language pathologists and audiologists. This is a responsibility of both practicing professionals and students. However, students may be in an especially awkward situation for fulfilling this responsibility. Practicing professionals and students should be aware of AAA (2011) and ASHA guidelines for reporting allegations of research misconduct as well as institutional policies.

Ethical issues and problems related to research were identified and discussed by Hoit (2005). These three issues were: self-plagiarism, conflict of interest, and authorship. For each ethical dilemma a resolution was provided, also issues and Ethical Principle and Rule, and concept.

Ethical misconduct in audiology and speech-language pathology has increased. This can be verified by reviewing the ASHA Leader which published sanctions for ethical misconduct of its members. According to the Office of Integrity (2010), ethical misconduct among Public Health Service research has increased from 163 in 1993 to 286 in 2010. Reynolds (2004) reported that "junior employees may bear the burden of sanction for scientific misconduct" (p. 509). The most frequent sanction was the requirement for a plan of supervision. Furthermore, research misconduct frequently involved all members of the research team not solely these at the doctoral level.

Research misconduct in any form threatens to undermine not only scientific progress and public support for science, but also has the potential to cause harm to those use the possible erroneous outcome(s) of this research. Those involved in research must specifically address this issue (Society for Clinical Trials, 2003).

Three types of legal perspectives have influenced selection of sanctions for research misconduct: (1) quasicontractual legal remedy of restitution; (2) philosophy of "just desserts" or retribution based on intuitive idea that the individual was who engages in criminal conduct deserves punishment; and (3) deterrence of misconduct (Dresser 1993).

Consequences for research misconduct include article retraction, private lawsuits, adverse personal actions, and administrative, civil, and criminal sanction. The names of individuals' guilty of research misconduct are listed in a federal database and published in federal print materials (Horner & Minifie, 2011).

Issues In Research Ethics

ASHA's 2010 Code of Ethics includes standards for reporting and publishing information. These standards contain expanded sections pertaining to authorship, adherence to basic ethical considerations for protection of human or animals in research, permission about copyrighted materials, dual commitment, and conflicts of interest. The most critical research issues identified by participants in a meeting sponsored by ASHA were authorship, peer-review, and handling allegations of research misconduct (Moss, 2006). Other issues include confidentiality, use of controlled groups, institutional review, and documentation. Research requires careful consideration of ethical issues. Recognition and discussion of these issues can reduce the risk of unethical misconduct.

Planning Research

Speech-language pathologists and audiologist design, conduct, and report research in accordance with recognized standards for ethical conduct of research. Research is planned so as to minimize the possibility that results will be misleading. Planning ethically responsible research involves application of basic ethical principles (beneficence, respect, justice) to research activities which are described in Table 2–3 (Sieber, 2992). In planning research, speech-language pathologists and audiologist consider the AAA (2011) and ASHA Code of Ethics (2010). If an ethical issue is unclear, speech-language pathologists and audiologists seek to resolve the issue through consultation with institutional review boards, the AAA and ASHA Board of Ethics, or other resources such as the *Publication of the American Psychological Association* (APA, 2010). Speech-language pathologists and audiologists take reasonable steps for ethical treatment of all those associated with the research: human and animal subjects, collaborators, assistants, students, and employees.

Table 2–3. Scientific Methods Based on Ethical Principles

Valid research design	Only valid research yields correct results: takes account of relevant theory, methods, prior findings (B, R)
Competence of researchers	Investigates capable carrying out procedures validity (B, R)
Identification of consequences	Assessment of risks and benefits; respected privacy, ensure confidentiality, maximize benefit, minimize risk (B, R, J)
Selection of subjects	Subjects must be appropriate to purpose of study, representative of population to benefit from research, appropriate number (B, R, J)
Voluntary informed consent	Obtained in advance
Compensations for injury	Researcher responsible for what happened to subjects. Federal law requires subjects be informed if harm compensated but does not require compensation (B, R, J)

B = beneficence; R = respect; J = justice.

Source: From *Planning Ethically Responsible Research: A Guide for Students and Internal Review Boards*, by J. E. Sieber, 1992, Thousand Oaks, CA: Sage. Copyright 1992 by Sage Publications, Inc. Reprinted by permission of Sage Publications, Inc.

Ethical issues that may arise during a study should be considered early, that is these issues should be considered before writing the research proposal (Creswell, 2003). These issues relate to all phases of research and include research sites and potential readers.

Confidentiality

Speech-language pathologists and audiologists have the ethical responsibility to maintain confidentiality in research activities including mentoring, reviewing manuscripts or research grants, consulting, or participating in research (Knapp & Van de Creek, 2006; Lansing, 2002; Lansing & Moss, 2003). Upholding participants' rights to confidentiality and anonymity is a central tenet of research. Speech-language pathologists and audiologists should also be aware of situations where they have access to confidential ideas such as hearing ideas during an informal conversation. Maintaining confidentiality in peer review is an ethical responsibility because a manuscript is a privileged communication and represents confidential information (Macrina, 1995). Reviewers of manuscripts have the ethical responsibility to maintain confidentiality. Speech-language pathologists increasingly are using the Internet for online experimentation, and chat rooms, and E-mail for collecting research data. This raises new issues of confidentiality, and informed consent that will probably require further consideration of existing codes of ethics (Meline, 2006).

Confidentiality is included in the ASHA (2010) Code of Ethics and is mentioned in Principles of Ethics 1, Rule 14, which states, "Individuals shall not reveal, without authorization, any professional or personal information about identified persons served professionally or identified participants involved in research and scholarly activities unless required by law to do so, or unless doing so is necessary to protect the welfare of the person or of the community or otherwise required by law" (p. 2). The AAA (2011) Code of Ethics also addresses confidentiality in Principle 3, "Members shall maintain the confidentiality of the information and records of those receiving services or involved in research" (p. 2).

HIPAA

The Health Insurance Portability and Accountability Act (HIPAA) has had an impact on research practices (Horner & Wheeler, 2005). Research involving the use of protected health information must adhere to both HIPAA's privacy rule and the U.S. Department of Health and Human Services' Common Rule. Information about both of these documents can be found in the U.S. Code of Federal Regulations.

HIPAA protects health coverage for workers and their families, provides standards for transmission of health care records, identification of providers, health care plans, and employer. It also addresses security and privacy (confidentiality of health care data. Although the Act was passed in 1996 the regulations (standards) were not implemented until 1999, and were not implemented in 2003 (Cornett, 2007).

Many aspects of HIPAA are relevant to research. The standards related to research are privacy, security, de-identification, and enforcement.

The Privacy Rule is intended to prevent using or disclosing individually identified health information without consent (Horner & Wheeler, 2005 November). Ness (2007) believes the intent of the Privacy Rule is, "to strike a balance between protecting the privacy of individual's identifiable health information and prescribing the legitimate use and disclosure of this information" (p. 2164).

The Privacy Rule addresses the use and disclosure of all protected health information, including paper and electronic that is related to the individuals' past, present, and future health conditions, treatment for these conditions, and financial history related to health care. A covered entity is a health plan, a health care clearing house, or a health care provider that transmits any health care information electronically in connection with a covered transmission (Horner & Wheeler, 2005). HIPAA compliance is required for all covered entities (Romanow, 2011).

Researchers are required to disclose certain information to all research participants. This information includes:

- Description of protected health information to be used or disclosed, identifying information in a meaningful, specific way
- Names or other detailed identification of the person(s) authorized to make the requested use of disclosure
- Names or other detailed identification of the person(s) to whom the

covered entity can make a requested use or disclosure

■ Description of every purpose of the requested use or disclosure
■ Authorization expiration date
■ Signature of participants and date. (Horner & Wheeler, 2005)

The Security Rule applies only to the protection of electronic health care information. It requires covered entities to meet three standards. The standards for compliance are administration, physical, and technical (Wikipedia, n.d.). Administrative standards are related to policies and procedures designed to cl describe how the entity complies with HIPAA. Physical refers to controlling physical access to content against inappropriate access to protected health information. Technical standards involve controlling access to computer systems and enabling covered entities to protect communication containing protected health information transmitted electronically over open networks from being intercepted by anyone other than the intended receiver.

De-identification of health information refers to individually identified information in which all individually identified information is removed. As an alternative to removing all individual identifiers, a researcher may use statistical methods to reduce the possibility that information will identify research participants (Horner & Wheeler, 2005).

The Enforcement Rule became effective in 2006. This rule established penalties for HIPAA violation related to civil violations and compliance. These violation and penalties are shown in Table 2–4.

There are possible changes in HIPAA related to privacy, business associates, and enforcement (Romanow, 2011). The privacy changes are related to the cov-

ered entity making a reasonable effort to resolve payment issue(s) prior to sending protected health information to the health plan. Business associates would be required to enter into a contract or their agreements with a subcontractor(s) to protect security of electronic protected health information. The proposed enforcement change addresses civil penalties, complaints, and compliance review. The civil monetary penalty will make a covered entity liable for acts of business associates which may require covered entities to conduct due diligence. Penalty(s) will also consider previous indications of violations, not just previous violation(s). The secretary of health and human services will attempt to resolve complaints when possible, but (Romanow, 2011) may directly proceed to formal enforcement without attempting informal resolution.

HIPAA has had considerable impact on research. Several obstacles have been identified in the peer-reviewed literature (Dunlop, Graham, Leroy, Glanzer, & Dunlop, 2007; Horner & Wheeler, 2011; Ness, 2007; Nosowsky & Giordano, 2006; O'Herrin, Fost, & Kudon, 2004; Wipke-Tevis & Pickett, 2008; Wolf & Benett, 2006). These obstacles to research include but are not limited to time, delay, cost, subject recruitment and retention, lesser user friendly, informed consent, and restricted use of databases. Some of the obstacles can be reduced by better education about HIPAA; researchers are working more closely with health care providers, and considering the role of researchers in health care (Gunn et al., 2004; Nosowsky & Giordano, 2006). Furthermore, Gunn and associates (2004) provided suggestions for reducing the negative impact of HIPAA on research. These suggestions include using deiden-

Table 2–4. HIPAA Violation and Penalties

Violation	Minimum Penalty	Maximum Penalty
Individual unknowingly violated HIPAA	$100 per violation $25,000 annual maximum	$50,000 per violation $1.5 million annual maximum
Reasonable cause, not due to willful neglect	$1,000 per violation Annual maximum $100,000 for repeated violations	$50,000 per violation annual maximum $1.5 million
Willful neglect but violation corrected within required time period	$10,000 per violation $250,000 annual maximum	$50,000 per violation $1.5 annual maximum
Willful neglect not corrected	$50,000 per violation $1.5 million annual maximum	$50,000 per violation $11.5 million annual maximum

Source: From *HIPAA Violations and Enforcement* by American Medical Association. Retrieved from http://www.ama-assn.org/ama/pub/physican-resources/sulutions-managing-our-practice/

tified health information or a limited dataset; requiring covered entity to develop authorization forms or requesting protected health information; if authorization is impractical seek an institutional review board/privacy board waiver; and/or be familiar with burdens the privacy rule imposes on covered entities.

Concern about HIPAA's impact on research is not universal; some believe that HIPAA has not gone far enough to protect privacy and security, especially ensuring patients' rights to control their health information both for research and health care (Nosowsky & Giordano, 2006).

Three factors related to HIPAA privacy standards will affect speech-language pathology and audiology research. These factors are: accessing data from a covered entity; and creating data, and disclosing data with a colleague from a different institution (Olsen, 2003).

HIPAA does not define electronic form but does define electronic media relative to storage and transmission. Storage means devices in computers (hard drives) and any removable transportable digital memory medium (magnetic tape or disk, optical disk, digital memory card). Transmission media is used to modify information already in electronic storage and includes internet extranet, dial up lines, leased lines, private networks, and physical movement of removable transportable electronic storage media (Romanow, 2011).

Informed Consent

Most research studies involve *informed consent* procedures that are designed to provide prospective participants with sufficient information to make a reasonable decision about the potential risks and benefits of participation (Polit & Beck, 2010). Informed consent should also be sought and documented if a treatment is experimental, that is if its efficacy has not been established empirically (Silverman, 1998b). According to the American Speech-Language Hearing Association (2005) the key component of informed consent are respect for participants, beneficial, and justice.

Informed consent requires that prospective participants sign a consent form. Obtaining informed consent may be complicated for several reasons: the most appropriate method of obtaining informed consent may not be clear, the competency of the patient is in doubt, participants are vulnerable because they are not competent to make an informed decision about participation, and circumstances make participants feel that free choice is constrained, or circumstances increasing their risk for harm. Children, adults with diminished cognitive ability, and individuals residing in institutions (nursing homes, orisons) are especially vulnerable. A major barrier to informed consent is problems with reading comprehension. Almost half the population in the United States reads at or below the 8th grade level, and some have little or no reading skills (Meline, 2006). Furthermore, special accommodations are needed for participants from different culture, ethnic, and socioeconomic groups to avoid misunderstanding. In addition, special accommodations are needed for individuals who are blind, deaf, or hard-of-hearing to ensure comprehension of informed consent.

The AAA (2011) Code of Ethics addressed informed consent in Principle 1, Rule A. The current ASHA (2010) Code of Ethics also contains references to informed consent in Principle 1, Rules 8 and 14 (see Appendix 2–B for the ASHA Code of Ethics).

Informed consent is usually considered as a means for protecting the rights of research participants (Silverman, 1998b). It also protects the rights of researchers and the institutions where the research is done. Informed consent provides researchers and institutions with some protection from research participants of alleged physical or mental harm.

Deception

One ethical issue that has been debated is the appropriateness of using deception (Mertens, 2005). The justification for deception is that the results of the study should be compromised without it because participants would modify their behavior if they knew what was being studied. Deception is supposed to be reduced by debriefing, misrepresentation, guaranteeing privacy, and obtaining fully informed consent.

Institutional Approval

Speech-language pathologists and audiologists should obtain prior approval for conducting research, and provide accurate information about their research proposals (APA, 2010). The research should be conducted consistent with the approved research protocol and consultation with the Institutional Review Board as needed. Many journals require information about the IRB status of a research report includes name of IRB and approval number.

Control Groups

The use of control groups has been a long-standing ethical issue. The most effective design for determining the effect of treatment is to compare subjects who receive treatment with those who receive no treatment or a sham treatment (Portney & Watkins, 2000). It is unethical to withhold treatment, that is, the control group should receive treatment (French, Reynolds, & Swain, 2001). Waiting list control groups are selected from persons on the waiting list for treatment. Furthermore, there is no basis for assuming that no treatment and waiting list control groups are equivalent (Lum, 2002).

Conflict of Interest

ASHA's Board of Ethics (ASHA, 2011) defines conflict of interest "as a situation in which personal and/or financial considerations have the potential to influence or comprise judgment in any clinical service, research, consultation, instruction, administration, or any other professional entity (e.g., clinical service, research, consultation, instruction, administration, etc.), or where the situation may appear to provide the potential for professional judgment to be compromised" (p. 1).

Both the AAA (2011) and ASHA (2010) Codes of Ethics address conflicts of interest. The AAA (2011) Code, Rule 4c indicates that, "Individuals shall not participate in activities that constitute a conflict of professional interest." ASHA's code of Ethics (2010) states that speech-language pathologists and audiologists "shall not participate in professional activities that constitute a conflict of interest." Speech-language pathologists and audiologists should also avoid the appearance of a conflict of interest, although there may not be an ethical violation. Appearance of a conflict of interest can damage the professional reputation of an individual,

and adversely affect his or her practice and profession (Diefendorf, 2003).

Conflicts of interest involve bias or influencing professional judgment or practice. Some conflicts of interest are obvious, whereas others may be subtle. These conflicts can be intellectual (non-financial) or financial and interfere with research conduct or reports. Examples of intellectual conflicts in interest include, but are not limited to, ego, professional advancement and beliefs (Ludlow, 2001). Financial conflicts include support for research, large honorariums, patents, agreements with industry, and product oriented research. Scientific conflicts of interest are the use of position to influence publication of manuscripts and review of grant applications (Bradley, 1995).

Conflict of commitment is another aspect of conflict of interest. Also referred to as dual loyalty or dual commitment, it refers to conflicting demands or speech-language pathologists and audiologists who have obligations to their patients and to others including students and other professionals (Beyrer, 2003). Multiple roles also can contribute to conflicts of interest (Sales & Lavin, 1995). Multiple roles are not unethical as long as they are not reasonably expected to have adverse effects. Speech-language pathologists and audiologists should be cautious about multiple roles. Guidelines and procedures for addressing personal and professional loyalty, *Dual Loyalty and Human Rights in Health Professional Practice*, have been developed by the International Dual Loyalty Working Group (2002).

Disclosure is often cited as the key to managing conflicts of interest (Association of American Medical Colleges, 1994; Korn, 2000). ASHA journals require disclosure of any real or potential conflict of interest that could be seen as having an influence on the research such as financial interests in a test or procedure, and funding by an equipment or materials manufacturer for efficiency research. In 2012, submission for the ASHA convention required a disclosure statement.

There are new disclosure requirements for presentation of courses offered for ASHA CEUs (ASHA 2012). These requirements are:

- Presenters must disclose financial or nonfinancial interest
- Focus on one method or device must indicate if information given about similar products
- Focus must be on science or contemporary practice not on sales or promotion
- Should not favor or use, promote, or purchase of product
- Acknowledge if presenting limited or no information about similar products or services
- Disclose of relevant financial and nonfinancial relationships or lack of attendees in each session.

Accurate outcome research aimed at assessing the efficacy of clinical services is essential to speech-language pathology and audiology. Product-oriented research increases the risk for conflict of interest (Sininger et al., 2004). Responsibility for conducting product efficacy research should be independent of the development and production of these products.

Mentoring

Mentoring is an important part of teaching research. Mentees not only learn scientific expertise from their mentors, but also learn about the reasonable conduct of research, preparing grant applications, interacting with colleagues, and preparing manuscripts for publication (Association of American Medical Colleges, 1994).

Unfortunately, sometimes the roles and responsibilities of mentees and mentors are misunderstood. The mentee may believe their role is passive, not active, and the mentors are responsible for the work. On the other hand, the mentor may view the mentee as inexperience labor. Therefore, it is important to understand the roles and responsibilities of both mentees and mentors.

Students usually select their mentor based primarily on which faculty member has research interests that most closely relate to their interests. Other factors that may be considered in selecting a mentor include the publication record of the faculty member, extramural financial support, national recognition, productivity of the department, atmosphere within the department, current positions of graduates, and opportunities for professional growth (Association of American Medical Colleges, 1994; Macrina, 1995a).

Both mentees and mentors should know what to expect from each other. It is reasonable for mentees to have expectations about the support and advice a mentor can provide. Mentors also have expectations such as the mentee will work independently and will be enthusiastic about their work.

Supervision is essential to maintaining and facilitating research integrity. Speech-language pathologists and audiologists often have dual roles as both a mentor and supervisor to students whom they also teach in class. It has been suggested that misunderstanding can be avoided by written agreement outlining the responsibilities of both the mentor and mentee. The agreement should also include authorship consideration, as well as the amount and type of supervision. It has been suggested that mentors set up periodic and specific meetings to provide mentees feedback, and maintain a record of supervision, including meeting times, issues discussed, and duties assigned.

Several problems related to mentoring have been identified. By Horner and Minifie (2011b). Among these problems were continued dependency, disparities of power, inadequate accountability, vulnerable subordinates, and failure to give appropriate credit. Recommendations for improving mentoring have been described by Shamoo and Resnick (2003). These recommendations included acknowledging mentors for effective mentoring, developing guidelines for amount and types of responsibilities and intellectual property, ensuring appropriate response to whistle blowing, establishing procedures for evaluating mentees, promoting adverse and nondiscriminatory environment safe from harm, and providing mentors with time for mentoring.

Documentation

Documentation is crucial to research (Macrina, 1995b). Documentation includes IRB approval, informed consent forms on all participants, participant encounters, research protocol, data collection and analysis, and research reports. Confidentiality is a major consideration in creating, storing, accessing, transferring, and disposing of records. According to the AAA (2011) Code of Ethics, "Individuals shall maintain documentation of professional services rendered, according to acceptable medical, legal, and professional standards and require-

ments." The ASHA (2010) Code of Ethics also addresses maintenance of records in Principle I Rule13 (See Appendix 2–B).

Referencing Sources

The AAA (2011) Code of Ethics has no specific reference to publication credit or authorship. The 2010 ASHA Code of Ethics states: "Individuals shall reference the source when using other person's ideas, research, presentations, or products in writing, and /or any other media presentations or summary."

Accurate and appropriate referencing of information even in slides and handouts prevent the appearance of plagiarism. Referencing of sources in ASHA journals is based on recommendations and guidelines of the *Publication Manual of the American Psychological Association* (APA, 2010). Speech-language pathologists and audiologists must accept the ethical responsibilities for appropriate referencing of sources.

Stealing ideas and/or plagiarism, is an issue at all levels of education, and has increased over the past 10 years (Young, 2003). Plagiarism is not giving credit to someone's ideas, results, or words. Plagiarism can take many forms and ranges from very obvious to very subtle. Some plagiarism involves direct verbatim copying of text or the text can be modified in ways that is not immediately recognizable from the source material (Association of American Medical Colleges, 1994). Other forms of plagiarism include lazy writing and redundant or duplicate publications. Lazy writing or patchwork plagiarism involves overreliance on direct quotations. Duplicate of self-plagiarism is repeated publication of previous results (Benninger, 2002). Duplicate publication is also inappropriate because ASHA journals require that submitted manuscripts have neither been previously published nor are currently under review elsewhere. In addition, information about any previous presentation of the data, whether at a professional meeting or in conference proceedings, book chapters, Web sites, or related media must be disclosed. Duplicate publications may also contribute to misrepresentation of publication credit, that is, a distorted in accurate record. Failure to acknowledge the contributions of colleagues, collaborators, or others, whether deliberate or not, can be viewed as a form of plagiarism (Association of American Medical Colleges, 1994). The widespread use of the Internet makes using information without acknowledging the source(s) easier. Cyber-cheating or online plagiarism enables cut and paste plagiarism and online paper mills.

Plagiarism frequently occurs as a result of ignorance about appropriate referencing. Ignorance is not an excuse for plagiarism. This can be avoided by learning and using guidelines for referencing sources such as the *Publication Manual of the American Psychological Association* (APA, 2010). Suspected plagiarism can be identified by Google's search engine for scholarship (http://scholar.google.com).

Copyright

Copyright is a legal concept protecting exclusive rights usually for a limited time, the creator of intellectual work. The American Medical Association (1998) defined copyright as providing "for the protection of rights of parties involved in the creation and dissemination of intellectual property" (p. 115). The Copy Right Act of 1976 is a comprehensive law related to permission for quoting, reproducing, or adapting published or unpublished information (American Psychological Association, 2010). Requirements for obtaining copyright permission vary. It is the author's responsibility to find out if permission is required from the copyright holder.

Exceptions from copyright permission are fair use and public domain (Blessing & Forister, 2012). Fair use provides for limited use of copyrighted materials. According to Homer and Minifie (2011) fair public domain applies to materials that can be used without permission but must be acknowledged. Additional, information about copyright is available in Silverman's (1999) Professional Issues in Speech-Language Pathology and Audiology.

Copyright Infringement is the use of published or unpublished information without permission. In other words, it is unauthorized use of information which includes computer software and programs published since 1976 (Blessing & Forister, 2012). Illegal copying of materials is not uncommon in educational and clinical activities. Test forms are often duplicated without authorization.

Authorship

Authorship is the basis by which university faculty are evaluated for employment, promotion, and tenure. Those faculties who do not publish may not be promoted or tenured. Therefore, these faculties may feel pressure to publish. Some faculty, however, believe publishing detracts from teaching and that resources and time are not available for publishing.

In addition, promotion and tenure there are other advantages in publishing research such as, staying current in professionally obtaining funds for research, networking, and collaborating with other professionals.

Authorship credit can be a problem because of the prevalence of honorary and ghost authorship as well as academia's competitive "publish or perish" (Bennett & Taylor, 2003; Macrina, 1995c; Mowatt et al., 2002). The different types of irresponsibility's are described in Table 2–5.

Several studies have confirmed that a substantial portion of authors listed in multi-authored publications did not meet criteria for authorship (Bennett & Taylor, 2003; Goodman, 1994; Mowatt et al., 2002; Shapiro, Wagner, & Shapiro, 1994). Some individuals who do not meet the criteria for authorship may be included or individuals who should be included as authors are omitted. Honorary or courtesy authorship is naming as an author an individual who does not meet authorship criteria. *Ghost authorship* is failure to name as an author an individual who has made substantial contribution that merits authorship or an unnamed individual who participated in writing the manuscript. Students are at

Table 2–5. Irresponsible Authorship: Types and Definitions

Types	Definitions
Coercion	Use of intimidation or bullying to gain authorship. The white bull effect.
Courtesy	Author who does not meet authorship criteria. Same as Gift, Guest, or Honorary.
Denial	Failure to include or acknowledge individual(s) who should be included as author. Same as Ghost or Silent author.
Duplicated	Publishing the same paper more than once. Sometimes referred to as self-plagiarism.
Gift	Same as Courtesy, Guest, or Honorary
Guest	Same as Courtesy, Gift or Honorary
Honorary	Same as Courtesy, Gift, or Guest.
Mutual support	Agreement by two or more authors to place each other's name on publication to give appearance of higher productivity. May or may not meet authorship criteria. Depending on the later may be a type of Courtesy, Gift, Guest, or Honorary.
White bull	Coercion or intimidation to obtain authorship

Sources: From "Why not just toss a coin?" by K. Strange, 2008, *American Journal of Physiology-Cell Physiology, 295*, pp. 567–575; and "The White Bull Effect: Abusive Co-Authorship and Publication Parasites" by L. S. Kwok, 2005, *Journal of Medical Ethics, 31*, pp. 554–556.

greater risk for not being given credit for authorship. Furthermore, students should be the principal author on any multiple-authored presentation or publication that is substantially based on the student's thesis or dissertation (Knapp & Van de Creek, 2006). Mere possession of an institutional position, such as Department Chair, does not justify authorship (APA, 2010). AAA's (2005a) guidelines for ethical practice address issues related to authorship in publication and presentation of research such as disclosure to avoid potential conflicts of interest and determination of authorship. ASHA's (2010) Code of Ethics provides some guidance about authorship: "Individuals shall assign credit only to those who have contributed to a publication, presentation, or product. Credit shall be assigned in purporting to the contribution and only with the contributor's consent" (ASHA 2010, P-IV, R-7). ASHA journal requires corresponding authors to affirm that all individuals listed in the byline have made appropriate contributions for authorship, have consented to the byline order, and have agreed to the submission of the manuscript in its current form. These contributions are outlined in Table 2–6.

The American Medical Association (2006) specifies three criteria for authorship: (1) substantial contributions to conception and design or acquisition of data, or analysis or interpretation of data; (2) drafting or revising the manuscript; and (3) final approval of the version to be published. Other responsibilities of author include; critical review and revision of manuscript; statistical expertise; administrative, technical or material support, and study supervision (Mowatt et al., 2002; Yedidia et al., 2003).

Table 2–6. Author Contributions

Study concept and design
Acquisition data
Analysis and interpretation of data
Drafting of the manuscript
Critical revision of the manuscript for important intellectual content
Obtained funding
Administrative, technical, or material support
Study supervision

The order of authorship also warrants consideration because disagreement about authorship can be very bitter and even result on legal action (Gabard & Martin, 2003; Kwok, 2005). Order of authorship should be in descending order based on level of contribution with the greatest contribution(s) made by the first author.

However, the order of authors may be considered relative to an author's university affiliation because some universities only consider first-author publications in determining promotion, tenure, and merit increases.

Journals do not have uniform criteria for designating authorship. For example, the American Speech Language Hearing Association (2011) requires a statement about authorship accompanies the manuscript submission. Specifically this affirms that all of the authors have made contributions appropriate for authorship. Furthermore, "the primary author is responsible for assuring that the list of authors include all and only those persons who have played significant roles in writing the manuscript, designing the study, preparing and executing the plan for data collection, and or interpreting the results in preparation for publication" (p. 4).

Some journals such as the Journal of the American Medical Association published the author contribution between the last section of a paper or report and the references.

Peer Review

Peer review has been a part of the scientific process for over 300 years, and researchers probably have complained about its shortcomings for nearly as long (Laine & Murlow, 2003). *Peer review* is the process by which the quality of research is assessed and involves multiple activities (Association of American Medical Colleges, 1994). First, there is the peer review of research proposals to assess the scientific merit of grant applications that is, funding decisions based on peer review. Second, professional journals and other publications use peer review to assess the quality of manuscripts, namely, publication decisions based on peer review. Thus, it is obvious that peer review is an essential component of research. High-quality reviews are those that provide constructive and substantiated comments about the importance and originality of the research, strengths and weaknesses, and an interpretation of results (Laine & Murlow, 2003).

Issues related to peer review include, but are not limited to, bias on the part of authors, editors, and reviewers, confidentiality; and plagiarism or theft of ideas (Macrina, 1995c; Olson et al., 2002; Scheetz, 2001). Reviewers and editors may be tempted to solicit the opinion of friends and colleagues with expertise in a particular area about a manuscript which may be a breach of confidentiality. The Scientific Research Society (1986) described several problems related to reviewers and editors. Among the reviewer problems were: obtaining a secondary citation for one's own publication in the guise of improving the manuscript; pirating the topic of the manuscript; providing criticism on a subsequent review; and excessive delay in review without explanation, and losing manuscript. Another problem is peer review failure that occurs when a peer reviewed paper contains several errors. Most journals do not have a policy for peer review failures other than "Letter to the Editor." Therefore, it becomes the individual reader's responsibility to identify and seek resolution of these failures in the form of a letter to the editor. The author of a quantitative paper usually has the option of publishing a reply to the Letter to the Editor. Peer review is such an important issue that there have been five International Congresses on Peer Review to discuss efforts to systematize reviews and improve reports of research. The first International Congress was in 1989 in Chicago, the second was in 1993 in Chicago, the third in 1999 in Prague, the fourth in 2001 in Spain (Rennie, 2002), and fifth, 2005 in Chicago. The topics of presentation included authorship, conflicts of interest, journal guidelines and policies, ethical concerns, peer review process, scientific misconduct, publication bias, and quality of journal articles.

Publication Correction

Research reports may be flawed because of errors in methodology, selective reporting of results, overuse and/or vague citation of references (Altman, 2002). Critical review of published reports and letters to the editor about inaccurate published reports are essential to the integrity of research (Getzsch, Delamothe, & Goodlec, 2010). Authors are sometimes reluctant to respond to critical reviews of their work. Editors should insist that the authors respond to criticism of their work. Speech-language pathologists and audiologists also have ethical obligations when their research is published. If authors discover or learn of errors in the published data, they are ethically obligated to promptly take reasonable steps to correct the error, retract the error, or use other appropriate publication means (APA, 2010).

Reports also may be retracted or withdrawn because of unsubstantiated or irreproducible data. According to Scheetz (2001), since 1992 findings of scientific misconduct have resulted in 63 revisions to the literature.

Several problems related to mentoring have been identified by Horner and Minifie (2011). Among these problems were continued dependency, disparities of power, inadequate accountability, vulnerable subordinates, and failing to give credit. Recommendations for improving mentoring have been described by Shamoo and Resnik (2003). These recommendations include acknowledge mentors for effective mentoring, develop guidelines for amount and type of responsibilities and intellectual property, ensure appropriate response to whistleblowers, establish procedures for evaluating mentees, promote a diverse and nondiscriminatory environment, secure an environment safe from harm, and provide mentors with time for mentoring.

More subtle issues of research ethics were identified by Rosenthal (1999).

These issues were related inadequate in research design, hyperclarity, data dropping, outlier rejection, self-censoring, and external censoring. *Hyperclarity* is suggesting that research is likely to achieve what it is unlikely to achieve. Closely related to hyperclarity is the tendency to imply a caused relationship when none has been established. Rosenthal (1999) believes bad science makes for bad ethics.

Reasons for retraction of a report include misconduct or presumed misconduct, significant reporting errors, and inability of author(s) to replicate (Horner & Minifie, 2011). If there are significant errors or ethical misconduct, published papers should be retracted and citation of retracted papers should not occur.

Evidence-Based Practice

Gupta (2003) believes there has been limited consideration of the ethical issues related to evidence-based practice. Ethical considerations are involved in evidence-based practice as well as in not practicing it. There are several areas for ethical concern. One concern is the potential for patients care to be manipulated by administrators to deprive persons of certain health services. Another area of concern is the effect that evidence-based practice has on the authority and power of health care providers. Evidence-based practice prioritizes certain types of research and, thus, increases the pressure for this research to be funded. There may be publication bias, that is, the publication of positive and/or statistically significant results. Another area for ethical concern is the uncritical and permissive attitude of evidence-based practice toward private funding of research. Other issues are related to control groups, randomization, need for research or treatment, meaning outcomes, setting (location) of research treatment, strategies for which evidence is not available, aid determining risks and benefits. Additional information about evidence-based practice is in Chapter 13.

AAA

The AAA (2011) Code of Ethics contains several specific statements related to research (see Appendix 2–A). AAA also has guidelines for ethical research; authorship in publication and presentations; adequacy of research design; security of data; and conflicts of interest in product-oriented outcome research (Sininger, March, Walden, & Wilber, 2004).

AAA's (2011) Ethical Practices Committee developed ethical guidelines that are commonly referred to as the "green book." The book focuses on a number of issues related to ethics in research. There is also an eight topic program for continuing education program (AAA, 2012).

ASHA

Standards for the Certificate of Clinical Competence (CCC) in Speech-Language Pathology (ASHA, 2009) require "knowledge of standards of ethical conduct" (p. 6). Standards for the CCC-Audiology (ASHA, 2011) also require knowledge about ethical conduct.

The ASHA (2010) Code of Ethics is central to the integrity of research (See Appendix 2–B). Twenty-one specific references to research are in the 2011 ASHA Code of Ethics (see Appendix 2–B).

Ethical responsibilities should be interpreted to include ethical treatment of all collaborators, assistants, and students associated with research (McCartney, 2002). The Issues in Ethics statement about research (ASHA, 2008), discusses and interprets the Code relative to ethics in research. It also provides guidance about teaching ethics to students. Other issues statements related to research are conflict of professional interest (ASHA, 2011), confidentially (ASHA, 2001), cultural competence (ASHA, 2004), and protection of human subjects (ASHA, 2005).

Sanctions for Ethical Misconduct

Three types of legal perspectives influence selection of sanctions for ethical misconduct: (1) quasicontractual legal remedy of restitution; (2) philosophy of "desserts" or retribution based on intuitive idea that the individual was engaged in criminal activity deserving punishment; and (3) detection of misconduct (Dresser, 1993).

Sanctions for ethical misconduct have been described by both AAA (2011) and ASHA (2010). Part II of the AAA (2011) Code of Ethics includes "procedures for the management of alleged violations." The sanctions are: educative letter; reprimand; probation of suspension; suspension of membership; and revocation of membership.

The fundamental purposes of ASHA's (2012) are: (1) penalize the person in violation; (2) serve as a mechanism to educate and rehabilitate; (3) protect the public; and (4) inform other ASHA members and certificate holders that the Association enforces its ethical standards

Table 2–7. ASHA's Research Integrity Supplement in JSLHR

Title	Authors
Research integrity in communication sciences and disorders	Moss (2011)
Research integrity in communication sciences and disorders: Preface	Horner & Minifie (2011a)
Research ethics I: Responsible conduct of research (RCR)—History and contemporary issues pertaining to human and animal experimentation	Horner & Minifie (2011a)
Research ethics II: Mentoring, collaboration peer review and data management and ownership	Horner & Minifie (2011b)
Research ethics III: Publication practices and authorship, conflict of interest, and research misconduct	Horner & Minifie (2011c)
Responsible conduct of research in communication sciences and disorders: Faculty and student perceptions	Minifie et al. (2011)
Ethical principles associated with the publication of research in ASHA's scholarly journals: Importance and adequacy of coverage	Ingham et al. (2011)

and alert them that there are penalties for engaging in professional misconduct. Typically more serious misconduct receives harsher sanctions. The sanctions from least to most severe are reprimand, censure, revocation membership and/or certification, suspension of membership and/or certification, withholding membership and/or certification, and cease and desist.

Institutional Review Board

An *Institutional Review Board* (IRB) is a committee mandated by the National Research Act, Public Law 93-348, to be established within each institution that conducts research involving human and animal subjects and needing needs for federal funding for research (Sieber, 1992). The IRB is a group of individuals who are affiliated with an institution who meet to review research proposals and monitor ongoing research relative to ethical standards. Responsibilities of the IRB include:

- Protecting the rights and welfare of subjects
- Ensuring protocols are presented by the sponsor(s)
- Ensuring sponsor(s) of a protocol disclosure(s) including areas of concern such as appearance of a conflict of interest and financial interests

■ Reviewing, monitoring, and approving research protocols

■ Ensuring that rights including privacy and confidentiality are protected

■ Ensuring that all research is conducted within current federal and state guidelines. (Pozar 2012)

The term "research ethics review board" not IRB has been suggested because of the focus is on ethics rather than the institution. HIPAA has had significant impact on IRB (see the HIPAA discussion earlier in this chapter).

IRBs are often viewed negatively by researchers because of delays and requirements that provide limited protection of subjects (Azar, 2002). However, delays and revisions can be reduced by using understandable language in the consent form, explicitly describing the research protocol submitted to the IRB, and by submitting all required documents (Sharp, 2001). Furthermore, many of the ethical problems related to research are resolved in the course of the IRB review, that is, appropriate risk-to-benefit rating, details about informed consent, and appropriateness of compensation (Jonsen, Siegler, & Winslade, 2006).

The IRB is responsible for making decisions about research plans at convened meetings. In making decisions, the following are considered: scientific merit; competence of the investigator(s); risk to subjects; feasibility based on identified reasons; procedures for selecting subjects; voluntary informed consent based on complete an understandable descriptions; and confidentiality. The required elements of informed consent are listed in Table 2–8. In addition, the informed consent must be written in lay language; that is, the language must be clear and

basic so that it can understand by the average participant (Portney & Watkins, 2009). Many believe that informed consent makes research ethical; however, informed consent is neither necessary nor sufficient for ethical research.

IRB members must be able to adequately review research proposals. The IRB must be composed of at least five members, and may not consist entirely of makes, females, or members of one profession. At least one IRB member must be primarily concerned with nonscientific areas; many are a lawyer, clergy, or ethicist. One member may not be affiliated with the institution where the research is to be conducted or be a member of the immediate family of a person who is affiliated with the institution (Polit & Beck, 2010; Sales & Folkman, 2000).

Many research plans require a full review by the IRB. For a full review, the IRB must meet with a majority of the members present. In order for the research plan to be approved, it must receive approval of the majority of IRB members present at the meeting.

IRBs are often viewed negatively by researcher and administrators. The major reasons for these negative views are increased delays, added costs, and limited protection of subjects. There have also been complaints about differences between federal regulations and IRBs (Azar, 2002). Several strategies have been suggested for improving IRBs. One strategy is modifying the local independent IRB system and replacement with a central ISRB plus local option out. Education and dissemination of guidelines about IRBs have also been suggested (Green, Lowe, Kowaoski, & Wysezewianski, 2006).

Delays and revisions of research protocol can be reduced by using understandable language in the consent form

Table 2–8. Elements of Informed Consent

Purpose	Clear explanation of research and its importance reason for selecting individual
Procedures	Clear explanation of what will be done to or by individual
Risks and discomforts	Truthful and inclusive statements
Benefits	Description of potential benefits to individual, general knowledge, or future of health care
Alternative to participation	Description of reasonable alternative procedures that might be used in treatment with treatment is being started
Confidentiality	Statement of procedures used to ensure anonymity for collecting, storing, and reporting information and who (persons or agencies) will have access to information
Request for more information	Statement that individuals may ask questions about or discuss study participation at any time, naming an individual to contact
Refusal or withdrawal	Statement that individual may refuse to participate or discontinue participation at any time without prejudice
Injury statement	Description of measures to be taken if injury occurs as direct result of research activity
Consent statement	Confirmation that individual consents to participation
Signatures	Participants; patient or guardian, assent of minor over age 7; witness

specific descriptions of the research methodology, and by submitting all associated documents (Sharp, 2001). Last, many problems are resolved in the course of the IRB review. These problems include risk to benefit, details about informed consent, and suitability of compensation (Jonsen, Seglar, & Wisslede, 2006).

Some research plans qualify for expedited review or exempted status. For certain types of research involving no more than minimal risk, the research plan may be expedited. An expedited review is conducted by the IRB chair or another IRB member designated by the chair. The advantage of an expedited review is that

it usually is completed in less time than a full review.

Research plans may be exempted from full review if there is no apparent risk. Surveys, interviews, or studies of existing records may be exempt from full review if data are collected so that subjects cannot be identified and the study does not involve sensitive issues such as criminal activity, drug abuse, or sexual behavior (Portney & Watkins, 2009).

Before implementing a study, the researcher must submit a research proposal to the IRB. An IRB can approve the proposed research plan, require restriction(s), or disapprove the plan. The main requirements governing IRB decisions are summarized in Table 2–9.

Recent issues about IRB include the cost of operation, local versus central IRB, and characteristics of IRB members. It was reported that high volume IRBs were more expensive than low volume IRBs but more economically efficient. The potential savings of large IRBs may encourage small IRBs to merge which could reduce local review, control, and oversight. Christian and associates (2002) advocate both central and local IRBs. Central IRBs review large national multicenter clinical studies whereas local IRBs continue to be a key compound of the review system. This approach preserves local autonomy and responsibility for local matters, reduces the workload of local IRBs, and eliminates duplication of effort. McWilliams and associates (2003) believe that there are serious differences in the review process between local and central IRBs for multicenter studies. Conversely, Rose (2003) opposed central IRBs and suggested that reviews by local IRBs could be improved by education, consultation, and funding. Campbell and associates (2003) studied the characteristics of medical school faculty members serving on IRBs. Faculty members serving on IRBs have research experience and knowledge but almost half of all faculty IRB members were consultants to industry, which raises the possibility of the potential for conflict of interest.

Teaching Research Ethics

Professional ethics begin on the college campus (DeRussy, 2003). Therefore higher education has a critical role in teaching ethics. Furthermore, ASHA's certification standards for speech-language pathology and audiology require training in research and ethics (ASHA, 2009, 2010). This involves integrating ethical principles in to research. This requires that students in speech-language pathology and audiology be able to understand and integrate ethical principles into research. Educational training programs must have curricula and experiences in the ethical conduct of research. This section addressed topics related to teaching research ethics. First, content is considered, and then methods for teaching about ethics in research. Goals for teaching ethics are listed in Table 2–10. Their goals should also be reviewed periodically by practicing speech-language pathologists and audiologists.

The goal of teaching research ethics is to apply ethical principles in making decisions about research.

Table 2–9. Major Requirements Governing IRB Decisions

Risks to participants minimized
Risks to participants reasonable in relation to anticipated benefits, if any, and importance of knowledge that may reasonable be expected to result
Equitable selection of participants
Informed consent appropriately documented
Adequate provisions for monitoring research to ensure safety of participants
Appropriate provisions to protect privacy or participants and confidentiality of data
When vulnerable subjects involved, appropriate additional safeguards to protect their rights and welfare

Table 2–10. Goals for Teaching Research

Examine and make distinctions between ethical concepts such as beneficence, nonmalfiecence, justice, fidelity, respect. Patient rights, confidentiality
Know that ethical certainty is often impossible but ethical reasoning about choice can be precise.
Serious consideration of personal and professional ethics
Identify ethical dilemmas and seek resolution of these dilemmas

Emanuel, Wendler, and Grady (2000) identified seven requirements for evaluating the ethics of research studies: (1) value—enhancement of health or knowledge must be derived from the research; (2) validity—methodological rigor; (3) fair subject selection—scientific objectives, not privilege or vulnerability, and potential for and distribution of risks and benefits should determine selection; (4) risk-benefit ratio within context of standard clinical practice and the research plan, risks must be minimized, potential benefits enhanced, and potential benefits to individual and knowledge gained for society must outweigh the risks; (5) independent review—unaffiliated individuals must review the research and approve, amend, or terminate it; (6) informed consent—individuals should be informed about the risks an provide voluntary consent; and (7) respect for enrolled subjects—subjects should have confidentiality protected, opportunity to withdraw, and their well-being monitored.

Content

The teaching of ethics cannot be separated from the Code of Ethics of AAA (2011) and ASHA (2010), which contain several references to ethics in research, (see Appendixes 2–A and 2–B). There is a wide range of information about the responsible conduct or research such as: (1) topic related to conduct and reporting of research; (2) ethical dilemmas presented by certain types of research; and (3) responses to research misconduct. Ingham and Horner (2004) identified 11 core areas for teaching the responsible conduct of research. These core areas are listed in Table 2–11.

In addition to the AAA (2011) and ASHA (2010) Codes of Ethics, it is helpful to beware of the ethical issues that may arise during a research study. These issues are usually related to: specifying the research problem; identifying a purpose statement and research questions; and collecting, analyzing, and writing up the results of the study (Creswell, 2003). By anticipating these issues in advance, ethical problems may be prevented or reduced. There is also need for information about research ethics in dissertations: Krellstrom, Ross and Fridland (2011) reported that ethical concerns about dissertations are often related to inadequate supervision. It was suggested

Table 2–11. Core Instructional for the Responsible Conduct of Research

Ethics and morality
Research misconduct
Human subjects protection
Publication practices and responsible authorship
Peer review
Mentor/trainee relationships
Conflict of interest and commitment
Data acquisition, management, sharing, and ownership
Collaborative research
Animal subjects protection
Guidelines and regulation

Source: From "Ethics and research," by J. Costello & J. Horner, 2004, *ASHA Leader*, Retrieved from http://www.asha.org

that ethical issues be emphasized in graduate and postgraduate studies.

Topics about conducting and reporting research are presented in Table 2–12. The second classification is related to ethical dilemmas associated with certain types of research that could become the focus of public debate.

These topics included the use of humans and animals in research. The third area addressed recognizing and responding to research misconduct such as plagiarism and fabricating or falsifying research data. This involves institutional policies and guidelines for the responsible conduct of research and guidance from the AAA (2011) and ASHA (2010) Codes of Ethics. The American Medical Association (Iverson et al., 1998) has guidelines for ethical and legal considerations in publishing papers. These topics and subtopics are listed in Table 2–13.

There is a need for information about ethical issues related to specific populations and work settings. Moss (2011) and Jakubowitz (2011) described ethical research practices in pediatric populations. Work settings such as the schools (Watson, Byrd, & Moore, 2011), and health care settings (Kummer & Turner, 2011; Larsen & McMillan, 2011) considered ethical research in multidisciplinary clinics.

A comprehensive survey of students and faculty in communication sciences and disorders by Minifie and associates (2011) found that students were not receiving adequate information about mentoring, research collaboration, conflicts of interest, and humane treatment of animals in research. These findings provide a basis for including and expanding this information.

There is also a need for continuing education about research ethics. Speech-language pathologists and audiologists need to periodically review and monitor information about professional ethics. The quality of instruction in ethics should be considered.

Ethical consultations are being used more frequently to resolve ethical dilemmas (Schneiderman et al., 2003). Lo (2003) suggests that ethics consultation fosters more effective education because it may identify areas needing improvement such as misunderstandings about ethics or limitations in communicating with patients and families. Kenny, Lincoln, and Balgain (2010) found that experienced speech-language pathologist more frequently used informal support networks to resolve ethical dilemmas than consulting work-based committees or their professional associates.

Table 2–12. Topics Related to Conducting and Reporting Research

Reasonable performance of research	Research design avoids subjectivity and minimizes bias
	Unbiased data selection and analysis
	Data management, storage, retrieval, ownership
	Sharing research methods, information
	Adherence to rules about safety, animal use, etc.
Responsible reporting of research	Authorship criteria
	Recognizing contributions of others
	Crediting previous work
	Duplicate and fragmented publication
	Avoidance of premature reporting or publishing
	Reporting in the public media
Ethical training practices	Fair performance evaluations, compensation, and benefit
	Responsibility to teach
	Responsibility to mentor
	Responsibility to give credit
	Avoidance of exploitation
Maintaining confidentiality	In reviewing submissions for publication
	In reviewing grant proposals
	In privileged personal communication

Source: Adapted from *Teaching the Responsible Conduct of Research Through a Case Study Approach*, by Association of American Medical Colleges, 1994, Washington, DC: Author.

Methods

There is literature available about a variety of methods for teaching ethics. These methods include role-playing, discussion groups, mentoring, case studies, self-directed learning, and computerized reference searched (American Speech-Language-Hearing Association, 2002; Association of American Medical Colleges, 1994; Bulger, 2001; Bulger, Heitman, & Reiser, 2002; Canter, Bennett, Jones, & Nagy, 1999; Davies 1999; Hamilton, 2002; Huffman, 2003; Jefferies & Bauer, 2003; Macrina, 1995a; Moss et al., 2003; Nagy, 2000). The National Institutes of Health have online training for protection of human subjects at no cost (http://cme.cancer.gov/clinicaltrials/learning/humanparticipants/protection.csp). Analysis and discussion about cases and situations are essential to teaching the responsible conduct of research (Heitman, 2002). Ethics courses and programs in many professions including speech-language pathology and audiology use the case study method to illustrate ethical issues in the field and to teach a system for ethical decision making professional practice.

Table 2–13. Ethical and Legal Considerations in Publishing

Authorship Responsibility	Authorship criteria
	Guest and ghost authors
	Unsigned editorials
	Number of authors
	Order of authorship
	Group/collaborative authorship
Acknowledgments	Permission to name individuals
Duplicate Publications	Secondary publication
	Editorial policy or preventions/handling allegations of duplicate publication
Scientific Misconduct	Misrepresentation
	Misappropriation
	Editorial policy for scientific misconduct
Conflict of Interest	Author's disclosure
	Peer reviewer's disclosure
	Editor's disclosure
	Editorial policy for failure to disclose financial interest
Copyright	Ownership and control of data
	Copyright
	Types of works; copyright duration
	Copyright assignment or licensure
	Copyright notice/resignation
	Copying, reproducing, adapting
	Publishing discussions from symposia, conferences
Reprint permissions, Intellectual Property	Standards for reprints
	Standards for licensed international editors
Ownership rights, Management	International copyright
	Moral rights
	Patent
	Trademark
	Peer review
	Allegation of scientific misconduct
Confidentiality	Selecting editors, editorial board members
	Legal petitions, claims privileged information

continues

Table 2–13. *continued*

Protecting Individual's Rights in Publication	Informed consent Patient's rights Rights to publish reports
Defamation Libel	Living persons, existing entities Public, private figures Statements of opinion Editorials, letters, reviews Works of fiction Republication, news reporting Defense against libel Other liability concerns
Editorial Freedom and Integrity	Policy on editorial freedom
Editorial Responsibilities, Procedures, Policies	Editor's responsibilities Rejection Acknowledging manuscript receipt Revisions Manuscript assessment Peer review Acceptance Correspondence column, corrections Disclosure of practices Audits, reviews Quality reviews
Advertisements, Suppliers Sponsored Supplements	Advertisements Criteria of advertisement Advertorials Sponsored suppliers Advertising, sponsorship Release of information to public Embargo Dealing with news media News release

Source: From *American Medical Association Manual of Style*, by C. Iverson, 1998, Philadelphia, PA: Lippincott Williams & Wilkins.

Another approach to teaching research ethics is on-site observation of ethical misconduct. This can be moeified and be based on role-playing or case-based observations (Oberman, Bosh-Missimov, & Ash, 2011).

Other resources for teaching research ethics are online print syllabi. McCarthy, Poole, and Solomon (2007) developed a model for teaching professional issues in university audiology and speech-language pathology training programs. The issues included ethical conduct and dilemmas and professional writing. Activities for these issues were based on Bloom's taxonomy ranging from one (knowledge) to seven (evaluation). A syllabus for research ethics committee training was developed by Cairoli and associates (2011). Training needs and competencies were identified. Funding for this training was reported to be a major problem. The University of Pittsburgh designed, implemented, and evaluated an institution with Web-based training for the responsible conduct of research (Barnes et al., 2006). The American Academy of Audiology (2012) also has a Web-based instruction based on the *Ethics Green Book.*

Current and Future Issues

There are several unresolved issues related to the responsible conduct of research. These issues should be recognized and appropriate strategy for resolution be developed. Two surveys have identified relevant issues (Ingham et al., 2011; Minifie et al., 2011). Ingham and associates (2011) completed a two-part survey of ASHA members about research principles of publishing research. Sev-

eral of the topics considered important were included in ASHA policy documents although some topics were not adequately addressed; recommendations were to have ASHA develop a single comprehensive publication policy document, implementation and enforcement of the policy, formal procedures for processing alleged ethical misconduct, and collaboration of communication sciences and disorders programs to design and implement long term educational programs about research ethics. Minifie and associates (2011) used a Web-based survey to assess students and faculty perceptions about the responsible conduct of research in communication science and disorders. Coverage of eight topics related to the responsible conduct of research was rated as adequate fabrication: falsification, reporting research misconduct, interpreting and reporting findings, confidentiality, protecting vulnerable subjects, alternative treatments, and data accuracy. Six topics did not receive adequate coverage: protection of electronic research information, recognizing and disclosing conflicts of interest. This information should be useful for improving instruction about the responsible conduct of research.

In a comprehensive review about research ethics, Minifie and associates (2011) identified "a host" of ethical issues. These issues were balance between risk and benefit; vulnerability and protection of subjects; conducting research with deceased subjects; protection of children; adequacy of federal regulations; appropriate limits of consent by parents and other legally authorized representatives; waive consent in intensive care; appropriate limitation of coercion and deception; representation of minorities; ethical and legal responsibilities of researchers; nature of research setting; social behavioral protection of subjects; harmful effect of randomization; and access to experimental pharmaceutical devices or alternative treatments when studies show no benefits.

Continuing Education for speech-language pathology or audiology licensure in Texas requires completion of two continuing education hours as part of the 20 hour minimum for two years (ASHA, 2011). Ingham and associates (2011) believe that "improved education of all aspects" of research ethics is needed (p. 394).

There is a need for professional universities and professional organizations to develop a consensus on the best ethical practices (Steneck & Bulger, 2007). There is also a need to assess the quality of ethical instruction and the effect of training.

Ethical training of students and professionals may be a way to decrease the need for regulation (Body & McAlister, 2009). Therefore, there should be increased self-assessment and monitoring.

Case studies should be detailed enough to provide meaningful ethical decisions but general enough for students to analyze from their own knowledge and experience. The goal of case studies is to determine an ethical resolution to the problem(s) pertinent to the case and to define appropriate action for resolving the problem(s). The basic steps of case study and analysis are outlined in Table 2–14. Yin (2003a, 2003b) provided extensive guidelines about the designing case studies. Case studies in research ethics are available in the Association of American Medical Colleges (1994), Hamilton (2002), Heitman (2002), Jonsen et al., (2006), and Macrina (1995).

Table 2–14. Steps for Case Study

1. Recognize and identify issues and specific ethical problems in the case.

2. Identify key facts, establish important definitions, and obtain other necessary information.

3. Identify professional ethical principles, standards or practice, and law relevant to ethical issues of the case.

4. Identify possible alternative courses and action, ethical arguments for and against implementation, and the likely outcome.

5. Choose the course of action best supported by the preceding analysis.

6. Evaluate the actions taken and the subsequent outcome.

Source: From *The Ethical Dimensions of the Biology and Health Science* (pp. 349–364), by E. Heitman, In R. E. Bulger, E. Heitman, & S. J. Reiser (Eds.), 2002, Cambridge, UK: Cambridge University Press.

Summary

Speech-language pathologists and audiologists face multiple ethical issues in planning, designing and implementing research. There is a need for ethical guidelines because research has not always been conducted ethically. There are three major types of research misconduct: (1) fabrication; (2) falsification; and (3) plagiarism. The Code of Ethics of AAA (2011) and ASHA (2010) have several standards related to responsible conducts of research and scholarly activities. The role and scope of the Institutional Review Board (IRB) and HIPAA are considered.

This chapter also included discussions of ethical issues related to research: (1) planning research; (2) confidentiality; (3) informed consent; (4) deception; (5) control group; (6) institutional approval; (7) conflicts of interest; (8) mentoring; (9) referencing of sources; (10) authorship; (11) copyright infringement and plagiarism; (12) peer review; (13) publication correction; and (14) evidence-based practice. Last, content and methods for teaching the responsible conduct of research and current and future issues are considered.

DISCUSSION QUESTIONS

1. Define the responsible conduct of research.
2. Explain the need for ethical guidelines
3. Trace the historical background of research conduct.
4. What is the impact of research misconduct?
5. How does research misconduct affect professional status?
6. Describe the major types of research misconduct.
7. Define fabrication, falsification, and plagiarism.
8. Explain ASHA's (2003b) ethical standards for reporting and publishing research.
9. Describe the ethical bases for the responsible conduct of research.
10. Why is confidentiality related to research?
11. Why does peer review fail?
12. How can confidentiality be maintained in research?
13. Why can obtaining informed consent be difficult?
14. How do professional codes of ethics address informed consent?
15. Define conflict of interest.
16. How can conflict of interest affect research?
17. What can be done to minimize conflicts of interest?
18. What factors should be considered in selecting a mentor?
19. Why should research records be maintained? For how long should they be maintained?
20. How can and why should plagiarism be avoided?
21. Why can authorship be a problem?
22. What is irresponsible authorship?

23. Describe the types of irresponsible authorship.
24. What is peer review?
25. What issues are related to peer review?
26. What should be done if authors discover or learn of errors in their published reports?
27. What guidelines for research are in the AAA (2011) Code of Ethics?
28. What guidelines for research are in the ASHA (2010) Code of Ethics?
29. What is IRB?
30. What are major responsibilities of an IRB?
31. What are the essential elements of informed consent?
32. What requirements affect IRB decisions?
33. What are the types of IRB reviews?
34. Discuss recent issues related to IRB.
35. How could these issues be resolved?
36. How can the ethics of research studies be evaluated?
37. What issues affect the content of teaching ethics?
38. Discuss the major topics related to conducting and reporting research.
39. Describe methods for teaching ethics.
40. How can case study and analysis be used to teach ethics?
41. What is the procedure for case study and analysis?
42. How can peer review fail?
43. What can be done to eliminate or resolve failed peer reviews?
44. What is copyright? Copyright infringement?
45. Why should and how can copyright infringement be avoided?
46. What is HIPAA?
47. How are HIPAA regulations enforced?
48. What are the penalties for violating HIPAA regulation?
49. List and briefly describe the three major HIPAA rules.
50. What is Protected Health Information?
51. How has HIPAA affected research?
52. What are the reasons for "Letter to the Editors?
53. What are the current issues relative to the responsible research?
54. How can these issues be resolved?

References

Altman, D. G. (2002). Poor quality medical research. *Journal American Medical Association, 287,* 2765–2767.

Ambrose, N. G., & Yairi, E. (2002). The Tudor study: Data and ethics. *American Journal of Speech Language Pathology, 11,* 190–203.

American Academy of Audiology. (2010). *The green book.* Retrieved from http://www.aaa.org./greenbook

American Academy of Audiology. (2011). *Code of ethics.* Retrieved from http://www.audiology.org

American Academy of Audiology. (2005a). *FAQs for publishing.* Retrieved from http://www.audiology.org

American Academy of Audiology. (2005b). *FAQs for understanding a research project.*

American Audiology Academy. (2012). *Ethics green book modules.* Retrieved from http://www.aaa.org/greenbook

American Medical Association. (1999). *Manual of style.* Chicago, IL: Author.

American Medical Association. (2011). *HIPAA violations and enforcement.* Retrieved from http://www.ama-assn.org/ama/pub/physician-resources/solutions-managing-your practice.

American Psychological Association. (2010). *Publication manual of the American Psychological Association.* Washington, DC: Author.

American Speech Language Hearing Association. (2001). *Conflict of interest.* Retrieved from http://www.asha.org

American Speech Language Hearing Association. (2005). *Protection of human subjects.* Retrieved from http://www.asha.org

American Speech-Language-Hearing Association. (2008). *Ethics in research and professional practice.* Retrieved from http://www.asha.org

American Speech-Language-Hearing Association. (2009). *Background information and standards and implementation for the Certificate of Clinical Competence in speech language pathology.* Rockville, MD: Author.

American Speech-Language-Hearing Association. (2010). *Code of ethics.* Retrieved from http://www.asha.org

American Speech-Language-Hearing Association. (2011). *Conflicts of professional interest.* Retrieved from http://www.asha.org

American Speech Language Hearing Association. (2011). *Cultural competence.* Retrieved from http://www.asha.org

American Speech Language Hearing Association. (2011). *Instruction for Authors.* Retrieved from http://www.asha.org

American Speech Language Hearing Association. (2011). *Standards and implementation for the Certificate of Clinical Competence in speech-language pathology.* Rockville, MD: Author.

American Speech Language Hearing Association. (2011). *Texas state characteristics of licensure law.* Retrieved from http://www.asha.org/Advocacy/state.into/TX/licensure/

American Speech Language Hearing Association. (2012). *How ASHA's Board of ethics sanctions individuals found in violation of the Coe of Ethics.* Retrieved from http://www.asha.org

American Speech Language Hearing Association. (2012, July 31). Presenter disclosure debut at convention. *ASHA Leader,* p. 19.

Annett, M. M. (2001). Article alleges 1939 study taught children to stutter. *ASHA Leader, 6*(13), 1, 17.

Association of American Medical Colleges. (1994). *Teaching the responsible conduct of research through a case study approach.* Washington, DC: Author.

Azar, B. (2002). Ethics at the cost of research? *Monitor on Psychology, 33*(2). Retrieved from http://www.apa.org/monitor/feb02/ethicscost.aspx

Bailar, J. C. (1995). The real threats to the integrity of science. *Chronicle of Higher Education,* pp. B1–B2.

Barnes, B. E., Fredkaj, C. P., Rosenberg, J. L., Russell, J., Beedle, A., & Levine, A. S. (2006). Creating an infrastructure for training in the responsible conduct of research. *Academic Medicine, 81,* 119–127.

Bennett, D. M., & Taylor, D. M. (2003). Unethical practices in authorship of science papers. *Emergency Medicine, 15*(3), 563–270.

Benninger, M. S. (2002). Duplicate publications in peer-reviewed journals. *Otolaryngology Head and Neck Surgery, 126*(2), 209–210.

Beyrer, C. (2003). Dual loyalty and human rights in health professional practice: Proposed guidelines and institutional mechanisms. *Journal of the American Medical Association, 290*(5), 671–672.

Blessing, J. D., & Forister, J. G. (2012). *Introduction to research and medical literature*. Burlington, MA: Barlett and Jones.

Blessing, J. D., & Forister, J. G. (2012). *Introduction to research and medical literature for health professionals*. Sudbury, MA: Jones and Bartlett.

Body, R., & McAllison, L. (2009). *Ethics in speech and language therapy*. West Susset, OK: Wiley & Blackwell.

Bradley, S. G. (1995). Conflict of interest. In F. L. Macrina (Ed.), *Scientific integrity* (pp. 166–188). Washington, DC: American Society for Microbiology.

Bulger, R. E. (2001). The ethics of teaching and learning. In American Speech-Language Hearing Association. *Promoting research integrity in communication sciences and disorders and related difficulties* (pp. 37–54). Rockville, MD: American Speech Language-Hearing Association.

Bulger, R. E., Heitman, E., & Reiser, S. J. (2002). *The ethical dimensions of the biological and health sciences*. Cambridge, UK: Cambridge University Press.

Cairoli E., Davies, H. T., Helm, J., Hooke, G., Knupfer, P., & Wells, F. (2011). A syllabus for research ethics committees: Training needs and resources in different European countries. *Journal of Medical Ethics, 10*, 136–138.

Campbell, E. G., Weissmen, J. S., Clarridge, B., Yucel, R. M., Causino, N., & Blumenthal, D. (2003). Characteristics of medical school faculty members serving on Institutional Review Boards: Results of a national survey. *Academic Medicine, 878*, 831–836.

Canter, M. B., Bennett, B. E., Jones, S. E., & Nagy, T. F. (1999). *Ethics for psychologists*. Washington, DC: American Psychological Association.

Christian, M. C., Goldberg, J. L., Killen, J., Abrams, J. S., McCabe, M. S., Mauer, J. K., & Wittes, R. E. (2002). A central institutional review board for multi-institutional trials. *New England Journal of Medicine, 346*(18), 1405–1408.

Cornett, B. S. (2007). Service delivery in health care settings. In R. Lubinski, L. A. Golpher,

& C. M. Frattali (Eds.), *Professional issues in speech-language pathology and audiology* (pp. 279–328). San Diego, CA: Plural.

Creswell, J. W. (2003). *Research design*. Thousand Oaks, CA: Sage.

Davies, P. (1999). Teaching evidence-based health care. In M. Daws, P. Davies, Gray, J. Mart, K. Seers, & R. Snowball (Eds.), *Evidence-based practice* (pp. 223–242). New York, NY: Churchill Livingstone.

DeRussy, C. (2003). Professional ethics begin on the college campus. *Chronicle of Higher Education*, p. B20.

Diefendorf, A. O. (2003). Ethics: Professionalism and conflicts of interest. *ASHA Leader, 25*. Retrieved from http://www.asha.org

Donaldson, T. M., Eistein, E., & Dunn, M. (2011). Case-based seminars in medical ethics education: How medical students define and discuss moral problems. *Journal of Medical Ethics, 36*, 816–820.

Dresser, R. (1993). Sanctions for research misconduct: A legal perspective. *Academic Medicine, 68*, S39–43.

Dunlop, A., Graham, T., Leroy, Z., Glanz, D., & Dunlop, B. (2007). The impact of HIPAA authorization on willing to participate in clinical research. *Annals of Epidemiology, 17*, 899–905.

Dyer, J. (2001, June 7). Ethics and orphans: The monster study. Part one of a Mercury News Special Report. *San Jose Mercury News*, p. 1A.

Dyer, J. (2001, June 11). Ethics and orphans: The monster study. Part two of a Mercury News Special Report. *San Jose Mercury News*, p. 1A.

Emanuel, E. J., Wendler, D., & Grady, C. (2000). What makes clinical research ethical? *Journal of the American Medical Association, 283*, 2701–2711.

Fifth International Congress on Peer Review. (2005). Retrieved from http://www.ama assn.org/public/peer/peerhome.htm

French, S., Reynolds, F., & Swain, J. (2001). *Practical research*. Boston, MA: Butterworth.

Gabard, D. L., & Martin, M. W. (2003). *Physical therapy ethics*. Philadelphia, PA: F. A. Davis.

Getzsch, P. O., Delamothe, T., & Goodlec, T. (2010). Adequacy of authors replies to critical or unfriendly electronic letters to the editor. *British Medical Journal, 3.*

Goldfarb, R. (2006). *Research ethics: A case study for fluency.* San Diego, CA: Plural.

Goodman, N. W. (1994). Survey of fulfillment of criteria for authorship in published medical research. *British Medical Journal, 309,* 1482.

Green, A., Lowery, J. C., Kowaiski, C. P., & Wyszewianski, L. (2006). Importance of institutional review board variation on observational health services research. *Health Science Research, 4,* 214–230.

Grodin, M. A., & Glantz, L. H. (1994). *Children as research subjects.* New York, NY: Oxford University Press.

Gunn, P. P., Fremont, A. M., Bottrell, M., Shuga, L. R., Galegher, L., & Biks, T. (2004). The Health Insurance Portability and Accountability Act Privacy Rule. *Medical Care, 42,* 321–327.

Gupta, M. (2003). A critical appraisal of evidence-based medicine: Some ethical considerations. *Journal of Evaluation of Clinical Practice, 9,* 111–121.

Halpern, S. A. (2004). *Lesser harms.* Chicago, IL: University of Chicago Press.

Hamilton, N. W. (2002). *Academic ethics.* Washington, DC: American Council on Education.

Heitman, E. (2002). Cases for discussion. In R. E. Bulger, E. Heitman, & S. J. Reiser (Eds.), *The ethical dimensions of the biological and health sciences* (pp. 349–364). Cambridge, UK: Cambridge University Press.

Heller, J. (1972, July 26). Syphilis victims in U.S. study without therapy for 40 years. *The New York Times,* pp. 1, 8.

Hoit, J. D. (2005). Write right. *American Journal of Speech-Language Pathology, 14,* 171.

Hornblum, A. M. (1998). *Acres of skin.* New York, NY: Routledge Press.

Hornblum, A. M. (2007). *Sentenced to science.* University Park, PA: Pennsylvania State University.

Horner, J., & Minifie, F. D. (2011a). Research ethics I: Responsible conduct of research (RCR)—History and contemporary issues pertaining to human and animal experimentation. *Journal of Speech, Language, and Hearing Research, 54,* S303–S329.

Horner, J., & Minifie, F. D. (2011b). Research ethics II: Mentoring, collaboration, peer review and data management and ownership. *Journal of Speech, Language, and Hearing Research, 54,* S330–S345.

Horner, J., & Minifie, F. D. (2011c). Research ethics III: Publication practice and authorship, conflict of interest, and research misconduct. *Journal of Speech, Language, and Hearing Research, 54,* S346–S362.

Horner, J., & Wheeler, M. (2005). HIPAA: Impact on clinical practice. *ASHA Leader.*

Horner, J., & Wheeler, M. (2005). HIPAA: Impact on research practices. *ASHA Leader,* pp. 8–9, 26–27.

Huffman, N. P. (2003). Ethics: Employers, employees, and ethics. *ASHA Leader, 23.* Retrieved from http://www.asha.org

Ingham, J, C., & Horner, J, (2004). Ethics and research. *ASHA Leader, 9,* 10–25.

Ingham, J. C., Minifie, F. D., Horner, J., Robey, R. R., Lansing, C., McCartney, J. C., . . . Moss, S. E. (2011). Ethical principles as associated with the publication of research in ASHA's scholarly journals: Importance and accuracy of coverage. *Journal of Speech, Language, and Hearing Research, 54,* S394–S416.

Institute of Society, Ethics and the Life Sciences. (1980). Applied ethics: A strategy for fostering professional responsibility. *Carnegie Quarterly, 28,* 1–7.

International Dual Loyalty Working Group. (2002). *Dual loyalty and human rights in health professional practice: Proposed guidelines and institutional mechanisms.* Cape Town, South Africa: University of Cape Town Health Sciences Faculty.

Iverson, C., Flanagin, A., Fontanarosa, P. B., Glass, R. M., Glitman, P., Lantz, J. C., . . . Young, R. K. (1998). *American Medical Association manual of style.* Philadelphia, PA: Lippincott, Williams, & Wilkins.

Jakubowitz, M. (2011). Ethical issues in a pediatric practice. *Seminars in Speech and Language, 32,* 347–356.

Jefferies, M., & Bauer, J. J. (2003, November). *Research ethics in graduate education.* Seminar presented at annual meeting of the American Speech-Language Hearing Association, Chicago.

Jones, J. (1982). *Bad blood,* New York, NY: Free Press.

Jonsen, A. R., Siegler, M., & Winsdale, W. (2006). *Clinical ethics.* New York, NY: McGraw Hill.

Journal of the American Medical Association. (2006). Instructions for authors. *Journal of the American Medical Association, 295*(1), 103–116.

Kenny, B., Lincoln, M., & Balardin, S. (2010). Experiencing speech-language pathologist response to ethical dilemmas. An integrated approach to ethical reasoning. *American Journal of Speech-Language Pathology, 19,* 121–134.

Knapp, S. J., & Van de Creek, L. D. (2006). *Practical ethics for psychologists.* Washington, DC: American Psychological Association.

Korn, D. (2000). Conflicts of interest in biomedical research. *Journal of the American Medical Association, 284*(17), 2234–2237.

Krellstrom, S., Ross, S. N., & Fridland, R. (2011). Research ethics in dissertations: Ethical issues complexity of reasoning. *Journal of Medical Ethics, 36,* 425–430.

Krogman, S. (2005). The Willowbrook hepatitis studies revisited. *Review of Infectious Disease, 8,* 157–162.

Kummer, A. W., & Turner, J. (2011). Ethics in the practice of speech-language pathology in health care settings. *Seminars in Speech and Language, 32,* 330–337.

Kwok, L. S. (2005). The white bull effect: Abusive co-authorship and publication parasitism. *Journal of Medical Ethics, 31,* 554–556.

Laine, C., & Mulrow, C. (2003). Peer review: Integral to science and indispensable to annals. *Annals of Internal Medicine, 139*(12), 1038–1040.

Lansing, C. R. (2002). Ethics: Loose lips: Confidentiality in relationships with colleagues. *ASHA Leader.* Retrieved from http://www.asha.org

Lansing, C. R., & Moss, S. (2003). Survey to determine knowledge of research ethics. *ASHA Leader, 18.* Retrieved from http://www.asha.org

Larsen, J., & McMillman, A. (2011). Ethical issues in the conduct of research at a multidisciplinary clinic. *Seminars in Speech and Language, 32,* 338–346.

Lo, B. (2003). Answers and questions about ethics consultation. *Journal of the American Medical Association, 290*(9), 1208–1210.

Ludlow, C. L. (2001). Responsible conduct of clinical research. In American Speech-Language Hearing Association, *Promoting research integrity in communication sciences and disorders and related disciplines* (pp. 29–45). Rockville, MD: ASHA.

Lum, C. (2002). *Scientific thinking in speech and language therapy.* Mahwah, NJ: Lawrence Erlbaum Associates.

Macrina, F. L. (1995a). Mentoring. In F. L. Macrina (Ed.), *Scientific integrity* (pp. 15–40). Washington, DC: American Society for Microbiology.

Macrina, F. L. (1995b). Scientific record keeping. In F. L. Macrina (Ed.), *Scientific integrity* (pp. 41–68). Washington, DC: American Society for Microbiology.

Macrina, F. L. (1995c). Authorship and peer review. In F. L. Macrina (Ed.), *Scientific integrity* (pp. 69–96). Washington, DC: American Society for Microbiology.

Mattick, K., & Blight, J. (2011) Teaching and assessing medical ethics: Where are we now? *Journal of Medical Ethics, 36,* 181–185.

McCarthy, M. P., Poole, K. L., & Solomon, B. (2007). Ethics: A model curriculum for teaching professional issues in university speech-language pathology and audiology programs. *Perspective on Administration and Supervision,* pp. 20–34.

McCartney, J. (2002). ASHA Code of Ethics and research. *ASHA Leader, 12.* Retrieved from http://www.asha.org

McWilliams, R., Hoover-Fong, J., Hamosh, A., Becik, S., Beaty, T., & Cuting, G. R. (2003).

Local vs. central Institutional Review Boards for multicenter studies — reply. *Journal of the American Medical Association, 290*(16), 2126–2127.

Meline, T. (2006). *Research in communication sciences and disorders.* Columbus, OH: Pearson.

Mertens, D. M. (2005). *Research and evaluation in education and psychology.* Thousand Oaks, CA: Sage.

Minifie, F. D., Robey, R. R., Horner, J., Ingham, J. C., Lansing, C., McCarthy, J. H., . . . Moss, S. E. (2011). Responsible conduct of research in communication sciences and disorders: Faculty, student perceptions. *Journal of Speech, Language, and Hearing Research, 54,* S363 –S393.

Moss, S. (2006). Researchers discuss integrity in publications practices. *ASHA Leader, 26,* 34.

Moss, S. E. (2010). Research integrity in communication sciences and disorders. *Journal of Speech, Language, and Hearing Research, 54,* S300–S302.

Moss, S. (2011). Promoting ethical research practices: Perspectives from pediatric populations. *Seminars in Speech and Language, 32,* 207–289.

Mowatt, G., Shirran, L., Grimshaw, J. M., Rennie, D., Flanagin, A., & Yank, V., . . . Bero, L. A. (2002). Prevalence of honorary and ghost authorship in Cochrane reviews. *Journal of the American Medical Association, 287*(21), 2769–2771.

Nagy, T. F. (2000). *Ethics in plain English.* Washington, DC: American Psychological Association.

Ness, R. B. (2007). Influence of the HIPAA privacy rule on health research. *Journal of the American Medical Association, 298,* 2164–2170.

Nosowsky, R., & Giordano, T. (2006). The Health Information Portability and Accountability Act of 1996 (HIPAA) privacy rule: Implication for clinical research. *Annual Reviews of Medicine, 57,* 575–590.

O'Herrin, J. K., Fost, N., & Kudson, K. A. (2004). The Health Insurance Portability and Accountability Act (HIPAA) regulations: Effect on medical record research. *Annual of Surgery, 239,* 772–778.

Oberman, A. S., Bosh-Missimov, T., & Ash, N. (2011). Medicine and the Holocaust: A visit to the Nazi death camps as a means of teaching ethics in the Israel Defense Forces' medical camps. *Journal of Medical Ethics, 36,* 826.

Office of Research Integrity. (2010). *Office of research integrity annual report.* Washington, DC: Office of Research Integrity.

Olsen, D. P. (2003). HIPAA privacy regulations and nursing research. *Nursing Research, 52,* 344–348.

Olson, C. M., Rennie, D., Cook, D., Dickerson, K., Flanagin, A. &, Magen, J. W., . . . Pace, B. (2002). Publications bias in editorial decision making. *Journal of the American Medical Association, 287*(21), 2825–2828.

Polit, D. F., & Beck, C. T. (2010). *Nursing research: Principles and methods.* Philadephia, PA: Lippincott.

Portney, L. G., & Watkins, M. P. (2009). *Foundations of clinical research.* Upper Saddle River, NJ: Prentice-Hall Health.

Pozar, G. D. (2012). *Ethical and legal issues for health professionals.* Sudbury, MA: Jones and Barlett.

Rennie, D. (2002). Fourth International Congress on peer review in biomedical publication. *Journal of the American Medical Association, 287*(21), 2759–2760. Retrieved from: http://www.audiology.org

Reynolds, S. M. (2004). ORI findings of scientific misconduct in clinical trials and public funded research 1992–2001. *Clinical Trials,* pp. 509–516.

Romanow, K. (2001). Bottom line: Patient information privacy bases. *ASHA Leader.*

Romanow, K. (2001). Bottom line: Possible HIPAA changes ahead. *ASHA Leader.*

Rose, C. D. (2003). Local vs. central Institutional Review Boards for multicenter studies. *Journal of the American Medical Association, 290*(16), 2126.

Rosenthal, R. (1999). Science and ethics in conducting, analyzing, and reporting psychological research. In D. N. Bergoff (Ed.), *Ethical conflicts in psychological* (pp. 127–

133). Washington, DC: American Psychological Association.

Rothman, D., & Rothman, S. (1984). *The Willowbrook Wars*. New York, NY: Harper and Row.

Sales, B. D., & Lavin, M. (2000). Identifying conflicts of interest and resolving ethical dilemmas. In B. D. Sales & S. Folkman (Eds.), *Ethics in research with human participants* (pp. 109–128). Washington, DC: American Psychological Association.

Scheetz, M. D. (2001). Research integrity issues in the publication of research. In American Speech-Language-Hearing Association, *Promoting research integrity in communication sciences and disorders and related disciplines* (pp. 46–54). Rockville, MD: ASHA.

Schneiderman, L. J., Glimer, T., Teetzel, H. D., Dugan, D. O., Blusten, J., Cranford, R., . . . Young, E. W. (2003). Effects of ethics consultations on nonverified life-sustaining treatments in the intensive care setting. *Journal of the American Medical Association, 290*(9), 1166–1172.

Shamoo, A. E., & Resnik, D. B. (2003). *Responsible conduct of research*. New York, NY: Oxford University Press.

Shapiro, D. W., Wenger, N. S., & Shapiro, M. F. (1994). The contributions of authors to multiauthored biomedical research papers. *Journal of the American Medical Association, 271*(6), 438–442.

Sharp, H. (2001). Issues in ethics: Institutional Review Boards. *Cleft Palate Newsletter, 274*(4), 8.

Sieber, J. E. (1992) *Planning ethically responsible research*. Thousand Oaks, CA: Sage.

Silverman, F. H. (1998a). The "monster" study. *Journal of Fluency Disorders, 13*, 225–231.

Silverman, F. H. (1998b). *Research design and evaluation in speech-language pathology and audiology*. Boston, MA: Allyn & Bacon.

Silverman, F. H. (1999). *Professional issues in speech-language pathology and audiology*. Boston, MA: Allyn and Bacon.

Sininger, Y., March, R., Walden, B., & Wilber, L. A. (2004). Guidelines for ethical practice in research for audiologists. *Audiology Today, 15*(6), 14–17.

Society for Clinical Trials. (2004). Lying, cheating and stealing in clinical research. *Clinical Trials, 1*, 475–476.

Steneck, N. H., & Bulger, R. E. (2009). The history, purpose, and future of instructions in the responsible conduct of research. *Academic Medicine, 82*, 829–833.

Strange, K. (2008). Authorship: Why not just toss a coin? *American Journal of Physiology-Cell Physiology, 295*, 567–575.

Washington, H. A. (2006). *Medical apartheid*. New York, NY: Random House.

Watson, J. B., Byrd, C. Y., & Moore, B. J. (2011). Ethics in stuttering treatment in the schools. *Issues and Instruction Seminars in Speech and Language, 32*, 319–329.

Wikipedia (n.d.). Health Insurance Portability and Accountability Act. Retrieved from http://wikipedial.org

Wikipedia (n.d.). Unethical human experiments in the United States. Retrieved from http://en.wikipedia.org/

Wipke-Tevis, D. D., & Pickett, M. A. (2008) Impact of HIPAA on subject recruitment on retention. *Western Journal of Nursing Research, 30*, 39–53.

Wolf, M. S., & Benett, C. L. (2006). Local perspective of the impact of the HIPAA privacy rule on research. *Cancer, 106*, 474–479.

Yedidia, M. J., Gillespie, C. C., Kechur, E., Schwarz, M. D., Oakene, J., & Chepaitis, A. E., . . . Lipkin, M. Jr. (2003). Effects of communications training on medical student performance. *Journal of the American Medical Association, 290*(9), 1157–1165.

Yin, R. K. (2003a). *Application of case study research*. Thousand Oaks, CA: Sage.

Yin, R. K. (2003b). *Case study research: Design and methods*. Thousand Oaks, CA: Sage.

Young, J. R. (2003). The cat and mouse game of plagiarism detection. *Chronicle of Higher Education, 47*(43), A26.

Appendix 2–A
American Academy of Audiology (AAA) Code of Ethics 2011

Highlighted Changes Effective April 2012

Preamble

The Code of Ethics of the American Academy of Audiology specifies professional standards that allow for the proper discharge of audiologists' responsibilities to those served, and that protect the integrity of the profession. The Code of Ethics consists of two parts.. The first part, the Statement of Principles and Rules, presents precepts that members (all categories of members, including Student Members) of the Academy agree to uphold. The second part, the Procedures, provides the process that enables enforcement of the Principles and Rules.

PART I. Statement of Principles and Rules

PRINCIPLE 1: Members shall provide professional services and conduct research with honesty and compassion, and shall respect the dignity, worth, and rights of those served.

Rule 1a: Individuals shall not limit the delivery of professional services on any basis that is unjustifiable or irrelevant to the need for the potential benefit from such services.

Rule 1b: Individuals shall not provide services except in a professional relationship, and shall not discriminate in the provision of services to individuals on the basis of sex, race, religion, national origin, sexual orientation, or general health.

PRINCIPLE 2: Members shall maintain high standards of professional competence in rendering services.

Rule 2a: Members shall provide only those professional services for which they are qualified by education and experience.

Rule 2b: Individuals shall use available resources, including referrals to other specialists, and shall not give or accept benefits or items of value for receiving or making referrals.

Rule 2c: Individuals shall exercise all reasonable precautions to avoid injury to persons in the delivery of professional services or execution of research.

Rule 2d: Individuals shall provide appropriate supervision and assume full responsibility for service delegated to supportive personnel. Individuals shall not delegate any service requiring professional competence to unqualified persons.

Rule 2e: Individuals shall not knowingly permit personnel under their direct or indirect supervision to engage in any practice that is a violation of the Code of Ethics.

Rule 2f: Individuals shall maintain professional competence, including participation in continuing education.

PRINCIPLE 3: Members shall maintain the confidentiality of the information and records of those receiving services or involved in research.

Rule 3a: Individuals shall not reveal to unauthorized persons any professional or personal information obtained from the person served professionally, unless required by law.

PRINCIPLE 4: Members shall provide only services and products that ate in the best interest of those served.

Rule 4a: Individuals shall not exploit persons in the delivery of professional services.

Rule 4b: Individuals shall not charge for services not rendered.

Rule 4c: Individuals shall not participate in activities that constitute a conflict of professional interest.

Rule 4d: Individuals using investigational procedures with human participants or prospectively collecting research data from human participants shall obtain full informed consent from the participants or legal representatives. Members conducting research with human participants or animals shall follow accepted standards, such as those promulgated in the current Responsible Conduct of Research (current edition, 2009) by the U. S. Office of Research Integrity.

PRINCIPLE 5: Members shall provide accurate information about the nature and management of communicative disorders and about the service and products offered.

Rule 5a: Individuals shall provide persons served with the information a reasonable person would want to know about the nature and possible effects of services rendered, or products provided or research being conducted.

Rule 5b: Individuals may make a statement of prognosis, but shall not guarantee results, mislead, or misinform persons served or studied.

Rule 5c: Individuals shall conduct and report product-related research only according to accepted standards of research practice.

Rule 5d: Individuals shall not carry out teaching or research activities in a manner that constitutes an invasion of privacy, or that fails to inform persons fully about the nature and possible effects of these activities, affording all persons informed free choice of participation.

Rule 5e: Individuals shall maintain accurate documentation of services rendered according to accepted medical, legal, and professional standards and requirements.

PRINCIPLE 6: Members shall comply with the ethical standards of the Academy with regard to public statements or publication.

Rule 6a: Individuals shall not misrepresent their educational degrees, training, credentials, or competence. Only degrees earned from regionally accredited institutions in which training was obtained in audiology, or a directory related discipline, may be used in public statements a-concerning professional services.

Rule 6b: Individuals' public statements about professional services, products, or research results shall not contain representations or claims that are false, misleading, or deceptive.

PRINCIPLE 7: Members shall honor the responsibilities to the public and to professional colleagues.

Rule 7a: Individuals shall not use professional or commercial affiliations in any way that would limit services to or mislead patients or colleagues.

Rule 7b: Individuals shall inform colleagues and the public in an objective manner consistent with professional standards abut products and services they have developed or research they have conducted.

PRINCIPLE 8: Members shall uphold the dignity of the profession and freely accept the Academy's self-imposed standards.

Rule 8a: Individuals shall not violate these Principles and Rules, nor attempt to circumvent them.

Rule 8b: Individuals shall not engage in dishonesty or illegal conduct that adversely reflects on the profession.

Rule 8c: Individuals shall inform the Ethical Practice Committee when there are reasons to believe that a member of the Academy may have violated the Code of Ethics.

Rule 8d: Individuals shall fully cooperate with reviews being conducted by the Ethical Practices Committee in any matter related to the Code of Ethics.

PART II. Procedures for the Management of Alleged Violations

Introduction

Members of the American Academy of Audiology are obligated to uphold the Code of Ethics of the Academy in their personal conduct and in the performance of their professional duties. To this end it is the responsibility of each Academy member to inform the Ethical Practice Committee of possible Ethics Code violations. The processing of alleged violations of the Code of Ethics will follow the procedures specified below in an expeditious manner to ensure that violations of ethical conduct by members of the Academy are halted in the shortest time possible.

Procedures

1. Suspected violations of the Code of Ethics shall be reported in a letter format giving documentation sufficient to support the alleged violation. Letters must be addressed to: Chair, Ethical Practice Committee

Source: American Academy of Audiology. (2011). *Code of Ethics.* Retrieved from http://www.audiology.org

Appendix 2–B

American Speech-Language-Hearing Association Code of Ethics 2010

PREAMBLE

The preservation of the highest standards of integrity and ethical principles is vital to the responsible discharges of obligations by speech-language pathologists, audiologists, and speech, language, and hearing scientists. This Code of Ethics sets forth the fundamental principles and rules considered essential to this purpose.

Every individual who is (a) a member of the American Speech-Language-Hearing Association, whether certified or not, (b) a nonmember holding the Certificate of Clinical Competence from the Association, (c) an applicant for membership or certification, or (d) a Clinical Fellow seeking to fulfill standards for certification shall abide by this Code of Ethics.

Any violation of the spirit and purpose of this Code shall be considered unethical. Failure to specify any particular responsibility or practice in this Code of Ethics shall not be construed as denial of the existence of such responsibilities or practices.

The fundamentals of ethical conduct are described by Principles of Ethics and by Rules of Ethics as they relate to the responsibility to persons served, the public, speech-language pathologists, audiologists, and speech, language, and hearing scientists, and to the conduct of research and scholarly activities.

Principles of Ethics, aspirational and inspirational in nature, form the underlying moral basis for the Code of Ethics. Individuals shall observe these principles as affirmative obligations under all conditions of professional activity.

Rules of Ethics are specific statements of minimally acceptable professional conduct or of prohibitions and are applicable to all individuals.

Principle of Ethics I

Individuals shall honor their responsibility to hold paramount the welfare of persons they serve professionally or who are participants in research and scholarly activities, and they shall treat animals involved in research in a humane manner.

Rules of Ethics

1. Individuals shall provide all services competently.
2. Individuals shall use every resource, including referral when appropriate, to ensure that high-quality services is provided.
3. Individuals shall discriminate in the delivery of professional services or the conduct of research and scholarly activities on the basis of race or ethnicity, gender, gender identity/gender expression, age, religion, national origin, sexual orientation, or disability.

4. Individuals shall not misrepresent the credentials of assistants, technicians, support personnel, students, Clinical Fellows, or any others under their supervision, and they shall inform those they serve professionally of the name and professional credentials of persons providing services.

5. Individuals who hold the Certificate of Clinical Competence shall not delegate tasks that require the unique skills, knowledge, and judgment that are within the scope of their profession to assistant, technicians, support personnel, to any nonprofessionals over whom they have supervisory responsibility.

6. Individuals who hold the Certificate of Clinical Compete may delegate tasks related to provision of clinical services to assistants, technicians, support personnel, or any other persons only if those services are appropriately supervised, realizing that the responsibility for client welfare remains with certified individual.

7. Individuals who hold the Certificate of Clinical Competence may delegate tasks related to provision of clinical services that require the unique skills, knowledge, and judgment that are within the scope of practice of their profession to students only if those services are appropriately supervised. The respobsibility for client welfare remains with the certified individual.

8. Individuals shall fully inform the persons they serve of the nature and possible effects of services rendered and products dispensed, and they shall inform participants in research about the possible effects of their participation in research conducted.

9. Individuals shall evaluate the effectiveness of services rendered and of products dispensed, and they shall provide services or dispense products only when benefit can reasonably be expected.

10. Individuals shall not guarantee the results of any treatment or procedure, directly or by implication; however, they may make a reasonable statement of prognosis.

11. Individuals shall not provide clinical services solely by correspondence.

12. Individuals may practice by telecommunication (e.g., telehealth/e-health), where not prohibited by law.

13. Individuals shall adequately maintain and appropriately secure records of professional services rendered, research and scholarly activities.

14. Individuals shall not reveal without authorization, any professional or personal information about identified persons served professionally or identified participants involved in research and scholarly activities unless doing so is necessary to protect the welfare of the person or of the community or is otherwise required by law.

15. Individuals shall not charge for services not rendered, nor shall they misrepresent services rendered products dispensed, or research and scholarly activities conducted.

16. Individuals shall enroll and include persons as participants in research or teaching demonstrations only if their participation is voluntary, without coercion, and with their informed consent.

17. Individuals whose professional services are adversely affected by substance abuse or other health-related conditions shall seek professional assistance and, where appropriate, withdraw from the affected areas of practice.
18. Individuals shall not discontinue service t those they are serving without providing reasonable notice.

Principle of Ethics II

Individuals shall honor their responsibility to achieve and maintain the highest level of professional competence and performance.

Rules of Ethics

1. Individuals shall engage in the provision of clinical services only when they hold the appropriate Certificate of Clinical Competence or when they are in the certification process and are supervised by an individual who holds the appropriate Certificate of Clinical Competence.
2. Individuals shall engage in inly those aspects of the professions that are within the scope of their professional practice and competence, considering their level of education, training, and experience.
3. Individuals shall engage in lifelong learning to maintain and enhance professional competence and performance.
4. Individuals shall not require or permit their professional staff to provide services or conduct research activities that exceed the staff member's competence, level of education, training, and experience.
5. Individuals shall ensure that all equipment used to provide services or to conduct research and scholarly activities is in proper working order and is properly calibrated.

Principle of Ethics III

Individuals shall honor their responsibility to the public by promoting public understanding of the professions, by supporting the development of services designed to fulfill the unmnet needs of the public, and by providing accurate information in all communications involving any aspect of the professionals, including the dissemination of research findings and scholarly activities, and the promotion, marketing, and advertising of products and services.

1. Individuals shall not misrepresent their credentials, competence, education, training, experience, or scholarly or research contributions.
2. Individuals shall not participate in professional activities that constitute a conflict of interest.

3. Individuals shall refer those served professionally solely on the basis of the interest of those being referred and not on any personal interest, financial or otherwise.

4. Individuals shall not misrepresent research, diagnostic information, services rendered, results of service rendered, products dispensed, or the effects of products dispensed.

5. Individuals shall not defraud or engage in any scheme to defraud in connection with obtaining payment, reimbursement, or grants for service rendered, research conducted, or products dispensed.

6. Individuals' statements to the public shall provide accurate information about the nature and management of communication disorders, about the professions, about professional services, about products for sale, and about research and scholarly activities.

7. Individuals statement to the public when advertising, announcing, and marketing their professional services; reporting research results; and promoting products shall adhere to professional standards and shall not contain misrepresentations.

Principle of Ethics IV

Individuals shall honor their responsibilities to the professions and their relationships with colleagues, students, and members of other professions and disciplines.

1. Individuals shall uphold the dignity and autonomy of the professions maintain harmonious interprofessional and intraprofessional relationships, and accept the professions self-imposed standards.

2. Individuals shall prohibit anyone under their supervision from engaging in any practice that violates the Code of Ethics.

3. Individuals shall not engage in dishonesty, fraud, deceit, or misrepresentation.

4. Individuals shall not engage in any form of unlawful harassment, including sexual harassment or power abuse.

5. Individuals shall not engage in any other form of conduct that adversely reflects on the professions or on the individual's fitness to serve persons professionally.

6. Individuals shall not engage in sexual activities with clients, students, or research participants over whom they exercise professional authority or power.

7. Individuals' shall assign credit only to those who have contributed to a publication, presentation, or product. Credit shall be assigned in proportion to the contribution and only with the contributor's consent.

8. Individuals shall reference the source when using other persons' ideas, research, presentations, or products in written, oral, or any other media presentation or summary.

9. Individuals' statements to colleagues about professional services, research results, and product shall adhere to prevailing professional standards and shall contain no misrepresentations.
10. Individuals shall not provide professional services without exercising independent professional judgment, regardless of referral source or prescription.
11. Individuals shall not discriminate in their relationships with colleagues, students, and members of other professions and discipline on the basis of race, or ethnicity, gender, gender identity/gender expression, age, religion, national origin, sexual orientation, or disability.
12. Individuals shall not file or encourage others to file complaints that disregard or ignore facts that would disprove the allegation, not should the Code of Ethics be used for personal reprisal, as a means of addressing personal animosity, or as a vehicle for retaliation.
13. Individuals shall have reason to believe that the Code of Ethics has been violated shall inform the Board of Ethics.
14. Individuals shall comply fully with the policies of the Board of Ethics in its consideration and adjudication of complaints of violations of the Code of Ethics.

Source: American Speech-Language-Hearing Association. (2010). *Code of Ethics* [Ethics]. Retrieved from www.asha.org/policy

3

Research Problems

LEARNING OBJECTIVES

Upon completion of this chapter the reader will be able to:

- Define and provide examples of independent and dependent variables

- Describe how variables and confounding factors may be controlled in a research project

- Describe how a topic can be selected for a research problem

- Discuss how to state a research problem, null hypothesis, and alternative hypothesis

- Describe what factors should be considered regarding the feasibility of a research project

- Discuss the six phases of budget preparation for a research project

- List the factors that may be included in a Charge Master.

Basic Concepts and Terms

Science is the search for knowledge. Schiavetti, Metz, and Orlikoff (2011) described *scientific method* as a method of efficiently or methodically generating knowledge by recognizing a problem capable of objective study, collecting data by observation or experimentation, and drawing conclusions based on analysis of the data. Silverman (1998) further described scientific method as a set of rules used for describing, explaining, and predicting "events" that are observable and occur over time.

The scientific method is an effective tool for answering the type of questions it was designed to answer. However, as Siegel (1987) points out, some questions in communication disorders (e.g., those involving social or personal values and attitudes) cannot be answered using pure methods of science.

Theoretically, studies can be classified as basic or applied experimental research. *Basic research* focuses on answering important questions or deciphering the laws of nature (Hegde, 2003; Shearer, 1982). *Applied research* employs the answers to the basic questions of further research to practical problems such as questions involving clinical practice.

Questions involving clinical management are answered using clinical or applied research models. Clinical research may be experimental or descriptive. Experimental studies involve the use of rigorous design in which variables are carefully controlled. Experimental research in speech-language pathology and audiology is often weakened somewhat statistically because some variables cannot be controlled (Shearer, 1982).

Variables are capable of change or modification. They may vary in quality or quantity. Examples of qualitative variables might include the sex of an individual, the disorder of speech or language an individual has been diagnosed as having, or the type of clinical management selected for particular patients. Quantitative variables such as intelligence can be measured quantitatively or numerically. *Discrete quantitative variables* are not expressed in decimals or fractions. Examples include the number of subjects in a study, scores on some tests, or the number of times a treatment is administered. *Continuous variables* can be expressed in any numerical value including fractions. Examples include age of subjects (i.e., 1.5 or 1½ years), scores on some tests that allow results to be expressed in whole numbers or in fractions, or height and weight data describing subjects. Variables describe the population investigated by a study. Variables that do not change from individual to individual (such as a diagnosis of stuttering) are called *constant variables.*

Research in speech-language pathology and audiology is designed to investigate the causes of disorders and the effect(s) of various phenomena on behaviors associated with disorders of communication. *Dependent variables,* or sometimes called the outcome variable, are the effect of unknown etiology(ies). An example of a dependent variable is a hyperfunctional voice disorder characterized by a rough voice quality and accompanied by frequent upper respiratory infections, coughing, allergies, and laryngitis. As illustrated, the dependent variable must be described in operational terms so that it is clear how the variable will be identified and measured for a particular study

(Hegde, 1994). An operational definition should have sufficient detail so another researcher can replicate the procedure or condition (Portney & Watkins, 2009).

Independent variables explain the dependent variables. For example, an individual's vocal habits (talking frequently, loudly, and excessive laryngeal tension) along with behaviors associated with a medical condition (laryngitis) might constitute identified independent variables explaining the dependent variable, a voice disorder defined according to description and accompanying medical condition. By manipulating independent variables, an investigator may change dependent variables involving disorders of communication. For example, reducing abusive vocal habits and medically testing the laryngitis may successfully effect a change in voice characteristics to a smooth, more relaxed and pleasant voice production.

Hegde (2003) described three types of independent variables in communication disorders research, those that:

1. Explain the cause of normal parameters of communication,
2. Explain the development of abnormal communication, or
3. Identify treatment techniques that create optimal changes in communication.

The independent variables that can be manipulated (e.g., vocal habits and medical condition of the larynx and surrounding tissues) are active variables (Hegde, 2003). Some independent variables may be impossible to change (e.g., a predisposition for laryngeal vulnerability to abusive vocal habits). These are called assigned variables (Hegde, 2003). They may play a role in determining out-

come but cannot be controlled by the researcher. The experimental researcher attempts to rule out assigned variables. For example, if patients identified as having a predisposition or vulnerability to some voice problems and those identified as less vulnerable both improve by changing voice habits and receiving medical intervention, the vulnerability variable may be ruled out as the assumption that it causes hyperfunctional phonation is reduced.

Control of Variables

According to Portney and Watkins (2009), "an extraneous variable is any factor that is not directly related to the purpose of the study, but may affect the dependent variable" (p. 153). When extraneous variables are not controlled, they can have a confounding influence on the independent variable. For example, if a patient has a history of sinus congestion and drainage, then this extraneous variable could influence vocal quality.

Complete control of all confounding variables is usually not possible. This may lead to results that are inconclusive and difficult to interpret. Portney and Watkins (2009), suggest several methods that may help control for extraneous or confounding variables such as random assignment of subjects, use of a control group, a well-defined research protocol, and blinding.

Random assignment of subjects involves that each subject has an equal chance of being assigned to any group and ensures that assignments will be independent of personal judgment or bias. However, in clinical research for speech-language pathology and audiology often using small numbers, randomization can result in groups with disparate differences on critical variables. Researchers may use statistical means of comparing groups on initial values in regard to the dependent variable to determine if the influence of any extraneous variable did balance out (Portney & Watkins, 2009).

Control groups are frequently used by researchers to rule out the influence of extraneous variables. In a classic experimental design, subjects in a control group receive no form of treatment. This is in contrast to the experimental group, which is targeted to receive the "new" treatment. This type of design strategy would lead the researcher to safely assume that if the treatment group is significantly different from the control group, then that is probably attributable to the influence of the "new" treatment.

Portney and Watkins (2000), state "the use of a control group is often unfeasible in clinical situations, for practical or ethical reasons" (p. 157). Because of such reasons, clinical researchers have a control group receive a "standard" form of treatment and the experimental group receive a "new" form of treatment. Without comparison of these two groups, it is difficult to conclude that any form of treatment is actually responsible for an observed change.

A well-defined research protocol usually ensures that many extraneous variables have been considered and controlled. The protocol needs to have each procedure explained and detailed in order for another researcher to critically analyze what was done, for IRB to make decisions, and to improve reliability. Research protocols should also include a description of all limitations in the study. Limitations would not prevent a study from being conducted, but recognize that other variables may not have been controlled which may have influenced results.

It is preferable that blinding be used in studies whenever possible to avoid the possibility of consciously or unconsciously influencing the performance of a subject or the recording of data by a researcher. According to Portney and Watkins (2000) *double-blind studies* are "where neither the subjects nor the investigators are aware of the identity of the treatment groups until after the data are collected" (p. 159). In some cases, *single-blind studies* can be conducted where only the investigator or research team is blinded. A further discussion about how these aspects of research control might influence validity and reliability of studies occurs later in this chapter.

Figure 3–1 demonstrates a model of the research process. Phases need to be completed in a sequential manner. This model is referenced in other parts of this text.

Selecting a Topic

Selecting a topic for a research project is influenced by many factors. First, it may be that a researcher or group of researchers shares a curiosity about a given topic. Second, it may be that a student must choose one to complete an academic requirement for a course or a degree. Third, a topic may be selected because clinical experiences have led a clinician to ask questions about the impact of various treatment protocols. Whatever the reason for selecting a topic, it is important that it be something the researcher(s) is very interested in doing. Intrinsic motivation and the willingness to know why or how something occurs will drive other decisions in the problem-solving process.

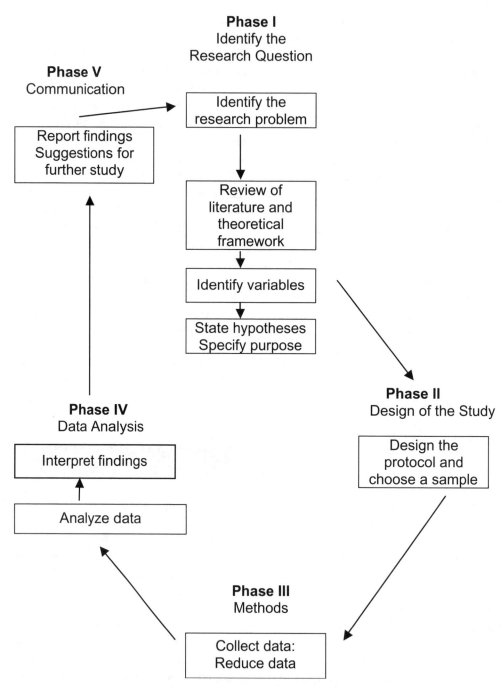

Figure 3–1. A model of the research process. From *Foundations of Clinical Research: Application to Practice* (2nd ed., p. 16), by L. G. Portney and M. P. Watkins, 2000, Upper Saddle River, NH: Pearson. Copyright 2000 Pearson Education, Inc. Adapted by permission.

There are numerous topics that may be selected and it may be challenging to determine which problem needs to be addressed first. Discussion with other researchers, faculty, and students should provide productive decision-making.

Selecting a Research Problem

Topics provide a general foundation to determine which area may be researched, but this then must be narrowed into a research question. A research question is usually answered in a single study (Portney & Watkins, 2000). The research question may start out very broad, but it does require refinement so that specific variables may be defined. The process of narrowing the research question can be facilitated by a review of the literature or "landmark" studies. Frequently, a review of studies relevant to the topic can provide good examples of the questions which have been asked and investigated.

The role of clinical experience may influence the type of research question that is asked (Maxwell & Satake, 2006). Clinicians often encounter situations with patients that are not easily explained. The clinician may believe it is important to explain unexpected results to the patient and/or family. Research questions have been generated based on everyday clinical experiences.

Research questions may result from working with different patient populations. For example, a clinician may find that a particular treatment protocol is very effective with one group of patients, but does not have a similar impact upon another group of patients. These situations can lead a clinician to question which variables differentiate the patients and necessitate the need to modify procedures.

Research is conducted to answer questions and is an increasingly important component of the field of communication sciences and disorders. In an effort to determine cause-and-effect relationships, researchers conscientiously apply scientific methodology to carefully control variables. Because of federal laws governing education of disabled children and the importance of documenting outcome measures for treatment, it is imperative that the scientific method be implemented in basic and applied research projects.

Johnson (2006) proposed that, when posing an answerable question, a key starting point for evidence-based practice (EBP), the method known as PICO should be used. PICO stands for P = patient/population, I = intervention/treatment/exposure, C = comparison, and O = outcome. Johnson (2006) stated "the following is a PICO question of possible relevance to childhood speech-language disorders: 'Does group, as compared with individual, language intervention result in greater expressive language growth for preschool children with delays in language production'" (p. 23). For this example, Johnson identified the following: "P = preschool children with delays in language production, I = group language intervention, C = individual language intervention, and O = expressive language growth" (p. 23).

Clinical theory is often used as a resource for developing research questions. Theories will guide and sometimes explain relationships between variables. Theories also may enhance the prediction of outcomes based on certain information (Portney & Watkins, 2009). Research will not "prove" that a theory is or is not correct. Research either will or will not support the theoretical principles. It is important that researchers carefully word the findings of a study in order to have any consumer of the research understand that nothing has been "proven," but can only support or refute a clinical theory.

Hypotheses and Theories

Hypotheses are often formulated for the purpose of testing theories which explain a phenomenon, event, or condition. Questions may be stated in the form of a formal or working hypothesis. The formal or null hypothesis to be accepted or rejected by a study is stated in negative terms. A *null hypothesis* states that there is "no statistically significant difference" or "no statistically significant relationship" between groups or variables. For example, to test the theory that phonological errors may be caused by the presence of a hearing loss, a null hypothesis attempts to eliminate bias from the hypothesis by declaring no relationship exists between the variables (Hegde, 2003). Thus, the researcher attempts to reject the null hypothesis that there is no relationship between phonological development and the presence of a hearing loss. Hegde (2003) cautions, however, that the null hypothesis does not eliminate or control for examiner bias. Objective interpretation of the results of a study requires objective, ethical research practices by a researcher with research education and experience, preferably initially in collaboration with experienced, objective researches.

A *working hypothesis*, or sometimes known as a research hypothesis, may simply ask a question: "Is there a difference" or "Is there a relationship" between groups or variables? When a researcher states in a hypothesis that there will be a change or describes a relationship in a certain direction this is known as a *directional hypothesis*. For example, if the hypothesis states "there is a high relationship" or "there is a low relationship," this would indicate the researcher would believe the results of the study will not only be statistically significantly different, but also in a certain direction.

Research hypotheses should include the description of the independent and dependent variables (Portney & Watkins, 2000). A *simple hypothesis* includes one independent variable and one dependent variable. A *complex hypothesis* contains more than one independent and dependent variables.

The acceptance or rejection of hypotheses (null, nondirectional, directional, simple, complex) based on the results of a study are always interpreted as tentative. The findings of current studies may be replaced or expanded by future findings based on new theories, different clinical practice procedures, or changes in research methods. Like the records set by athletes, research findings often do not withstand expansion and changes in the knowledge bases. As Silverman (1998) stated, "The final aspect of the scientific approach is being aware of the *tentative* nature of answers and hypotheses because it indicates that no answer to a question or test of a hypothesis is *final*. In other words, 'the data is [*sic*] never all in'" (p. 14). Thus, the language used to convey the conclusions reached by a researcher conducting any study revolves around the words "suggest," "support," or "refute" rather than "prove."

Feasibility of a Research Project

Feasibility of a research study needs to be considered very early in the research process (Portney & Watkins, 2000). Any research project that is worthy of investigating and investing of time and resources must undergo a "feasibility" test. The researcher may need to consider several factors when determining feasibility (Johnson, 2004).

■ What previous experience does the researcher have with this topic?

■ What are the risks/benefits for the subjects?

■ What is the duration of the project?

■ Does a "pilot study" need to be conducted? Will subjects require screening?

■ Will an Institutional Review Board (IRB) approve the protocol?

■ Will the consent form need to be translated for non-English speakers? What about consent for subjects with mental disabilities or learning disabilities?

■ Can the research protocol be adequately integrated with routine standards of care?

■ Is specialized equipment required? If so, how will it be calibrated and maintained?

■ Is outside personnel required to conduct special procedures or efficacy measures?

■ What is the frequency and severity of an Adverse Event (AE)?

■ Are the inclusion/exclusion criteria reasonable to meet enrollment?

■ Will these factors impede enrollment: age, duration of participation, frequency of visits, and procedural discomfort?

■ Will extended hours be required? Is current staffing adequate to conduct the protocol?

■ Will personnel requirements compete with other research projects?

■ How much funds will be necessary to conduct the project? Who will pay for them? What about personnel time? What if there is a long lag between getting budgetary figures and actually initiating the study? Will subjects need to be paid for their time?

Feasibility of a research study needs to be carefully discussed with all parties during the planning phase. After several discussions with key personnel then a "go/no go" decision is made by all parties. The next phase involves the development of a budget which includes several phases.

Budgetary Considerations and Preparation

Rowell (2004) suggests that there are six phases when developing a research budget (Figure 3–2). Phase one includes the preparation phase. During this time, the researcher(s) should have a good idea of what they can or cannot do, know the costs of services that will be necessary to complete the budget and develop a "charge master." It is important to determine start-up costs by considering IRB fees, IRB preparation, protocol review time, copies, equipment (and any upgrades), chart reviews, database

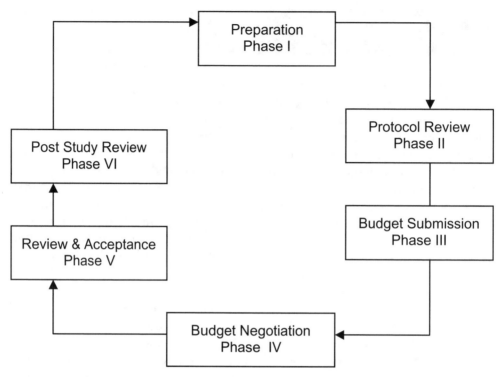

Figure 3–2. The six phases of a research site budget. From *Clinical Research Workshop,* by J. Rowell, 2004, LSU School of Medicine, Division of Research and Department of Pediatric/Section on Clinical Pharmacology. Copyright 2004 LSUHSC-Shreveport. Adapted by permission.

reviews, prestudy visits, pharmacy and lab setups, administrative oversight, and regulatory requirements.

When considering the per-patient cost, it important to figure *direct cost* (what will be involved with direct subject contact), variable costs (charges that depend on things the subject may or may not require), and time for the researcher to conduct the experiment. Rowell (2004) states that time is the most underestimated value when considering per-patient costs. This may not only include salary, but fringe benefits that must be paid for a researcher. Close-out costs need to be considered and include administrative costs, closing out records, and long-term storage of records.

Phase two involves the protocol review phase. It is important that the principal investigator (PI) choose realistic timelines for completion of the study. Time is one variable that can be easily under or overestimated. During this phase, it is important to consider the amount of time for the following:

- Consent process—may take 45 minutes to 1 hour including a discussion about the *Health Insurance Privacy and Portability Act* (HIPAA)
- Screening failure compensation— if a subject doesn't meet criteria for inclusion how is the subject compensated

- Payments for unscheduled procedures such as adverse events, tests, and failures
- Advertising for subjects including print and electronic media
- Costs that may be necessary if the study runs longer than expected
- Time for the "coordinator" or someone who has administrative oversight of the project that includes protocol revisions, meetings, consent or re-consent, audits, training, travel, faxing, and preparing source documents.

Phase three includes the budget submission to the funding source. There are various ways this may be done including flat rate (nonnegotiable), small up-front payments, competitive bidding, high performance, and speedy enrollment performances. Rowell (2004) suggests that requesting more funding than may be expected is possible. However, any sponsor or supporter of the research may require a single cost figure per patient and justification for each cost.

Phase four includes budget negotiation. In some instances, a sponsor or funding source may allow for some negotiation before support will be provided. It is important that during negotiation the sponsor understand the conviction of the researcher toward the project. Enthusiasm and dedication can lead a sponsor or funding agency to support the project at the level required to be successful. If adjustments are necessary by the researcher, it is important that they be carefully considered so as not to jeopardize the completion of the protocol or violate IRB rules and regulations.

Phase five of the process includes the review and acceptance of the budget. During this time, be sure to use your Charge Master (spreadsheet) to determine that all charges are accurate. Carefully review the contract and seek legal counsel when necessary. Does the contract state a start-up date? How will the contract be paid? What are the milestones for payment? Payment can vary but it may include one-fourth of the budget to cover start-up and screening costs or payment when one-half of the enrollment target is made.

Phase six is also called the "poststudy" phase of the budget. This phase takes place when all obligations have been met and all payments have been received. At this time, the researcher(s) should review the Charge Master to see if it was indeed accurate. Did the budget reflect the work performed? Have all fees been paid? Were there extra procedures that were not requested in the original budget?

Budgetary issues should not be an afterthought. Careful planning of time, supplies, administrative costs, and site preparation need to be included early when discussing feasibility of a study. Failure to carefully consider these issues could result in some projects being started, but not completed, thus, resulting in a waste of time and resources. Furthermore, all subjects should clearly understand any type of compensation that is due and what is not to be paid.

Summary

By the time a research project is published, it has been organized and presented in established, straightforward format. However, the actual process of doing research is not as organized as one might think after reading numerous published articles that have been repeatedly edited. Hegde (2003) described a formative view of research as an evolving process. After much discussion and pondering, numerous false starts, and repeated attempts, a project may emerge and develop. Many worthy projects are abandoned in the process. Braddom (1990) provides an in-depth outline or guide to assist in identification of specific omissions or errors in the major sections of a completed research project.

Some significant findings in science over the years have been based on accidental discoveries. Hegde (2003) refers to serendipity in research as evidence that worthwhile projects are not always carefully planned. Accidental discoveries may be the reward for flexibility and a creative sense of inquiry on the part of observers when conducting a research project.

DISCUSSION QUESTIONS

1. What is an independent variable? Provide an example of it in research.
2. What is a dependent variable? Provide an example of it in research.
3. What is meant by experimental control? What are some examples of things that can be controlled in a research project?
4. What is the purpose of a control group? Why might it be difficult to have a control group during clinical research?
5. How might a researcher decide upon a topic? How might the researcher decide upon a specific problem to study?
6. What is the difference between a null hypothesis and a research hypothesis? Provide an example of each.
7. Why would a conclusion from a hypothesis only "suggest" rather than "prove" something?
8. What are some variables to consider when determining feasibility of a study? When is feasibility determined? Who makes the decision for "go/no go"?
9. What are the six phases of planning a budget?
10. What is a Charge Master? What variables might be included in it?

References

Braddom, C. (1990). A framework for writing and/or evaluating research papers. *American Journal of Physical Medicine*, *69*, 333–335.

Hegde, M. N. (2003). *Clinical research in communicative disorders* (3rd ed.). Austin, TX: Pro-Ed.

Johnson, C. J. (2006). Getting started in evidence-based practice for childhood speech-language disorders. *American Journal of Speech-Language Pathology*, *15*, 20–35.

Johnson, V. A. (2004). *Feasibility and risk management in clinical trials*. Paper presented at the Clinical Research Workshop, Louisiana State University Health Sciences Center, Shreveport, LA.

Maxwell, D. L., & Satake, E. (2006). *Research and statistical methods in communication sciences and disorders*. Clifton Park, NY: Thomson Delmar.

Portney, L. G., & Watkins, M. P. (2000). *Foundation of clinical research: Applications to practice*. (2nd ed.). Upper Saddle River, NJ: Prentice-Hall Health.

Portney, L. G., & Watkins, M. P. (2009). *Foundation of clinical research: Application to practice* (3rd ed.). Upper Saddle River, NJ: Prentice-Hall Health.

Rowell, J. P. (2004, March). *The six phases of a successful research budget*. Paper presented at the Clinical Research Workshop, Louisiana State University Health Sciences Center, Shreveport.

Schiavetti, N., Metz, D. E., & Orlikoff, R. F. (2011). *Evaluating research in speech pathology and audiology*. Boston, MA: Pearson.

Shearer, W. S. (1982). *Research procedures in speech, language, and hearing*. Baltimore, MD: Williams & Wilkins.

Siegel, G. M. (1987). The limits of science in communication disorders. *Journal of Speech and Hearing Disorders*, *52*(3), 306–312.

Silverman, F. H. (1998). *Research design and evaluation in speech-language pathology and audiology* (4th ed.). Needham Heights, MA: Allyn & Bacon.

4

Locating, Accessing, and Assessing Information

LEARNING OBJECTIVES

Upon completion of this chapter the reader will be able to:

■ Discuss the methods involved in a successful literature search

■ Describe speech-language pathology and audiology journals that allow online access

■ List some commonly used databases

■ Describe the content of critical appraisal of topic or paper (CAT or CAP)

■ List the advantages and disadvantages of using a CAT or CAP.

Introduction

Locating information for a research project can be done efficiently and effectively if the speech-language pathologist or audiologist applies some basic principles regarding literature searches. Furthermore, after the literature is obtained it is important that assessment of the research reports involves a systematic approach to summarizing and organizing the evidence. *Critical appraisal topics or papers* (CATs or CAPs) are the preferred format for organizing evidence-based information. This chapter provides information about locating, accessing, rating, classifying, and reporting levels of evidence that can be used for clinical practice. It also provides an example of a CAT.

Locating Information

Speech-language pathologists (SLPs) and audiologists (AUDs) should utilize a variety of methods when locating information for research and consumer health materials. As computers and various databases are now available for professionals to utilize it is not possible to know *all* information that has been published. For example, the Cumulative Index to Nursing and Allied Health Literature (CINAHL) has a Subject Heading List of over 11,000 headings, of which 4,526 terms are unique, covering nursing and allied health topics (Levy, 2005). According to Portney and Watkins (2009), there are numerous sources such as indexes and abstracts that provide bibliographic listing of several thousand articles and conference proceedings.

Clinicians and students conducting research are busy and need strategies to locate and access critical information. Furthermore, more researchers are expecting full text online articles after completing the bibliographic search. It is important that a researcher utilize all sources of information when locating sources. A reference librarian at a university library is a very valuable resource in learning to conduct effective and informative literature searches. The reference librarian will help guide literature searches and provide instruction about using the various databases that include research in health sciences. It is important that any researcher have a topic and utilize the strategies presented in Chapter 3 to determine a topic of interest. Specificity about a topic facilitates any literature search and provides the reference librarian with key word information.

In Figure 4–1, CINAHL (2001) provides a strategy for a successful literature search that should be used when locating resources. Figure 4–1 emphasizes the importance of using a logical sequence when conducting literature searches. Subject headings need to be carefully worded utilizing key words that will allow the search process to specifically pull articles, abstracts, or books relevant to the topic. If a literature search utilizing an online system is not successful in retrieving information, then it may require rephrasing the heading or reconsidering the topic (CINAHL, 2001).

Databases

Numerous databases can assist the researcher when locating information. These databases may include literature

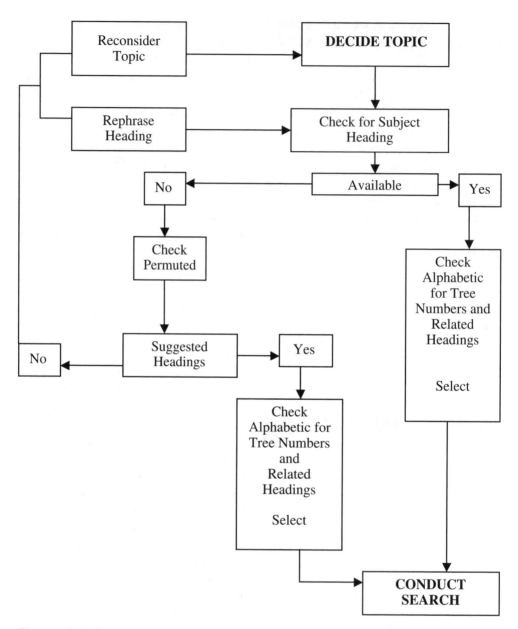

Figure 4–1. Strategies for a successful literature search. From *Strategies for a Successful Literature Search*, 2001, Glendale, CA: Cinahl Information Systems. Flow Chart Copyright © 2001 Cinahl Information Systems. Reprinted with permission. http://www.cinahl.org

from around the globe and some allow for online access. Johnson (2006) also provides a list of databases that may be utilized regarding children with speech and language disorders. Table 4–1 lists some commonly used indexes and databases for references and abstracts in science and related areas.

Table 4–1. Commonly Used Indexes and Databases for References and Abstracts in Science and Related Areas

Database	Description
Academic Search Premier	A multidisciplinary database that covers scholarly journals in biomedical fields, social sciences, humanities, education, physical sciences, and engineering.
CINAHL: Cumulative Index to Nursing & Allied Health Literature	Available from several vendors, CINAHL indexes journals in nursing and allied health. Some versions provide full text of many articles.
Cochrane Library	The Cochrane Library is a collection of databases created to supply evaluated, high-quality information in support of evidence-based medicine. Although its focus is necessarily broader, it does contain material relevant to communication disorders.
Dissertation Abstracts	A bibliographic database that indexes doctoral dissertations and master's theses from about 1,000 graduate schools and universities. About 47,000 new dissertations and 12,000 new theses are added annually.
ERIC (Educational Resources Information Center)	ERIC indexes information from education journals, including articles on communication disorders in an educational context.
JSTOR	A series of full-text archives covering scholarly journals. Subscriptions are available for discipline-specific or multidisciplinary subsets of the archive, some of which contain journals relevant in communication disorders.
Linguistics & Language Behavior Abstracts	This database indexes and provides summaries of journal articles in the language sciences including communication disorders as well as broader subjects such as linguistics.
PsycINFO	PsycINFO contains over two million citations and abstracts of journal articles, book chapters, books, and dissertations. More than 65,000 new records are added each year.
PubMed	PubMed, produced by the National Library of Medicine and available to the public without charge, indexes about 4,000 journals covering all aspects of the health sciences. Much of this content is also licensed to commercial vendors for use on their database platforms for a fee.
Web of Science	A bibliographic database that covers many scholarly journals in the sciences.

Data Mining

Data mining, generally, is the process of analyzing data from different perspectives and discovering new patterns from large data sets involving the intersection of several areas of science procedures and related databases ("Data mining," 2012). This term is also called data fishing and data snooping.

Technically, data mining can be used to find correlations or patterns in field in large relational databases. Data mining can be conducted in a variety of different ways with the use of more advanced software and machine learning. In general the relationships are sought among the following areas: (1) Classes: stored data in predetermined groups. For example, a researcher may be concerned with the variables of individuals with stuttering and perceptions by potential employers have towards such individuals. (2) Clusters: data items are grouped according to logical relationships and determine potential markets. For example, an audiologist may be interested in determining which groups are best for dispensing hearing aids. (3) Associations: data can be used to identify associations such as the relationship between hearing loss and the development of phonological development in children. (4) Sequential patterns: data is used to anticipate behavior patterns and trends. For example, a researcher may study the identification of hearing loss and how many batteries are purchased in a month by various clients. (Frand, 2012)

The use of data mining methods in communication sciences and disorders is an emerging field of interest. A study by Danubianu, Pentiuc, Tobolcea, and Schi-por (2010) has utilized the association portion of data mining with a case study. The authors used associative data mining with a method of speech-language treatment. They used the database developed from a single-subject case study to answer the following questions: What is the predicted final state for a child or what will his or her state at the end of various stages of therapy? Which are the best exercises for each case? Which factors might be associated with certain family characteristics and the success of therapy? In general, the authors determined that associative data mining can be used in communication sciences and disorders. However, more research is needed to explore the use of data mining in the use of finding effective assessment and treatment procedures.

The application of data mining has occurred frequently in business with WalMart® pioneering massive amounts of datasets to transform its supplier relationships. Data mining is also being used in sports, gaming, and health care. The more data being processed and the more complex the queries to do data mining requires a more powerful system (Frand, 2012).

Online Journals

Online journals may or may not be free. The American Speech-Language-Hearing Association (ASHA) offers online access to its membership at http://www.asha.org. Access to online journals is sponsored by ASHA and some date back from 1980 to the present. These include *American Journal of Audiology (AJA)*, *American Journal of Speech-Language*

Pathology (AJSLP), Journal of Speech-Language-Hearing Research (JSLHR), Language, Speech, and Hearing Services in the Schools (LSHSS), and *ASHA Leader Online.* In addition, ASHA members may now receive E-mail alerts (i.e., eTOCS) with a full table of contents. "CiteTrack" provides E-mail alerts when new content is published that matches specific selected parameters, quick and advanced searches from http://www.highwire.org, improved "Googling," and personal folders (ASHA Leader, 2006). The American Academy of Audiology (AAA) allows access to the *Journal of the American Academy of Audiology* online at http://www.audiology.org and it does not require membership in AAA.

Many journals are subject to a publication embargo. This means that access to the full text becomes available only after a specified period: generally 6 to 12 months, but up to 2 years for a few journals (LSUHSC, 2005). Most databases that contain free journal access online are identified by the "free" icon.

Use of the World Wide Web

The World Wide Web (WWW) is frequently one of the first sources that researchers and/or consumers of health information utilize when locating information. Although, the WWW provides an excellent source of information, it "must be recognized that this resource cannot replace the quality materials accessible from professional organizations, peer-reviewed health care journals, the Cochrane Library, etc." (Levy, 2002, p. 1).

O'Brien (2001) made the point that "information on the WWW needs to be evaluated because, while some of it is accurate, some of it can be potentially dangerous as there can be a lack of peer review or regulation and because the information can be inaccurate and misleading" (p. 42). Levy (2002) provides a credibility checklist that can be utilized when evaluating research on the WWW. These include the following:

- Look at the URL. These include .gov for government sites, .edu for educational sites, or .org for not-for-profit organizations (O'Brien, 2001).
- Look for information from trained and licensed health professional. Cooke (1999) suggests that affiliations be noted.
- The mission and objectives of any organization should be given at the Web site so conflicts of interest and advertising can be considered. (Cooke, 1999; O'Brien 2001).
- Statements about any Web site limitations, scope, or purpose should be carefully considered (Cline & Haynes, 2001).
- Be certain that the information has been peer-reviewed. Review the credentials of the reviewers and determine if conflicts of interest might be present (Levy, 2002).
- Although the Web site may look professional, be sure that references and sources are clearly listed. Also, check when the site was last updated.

It is important for researchers and consumers of health care research to understand that the acceptance rate on the WWW for information is probably 110%. Therefore, all information should be carefully scrutinized when reviewing information from any Web site. The use of the WWW may be one of the first resources used, but it certainly should not be the only one.

Interlibrary Loan

Interlibrary loan is one method of obtaining information that may not be available in electronic format or books that may have limited editions. A reference librarian can help when making requests for an interlibrary loan. Charges for the interlibrary loan may or may not exist depending on the agreement the libraries have with each other. Many libraries allow for online requests for interlibrary loan through the ILLiad system. Many loans can be delivered to the user's desktop, depending on the delivery method used by the library that filled the request (LSUHSC, 2005).

Manual Searches

Manual searches involve going to the periodical sections of a library and reviewing articles that are bound into annual issues. This method may seem somewhat antiquated compared to the use of computerized databases, but it still provides an excellent method to review literature. Probably the most useful aspect of a manual search includes the review of more "classic" studies and other types of research that have not been transferred to electronic formats. Furthermore, photographs and other types of visual information which may not be available in online searches can be reviewed during a manual search. It

is important that any researcher not be limited to publications that are available only in electronic format. According to Galvan (2006), landmark studies and theorists with historical importance in developing an understanding of a topic or problem can be achieved by utilizing a manual research.

Social Media

The use of social media such as E-mail, message boards, Skype, and Facebook is developing a method for expanding research. The use of these methods for communication has increased dramatically within the last few years (Mershon, 2011). Quinnell (2011) discussed that using social media for research and researcher development allows for collection of data from a wide range of stakeholders. This author conducted interviews using asynchronous message boards, Skype and E-mail conversations. In addition, this author was able network with other policy-makers and organizations on a variety of topics and related issues. There are ethical and logistical issues associated with the use of these types of social media that must be considered.

Evaluating Research

Evaluating research evidence is important for several reasons. First, sources of evidence are heterogeneous; in other words, not all sources or evidence are equal. Second, the quality of clinical services is related to evidence and the manner in which it was obtained and presented.

Third, application of research to clinical practice is related to the level of evidence (Finn, Bothe, & Bramlett, 2005). Last, the use of high level of evidence in making clinical decision is an ethical responsibility, that is, evidence-based practice is fundamental to ethical practice.

There is a need for SLPs and AUDs to utilize evidence-based results to make clinical decisions. Unfortunately, this is not always the case. Zipoli and Kennedy (2005) found that SLPs used clinical experiences and opinions of colleagues more frequently than research studies or clinical practice guidelines to make clinical decisions. Utilization of research reports can be facilitated by a step-by-step process. These steps include: (1) asking a question(s); (2) finding the highest level of evidence; (3) critically appraising the evidence; (4) integrating the evidence with clinical experience and client values; and (5) evaluating the decision-making process (Boswell, 2005; Johnson, 2006; Kully & Langeven, 2005). Evaluating research reports requires critical analyses. Methods of evaluating research reports can be classified as traditional, evidence-based (levels of evidence), and criterion-based in distinguishing between science and pseudoscience. Critically appraised topics or papers (CATs or CAPs) are a format for organizing evidence-based information.

Several systems have been developed for classifying levels of evidence (Agency for Health care Research and Quality, 1999; ASHA 2004; Hadorn, Baker, Hodges, & Hicks, 1996; Ottenbacher, 2002; Queensland Center, 2002). The systems are generally based on levels of evidence according to quality and credibility from highest/most credible to lowest/least credible.

Rating the Evidence

Rating the level of evidence is challenging (Yorkston, Spencer, Duffy, Beukelman, Golper, Miller, et al., 2001). Hadorn and associates (1996) believe that it is not clear as to what counts as evidence and even less clear, what weight to assign to different types of evidence. Four questions are usually considered in evaluating the literature for strength of evidence. These questions and more description of the criteria are in Table 4–2 (Yorkston et al., 2001).Chambless and Hollon (1998) rated the level of evidence based on guidelines of the American Psychological Association. Three questions were considered: (1) Has the treatment been shown to be beneficial in controlled research? (2) Is the treatment useful in applied clinical settings and, if so, with what patients and under what circumstances? and (3) Is the treatment efficient in the sense of being cost-effective relative to other alternative treatments? Dawes, Davies, Gray, Mant, Seers, and Snowball (1999) also described questions that are important when reviewing a paper on treatment. These questions are listed in Table 4–3.

Levels of Evidence

It is important to recognize the level of evidence in evaluating research. Typically, research evidence is classified according to levels based on the type and quality of research (ASHA, 2004). The earliest evidence scale was published in 1994 by the American Academy of Neurology. This evidence scale

Table 4–2. Four Questions Used in Evaluating Literature for Strength of Evidence

How well were the subjects described?

How well was the treatment described?
- Rationale for treatment
- Replication of treatment

What measures of control were used in the study?
- Reliability and stability of outcome measures (inter- or intrarater reliability, dispersion of scores)
- Support for internal validity (outcome measures obtained with or without treatment; improved performance with treatment in progressive disorders)
- Presence of comparison or control group

Are the consequences of the treatment well described?
- Outcome measures at levels of impairment, activity limiting, restriction in participation
- Risks and complication of treatment

Table 4–3. Important Questions When Reviewing a Paper on Treatment

Did the authors answer the question(s)?

Were groups of patients randomized?

Are the comparison groups similar?

Were patients "blinded"?

Was it placebo-controlled?

Was evaluation of efficacy "blinded"?

Was the length of study appropriate?

What was the follow-up rate?

Are there clear measures of outcomes?

Source: Reprinted from *Evidence-Based Practice* (p. 52), by M. Dawes, P. Davies, A. Gray, J. Mant, K. Seers, and R. Snowball, 2005, Edinburgh, Scottland: Elsevier Churchill Livingstone. Copyright 1999, with permission from Elsevier.

has a hierarchy of three levels of evidence. These levels of evidence are on a continuum of hierarchy, based on study design, that is, evidence based on opin-ion of respected authorities, evidence from case-controlled studies, and evidence from randomized controlled clinical trials. Class III, the lowest level of evidence, is evidence provided by expert opinion, case studies, case reports, and studies with historical controls. Class II evidence is that provided by at least one or better designed observational, clinical studies with concurrent controls, that is, single case control or cohort control studies. Class I, the highest level of evidence, is provide by at least one well-designed, randomized controlled clinical trial (ASHA 2005; Wertz, 2002).

Hadorn and associates (1996) described a hierarchy of seven levels of evidence based on study design (Table 4–4). The seven levels of evidence were collapsed into three levels: A, B, and C. "A" level evidence consisted of levels one through three; "B" level evidence consisted of levels four through six; and "C" level evidence was seven or expert opinion. "A" is most rigorous and "C" is least rigorous. Four levels (A–D) of evidence for intervention were described by Otten-

Table 4–4. Hierarchy of Seven Levels of Evidence Based on Study Design

1. Supportive evidence from well-conducted randomized controlled trials that included over 100 patients or more.

   a. Evidence from a well-conducted multicenter trial

   b. Evidence from a meta-analysis that incorporated quality ratings in the analysis and included a total of 100 patients in its estimates of effect size and confidence intervals.

2. Supportive evidence from well-conducted randomized controlled trials that included fewer than 100 patients.

   a. Evidence from a well-conducted trials at one or more institutions

   b. Evidence from a meta-analysis that incorporated quality ratings in the analysis and included fewer than 100 patients in its estimate of effect size and confidence intervals

3. Supportive evidence from well-conducted cohort studies

   a. Evidence from a well-conducted prospective cohort study or registry

   b. Evidence from a well-conducted retrospective cohort study

   c. Evidence from a well-conducted meta-analysis of cohort studies

4. Supportive evidence from a well-conducted case-control study

5. Supportive evidence from poorly controlled or uncontrolled studies

   a. Evidence from randomized clinical trials with one or more major or three or more minor methodological flaws that could invalidate the results

   b. Evidence from observational studies with high potential for bias (such as case studies with comparison to historical controls)

   c. Evidence from case studies or case reports

6. Conflicting evidence with the weight of evidence supporting the recommendation

7. Expert opinion

Sources: From "Rating the Quality of Evidence for Clinical Practice Guidelines," by J. S. Hodges and N. Hicks, 1996, *Journal of Clinical Epidemology, 49*(7), pp. 749–754; and "Identification and Nursing Management of Dysphagia in Adults with Neurological Impairment," by the Queensland Center of the Joanna Briggs Institute, 2000, *Best Practice Information Sheets for Health Professions, 4*(2). Retrieved October 10, 2002 from http://www.joannabriggs.edu/ BPFSdysl.html

bacher (2002). Minor and major flaws were identified for eight aspects of study methodology; selection of patients; allocation of patients to treatment groups, treatment regimen; study administration; withdrawal from the study; patient blinding (randomized clinical trials only); outcome measurement; and statistical analysis. Minor flaws include deviations from good practice that do not create a potential for bias large enough to cast doubt on the validity of a study. Major flaws create a potential for bias large enough to question a study's results.

Critical Appraisal

Unfortunately, published papers can have flaws which may occur anywhere along the publication process (Dawes et al., 1999). Critical appraisal is important in examining the rigors with which a study was conducted, and thus the amount of confidence placed in the findings. SLPs and AUDs should read and critique the literature to stay current on prevailing clinical research findings, and apply what is known to clinical practice (Frattali & Worrall, 2001). Critical appraisal involves the application of knowledge about research design to the literature (Gallagher, 2001).

A Critical Appraisal Topic or Paper (CAT or CAP) is a summary of a critical review of the best evidence on a specific topic (Worrall & Bennett, 2001). It is a written outcome of the evidence-based practice (EBP) process. A CAT begins with a declarative title and then indicates a "clinical bottom line" which describes the clinical action that results from the report (Sackett, Strauss, Richardson, Rosenberg, & Haynes, 2000). There are five major types of CATs: (1) diagnosis/screening; (2) progress; (3) evaluating risk and harm in case-controlled studies; (4) evaluating risk and harm in a control study; and (5) intervention (treatment, prevention, screening) (Law, 2002). An example of a CAT on treatment of voice problems of teachers is shown in Table 4–5. Another example of a critical review based format is presented in Table 4–6. Johnson (2006) suggests the development of collaborative working groups to develop a system for developing a large database of CATs. For more examples of CATs, see http://www.otcats.com/ (Johnson, 2006).

Critical appraisals are not without critics. Several problems have been identified that warrant discussion (Woolf, 2000;

Table 4–5. Example of a Critically Appraised Topic (CAT) on Treatment of Teachers with Voice Problems

Clinical Bottom Line:	Amplification for teachers with voice problems yields better outcome than vocal hygiene instruction for six weeks.
Citation:	Roy, N., Weinrich, B. Gray, S. P., Tanner, K., Toledo, S. W., Dove, H., Corbin-Lewis, K., & Stemple, J. C. (2002). Voice amplification versus vocal hygiene instruction for teachers with voice disorders: A treatment outcomes study. *Journal of Speech-Language-Hearing Research, 45*, 625–638.
Clinical Question:	Which is more effective for treatment of teachers with voice problems, voice amplification (VA) or vocal hygiene (VH) instruction?
Search Terms:	Voice disorders, treatment, teachers, voice amplification, vocal hygiene.
Design:	Prospective, randomized control group.

Table 4–6. Example of a Critical Review-Based Format

Study:	Class I
Study Title:	Voice amplification versus vocal hygiene instruction for teachers with voice disorders: A treatment outcomes study.
Authors:	Roy, N., Weinrich, B., Gray, S. D., Tanner, K., Toledo, S.W., Dove, H., Corbin-Lewis, K., & Stemple, J. C.
Year of Publication:	2002
Source:	*Journal of Speech-Language-Hearing Research, 45,* 625–638.
Design:	Prospective, randomized clinical trial
Subjects:	44 voice disordered teachers randomly assigned to one of three groups: voice amplification (VA, n = 15); vocal hygiene (VH, n = 15), nontreatment control group (n = 14).
Treatment:	VA consisted of using Chatter Box portable amplifier. VH program was adapted from Morrison et al.'s (1994) program
Duration and Intensity of Treatment:	6 weeks
Outcome Measures:	Voice Handicap Index; voice severity self-rating scale; audio recording for later acoustic analysis
Analysis:	Descriptive statistics
Results:	Clearly support clinical validity of amplification as alternative for treatment of voice disorders in teachers

Yorkston et al., 2001). First there is frequent reliance on a single indicator of study quality, that is, marked emphasis on one type of research, randomized controlled trials. Second, individuals are strikingly heterogeneous despite common diagnostic categories. Third, there is an incomplete base of evidence, that is, the research literature is not sufficiently current and complete to answer all clinical questions; there are important gaps in evidence. Fourth, not all sources of information are readily available through electronic searches. Excessive and inadequate critical appraisal can lead to premature adoption or abandonment of treatment and result in overlooking potential harms of more effective treatment alternatives. In addition, critical appraisal can do harm if valid evidence is rejected. Last, critical appraisal lacks systematic application. Criteria to determine which studies are rated "bad" or "good" should be specific and consistent.

Another criticism is the amount of time to write and apply CATs. Worrall and Bennett (2001) suggested that CATs can be undertaken by groups of speech-language pathologists and audiologists. Students and practicing professionals are involved with interest groups and journal clubs. Resources and expertise can be shared in developing CATs. CATs can be the product of one individual or a small group of individuals, and may be subject to error, bias, and other limitations inherent in non-peer-reviewed materials (Law, 2002). CATs can also be flawed because of the speed in which they are created.

Summary

Locating, accessing, and assessing the evidence is an essential part of evidence-based practice. Appropriate clinical decisions require systematic evaluation and integration of evidence from published research reports. It is important to summarize the results of critical appraisal and share information with SLPs and AUDs.

DISCUSSION QUESTIONS

1. Describe the strategy for a successful search.
2. Discuss how databases are utilized for literature searches.
3. What are some of the types of data mining being used for research? How might these be used for communication sciences and disorders?
4. Discuss some use of social media that can be used for research and researcher development.
5. What are some journals that are available online? Are these always free?
6. Who is the person in a library that will probably help the most when doing a literature search?
7. Why is rating the level of evidence from a body of literature difficult?
8. What are some key questions to ask when rating the strength of evidence?
9. How can evidence be classified?
10. What is a critical appraisal?
11. What are the key components of a critically appraised topic or paper?
12. Discuss the relative advantages and disadvantages of using CATs.

References

Agency for Health care Research and Quality. (1999). *Diagnosis and treatment of swallowing disorders (dysphagia) in acutecare stroke*. Retrieved from http://ahrp.gov/clinic/spcsums/dysphsum.htm

American Speech-Language-Hearing Association. (2004). *Evidence-based practice in communication disorders: An introduction* [Technical report]. Retrieved from http://www.asha.org/members/deskref -journals/deskref/default

American Speech-Language-Hearing Association. (2005). *Evidence-based practice in communication disorders* [Position statement]. Retrieved from http://www.asha .org/members/deskrefjournals/deskref/ default

American Speech-Language-Hearing Association. (2006). Online access expands for journals. *ASHA Leader*. Retrieved from http://www.asha.org/about/publications/ leader-on-line/archives/2006/060411b .htm

Boswell, S. (2005). Finding the evidence for school-based clinical decision making. *ASHA Leader*, pp. 26–27, 39.

Chambless, D. L., & Hollon, S. D. (1998). Defining empirically supported therapies. *Journal of Consulting and Clinical Psychology, 66*(1), 7–18.

Cline, R. J. W., & Haynes, K. M. (2001). Consumer health information seeking the Internet: The state of the art. *Health Education Research, 16*(6), 671–692.

Cooke, A. (1999). Quality of health and medical information on the Internet. *British Journal of Clinical Governance, 4*(4), 155–160.

Cumulative Index in Allied Health Literature® Information Systems. (2001). *Strategies for a successful literature search*. Glendale, CA: CINAHL Information Systems.

Danubanu, M., Pentiuc, S. G., Tobolcea, I., & Schipor, O. A. (2010). Advanced information technology-support of improved personalized therapy of speech disorders. *International Journal of Computers Communications and Control, 5*, 684–692.

Dawes, M, Davies, P., Gray, A., Mant, J., Seers, K., & Snowball, R. (1999). *Evidence-based practice*. New York, NY: Churchill Livingstone.

Finn, P., Bothe, A. K., & Bramlett, R. E. (2005) Science and pseudoscience in communication disorders. *American Journal of Speech-Language Pathology, 14*, 172–186.

Frand, J. (2012). *Data mining: What is data mining?* Retrieved from http://www .anderson.ucla.edu/faculty/Jason.frand/ teacher/technologies/palace/datamining

Fratalli, C., & Worrall, L. E. (2001). Evidence-based practice: Applying science to the art of clinical care. *Journal of Medical Speech-Language Pathology, 9*(1), ix–xi.

Gallagher, T. M. (2001). Implementation of evidence-based practice communication disorders course work and practicum. In P. Hargrove, R. McGuire, C. O'Rourke, & W. Swisher (Eds.), *Proceedings of the Council of Academic Program in Communication Sciences and Disorders* (pp. 29–45). Sarasota, FL.

Galvan, J. L. (2006). *Writing literature reviews* (3rd ed). Glendale, CA: Pyrczak

Hadorn, D. C., Baker, D., Hodges, J. S., & Hicks, N. (1996). Rating the quality of evidence for clinical practice guidelines. *Journal of Clinical Epidemiology, 49*(7), 749–754.

Johnson, C. J. (2006). Getting started in evidence-based practice for childhood speech-language disorders. *American Journal of Speech-Language Pathology, 15*, 20–35.

Kully, D., & Langeven, M. (2005). Evidence-based practice in fluency disorders. *ASHA Leader*, pp. 10–11, 23.

Law, M. L. (2002). *Evidence-based rehabilitation*. Thorofaare, NJ: Slack.

Levy, J. R. (2002). Searching the CINAHL® database Part 4: Accessing consumer health information and patient education materials. *CINAHLnews, 21*(4), 1–3.

Louisiana State University Health Sciences Center, Shreveport Medical Library. (2005).

Library information for new faculty. Shreveport: LSUHSC Medical Library.

Meshon, P. (2011). *How to grow social media leads: New research.* Retrieved from http://www.socialmediaexaminer.com/how-to-grow-social-media-leads-new-research

O'Brien, K. (2001). The World Wide Web and consumer health information. *Collegian, 8*(4), 42.

Ottenbacher, K. J. (2002, June). *Critical appraisal of evidence-based intervention.* Paper presented at the Boston University Faculty Summer Institute, Boston, MA.

Portney, L. G., & Watkins, M. P. (2009). *Foundations of clinical research: Applications to clinical practice* (2nd ed.). Upper Saddle River, NJ: Prentice-Hall Health.

Queensland Center for the Joanna Briggs Institute. (2000). *Identification and nursing management of dysphagia in adults with neurological impairment. Evidence-Based Practice Information Sheets for Health Professions.* Retrieved from http://www.joannabriggs.edu/au/BP/Syds1.htm

Quinnell, S. L. (2011). *Using social media for research and researcher development.* Retrieved from http://www.phd2published.com/2011/04/26/using-social-media-for-research-researcher development

Sackett, D. L., Strauss, S. E., Richardson, W. S., Rosenberg, W., & Haynes, R. B. (2000). *Evidence-based medicine.* New York, NY: Churchill Livingstone.

Wertz, R. T., (2002). Evidence-based practice guidelines: Not all evidence is created equal. *Journal of Medical Speech-Language Pathology, 10*(3), xi–xv.

Wikipedia. (2012). *Data mining.* Retrieved from http://en.wikipedia.org, wiki/Data_mining

Woolf, S. H. (2000). Taking crtical appraisal to extremes. *Journal of Family Practice, 49*(12), 1081–1085.

Worrall, L. E., & Bennett, S. (2001). Evidence-based practice: Barriers for speech-language pathologists. *Journal of Medical Speech-Language Pathology, 9*(2), xi–xvi.

Yorkston, K. M., Spencer, K., Duffy, J., Beukelman, D., Golper, L. A., Miller, R., . . . Sullivan, M. (2001). Evidence based medicine and practice guidelines: Application to the field of speech-language pathology. *Journal of Medical Speech-Language Pathology, 9*(4), 243–256.

Zipoli, R. P., & Kennedy, M. (2005). Evidence-based practice among speech language pathologists: Attitudes, utilization, and barriers. *American Journal of Speech-Language Pathology, 14*(3), 208–220.

5

Literature Review

CHAPTER OUTLINE

Organizing Literature Reviews
Formulating Questions
Narrative Reviews
Systematic Reviews
  Difference Between Narrative
    and Systematic Reviews

Meta-Analysis
Best-Evidence Synthesis
Clinical Practice Guidelines
Summary
Discussion Questions
References

LEARNING OBJECTIVES

Upon completion of this chapter the reader will be able to:

- Prepare and organize a literature review
- Explain the limitations of narrative reviews
- Know the difference between narrative and systematic reviews
- List and describe the parts of a systematic review
- Explain why meta-analysis is a strong basis for clinical decisions
- Define best evidence synthesis
- Beware of the limitations of practice guidelines
- Select best available practice guidelines.

Literature reviews are essentially at the heart of any research. They may serve as the background for a research project or be an end in themselves, either to improve practice or to provide a comprehensive understanding about what is known about a topic (Mertens, 2005). In other words, reviews are research in themselves. Sometimes they are referred to as tutorials (APA, 2001). There are several types of reviews: narrative or traditional; systematic; meta-analysis, best evidence synthesis; and practice guidelines. All have potential limitations, many of which can be overcome by using an evidence-based approach. The more rigorous the method of reviewing the literature and the quality of the primary research that is reviewed, the more evidence-based the review is likely to be (Cook, Greengold, Elrod, & Weingarter, 1997).

Reviewing the literature involves consideration of potential biases related to publication practices, variable quality of the studies involved in the review, and inclusion-exclusion criteria (Mertens, 2005). There is a tendency for research which statistically significant results to be published. Conversely, research studies that show no difference are published less frequently because they either are not submitted or are rejected more frequently. Literature reviews can be biased by data exclusion that is methodologically questioned, or subjective selection of studies for selection.

Organizing Literature Reviews

A number of steps are involved in preparing and organizing a literature review as summarized in Figure 5–1. As the figure shows, after identifying potential sources, references need to be located and screened for relevancy to the topic being reviewed. References that seem appropriate are read and notes taken, and inappropriate references are discarded.

One reference may provide citations to several other relevant references. After all relevant references have been reviewed; they are organized, analyzed, and synthesized. Organization facilities analysis and synthesizes the literature. Information can be organized into four categories based on relevance: A-pile: highly relevant; B-pile: somewhat relevant; C-pile: might be relevant; and X-pile: not relevant (DePoy & Gitlin, 2011). There are several ways literature can be organized to provide a visual summary of research and is typically represented as a table or figure (Creswell, 2003).

One approach to organizing and integrating the literature is a chart summarizing each study (DePoy & Gitlin, 2011; Polit & Beck, 2010). These charts are sometimes referred to as evidence tables (Golper et al., 2001). A chart is used in considering the literature as a whole, and critically evaluating and identifying research gaps. An example of a literature review table is presented in Table 5–1.

Another approach to organizing the literature is a concept/construct matrix in which information is organized by key concept (x-axis) and source (y-axis). A matrix helps in identifying specific concepts that need to be discussed in the written report (DePoy & Gitlin, 2011). This approach can be a preliminary step in developing a concept map which is described in Chapter 11.

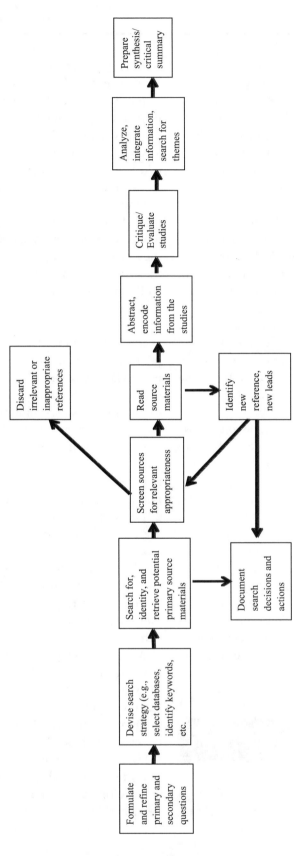

Figure 5–1. Steps in preparing a literature review. From *Nursing Research: Principles and Methods* (p. 105), by D. F. Polit and C. T. Beck, 2004, Philadelphia, PA: Lippincott Williams & Wilkins. Reprinted with permission from Lippincott Williams & Wilkins.

Table 5–1. Literature Review Table

Type of Study	Primary Focus	Number of Subjects	Measures	Conclusions
Randomized Clinical Trials	Voice amplification resonance therapy	6+	Voice Handicapped Index Voice Severity Self-Rating	Voice resonance therapy group improved

Formulating Questions

Formulating a question is the first step in a systematic review. This involves determining the type of question is it, background or foreground? Background questions ask for general information about a condition or process, who, what, when, and so forth. Foreground questions focus on a specific information about clinical decisions or recommendations. Background questions are usually asked because of the need for basic information. Typically, background questions are not asked because of a need to make a (Nursing Library and Information Resources, n.d.).

The first step evidence-based practice and systematic reviews is formulation of clinical guidelines questions. Two methods for formulating clinical questions have been described in the literature. PICO and PESICO. Each letter in the acronyms stands for its components.

PICO stands for population, intervention, comparison, and outcome. Descriptions for each component are listed in Table 5–2.

It was first described in 1995 by Richardson, Wilson, Nishikawa, and Haywood. PICO has been used in evidence-based medicine and has been adopted for use in speech-language pathology.

The adequacy and stability of PICO was evaluated by Huang, Lin, and Demner-Fushman (2006). It was reported that PICO primarily focused on questions and was less suitable for clinical questions related to diagnosis, prognosis, and etiology. A Web-based tutorial for understand PICO and answering questions, accessing and assessing the evidence, was developed by LaRue, Draus, and Klem (2009). PICO can be used to answer clinical questions such as:

1. What intervention I studied?
2. What outcome is measured?
3. What is studied?
4. Who are the researchers?
5. What are the results?
6. What is the final analysis/practical application?

PESICO was described by Schlosser, Koul, and Costello (2007). The six components of PESICO are person, environments, stakeholders, intervention, comparison, and outcomes. Table 5–3 summarizes the PESICO framework.

It has also been applied in other disciplines including occupational therapy and physical therapy (Jewell, 2011; Portney & Watkins, 2009).

There are differences between PICO and PESICO. PICO is the more frequently

Table 5–2. Description of PICO Components

Component	Description
Patient Population	**Patient population or disorder of interest** Age Gender Ethnicity
Intervention	**Intervention or range of interventions** Exposure to disorder Prognostic factors Risk(s)
Comparison	**Comparison of intervention** No disorder Placebo or no intervention Prognosis Absence of risk factor(s)
Outcome	**Outcome of interest** Risk of disorder Accuracy of diagnosis Rate of occurrence of adverse outcome

Source: From *Evidence-Based Practice* (pp. 25–37), by R. Nolan, E. Fineout-Overholt, and P. Stephenson, In B. A. M. Melynk and E. Fineout-Overholt (Eds.), 2005, Philadelphia, PA: Lippincott Wilkins & Wilkins.

used framework for formulating questions. PESICO has two additional components: environments and stakeholders. It may be that PICO does not include these two components because it is based on a medical model that focuses less on environmental and stakeholder issues (Schlosser et al., 2007).

Narrative Reviews

Traditional *narrative reviews* are nonsystematic reviews of the literature. Narrative reviews have been the most prevalent approach to synthesizing the speech-language pathology and audiology literature, although this is changing. Narrative reviews are particularly useful for topics with limited evidence such as emerging clinical issues (The Editors, 2005). There are three major disadvantages or narrative reviews: (1) the sources and identification of studies are not described; (2) the search terms are not specified; and (3) the criteria for including and excluding studies are not specific (Schlosser, 2000). In addition, narrative reviews do not provide a detailed description of each study. Typically, narrative literature reviews are at risk for subjectivity

Table 5–3. PESICO Framework

Component	Description
Person or problem	Age
	Gender
	Ethnicity
	Risk
	Diagnosis or classification
	Sensory status
	Motor status
	Cognitive status
	Communication competence
Environments	Current
	Future
	Communication
Stakeholders	Direct (person)
	Secondary (others)
	Perception of problem
Intervention	Comparison of options
Outcomes	Effectiveness (acquisition, generalization maintenance of skills)
	Efficiency
	Communication partners
	Self-determination
	Quality of life
	Stakeholders

Source: From "Asking well-built questions for evidence-based practice in augmentative and alternative communication," by R. W. Schlosser, R. Kuol, and J. Costello, 2006, *Journal of Communicative Disorders, 40,* pp. 225–238.

in selecting, evaluating, and interpreting studies. For example, Meline (2006) pointed out that narrative reviews are prone to different interpretations by different authors. Two authors may review the same literature, but reach different conclusions. The adequacy of a narrative literature review is based on three criteria: (1) the selection of the literature, (2) the summary and analysis of the literature, and (3) the relevance of the literature to the topic (McMillan & Schulmacher, 2010).

Systematic Reviews

Melnyk and Fineout-Overholt (2005) define *systematic reviews* as "a summary of evidence, typically conducted by an expert or expert panel on a particular topic that uses a rigorous process (to minimize bias) for identifying, appraising, and synthesizing studies to answer a specific clinical question and draw conclusions about the data gathered" (p. 594).

Systematic reviews are the basis of evidence-based practice (Pring, 2004). These reviews are a source of evidence to guide practice and identify the need for further research (Bannigan, Droogan, & Entwistle, 1997). In addition, systematic reviews have the potential for facilitating the transfer of research evidence into clinical practice and for helping readers understand generalization and consistency of research findings (McCauley & Hargrove, 2004). Parts of a systematic review are listed in Table 5–4. There is the challenge of including gray literature in systematic reviews (Hartling et al., 2005) Gray literature includes unpublished study's or services that are not published in peer-reviewed journals (Portney & Watkins, 2009).The reports gray literature is difficult to locate or retrieve by using electronic databases. The gray literature is heterogeneous and varies substantially in design and quality.

A systematic review is a method for locating, appraising, and synthesizing evidence (Petticrew, 2001). A number of steps are involved in preparing a systematic review as summarized in Table 5–5. The initial steps are related to finding evidence and later steps focus on using evidence. These are essentially the same steps that are involved in development of meta-analysis and evidence-based guidelines.

The last step of research is writing a report. The report should be concise, confirm to standards for professional writing, and provide a critical analysis/ synthesis of current information related to the topic. Additionally, the report should identify gaps in knowledge and research needs. It should not simply list what research has been done on the topic. The report should provide the confirming and contradictory evidence

Table 5–4. Systematic Review Template

Abstract
- Purpose
- Method
- Conclusion

Introduction
- Background/Need
- Purpose/Question

Method (Source Selection)
- Inclusion Criteria
- Exclusion Criteria

Sources
- Electronic databases
- Key words

Total Number of Sources Identified
- Number of sources excluded
- Number of sources included

Discussion
- Quantitative analysis
- Qualitative analysis

Conclusion
- Criterion-based recommendations
- Limitations
- Clinical Implications
- Future Research

References

Tables
- Table 1 Reference levels
- Table 2 Evidence table (appraisal summary of studies)

Table 5–5. Steps in Conducting a Systematic Review

Problem Formulations
Information search and retrieval
• Search terms (Key words)
• Search electronic and manual
– Level of evidence
Analysis and synthesis of evidence
• Grades for recommendation of use
Report results

Source: From *Foundation of Clinical Research*, by L. G. Portney & M. P. Watkins, 2009, Upper Saddle River, NJ: Pearson; and *Research in Education*, by J. H. McMillian & S. Schumacher, 2010, Boston, MA: Pearson.

about possible explanations of findings (APA, 2010; DePoy & Gitlin, 2011; Polit & Beck, 2010

A template was designed for writing reviewing or teaching systematic reviews. The template is shown in Table 5–4. It can be used in developing or writing a systematic review, as a checklist for evaluating systematic reviews, or a method for teaching about systematic reviews. The template can be used in electronic or paper format.

There are several reasons for undertaking a systematic review. Among the reasons are to: (1) summarize large amounts of information; (2) provide decision-makers with synthesized information; (3) explain consistency and inconsistency of data; (4) identify conflicts; (5) increase power and precision in estimates of risk or effect size; (6) identify gaps in knowledge; and (7) improve treatment (Seers, 2000).

Systematic reviews vary in quality and should be critically appraised. Some systematic reviews are misleading because the quality of the review is poor or biased. In other words, a systematic review may not present accurate analysis-synthesis of about research reports. Criteria for evaluating and making recommendations about systematic reviews are presented in Tables 5–6 and 5–7. L. Johnston (2005) suggests a rapid checklist for appraising a systematic review, which consist of three questions: (1) are all relevant peers identified? (2) how is the quality of peers assessed? and (3) how are results summarized?

Systematic reviews are available from the Web sites of the Academy of Neurologic Communication Disorders and Sciences, American Academy of Audiology, American Speech Language Hearing Association, and the Cochrane collections. These reviews can also be located by manual searches of of professional journals. Systematic reviews have been published in a variety of journals in speech-language pathology and audiology. ASHA (Evidence-based practice tool available, 2006) recently developed a registry of systematic reviewing and evidence-based guidelines. Guidelines have been developed to help in the critical appraisal and application of systematic reviews such as the criteria described in Tables 5–6 and 5–7.

There are several myths and misunderstandings about systematic reviews which Petticrew (2001) identified. Two of the more common misconceptions are: (1) systematic reviews are not research but are something that should be done without training or funding, and (2) they are solely for making clinical decisions, which understates wider uses. Other myths are: (1) same as ordinary reviews, only bigger; (2) only include randomized controlled trials; (3) require adaption of

Table 5–6. Criteria for Evaluating Systematic Review

Grade Recommendations	Criterion
A. Good evidence for inclusion	There is good peer-review evidence supporting consideration of use for the treatment
B. Fair evidence for inclusion	There is fair peer-review evidence supporting consideration of use for the treatment
C. Insufficient evidence	There is insufficient peer-review evidence for inclusion supporting consideration of use for treatment although recommendations for use are possible on other grounds
D. Fair evidence for exclusion	There is fair peer-review evidence supporting that the treatment should be excluded from consideration of use
E. Good evidence for exclusion	There is good peer-review evidence supporting that the treatment should be excluded from consideration

Source: From "Evidence-Based Practice in Schools: Integrating Craft and Theory with Science and Data," by L. M. Justice and M. E. Fey, 2004, *ASHA Leader, 9*(4–5), pp. 30–32. Copyright 2004 by American Speech-Language-Hearing Association. All rights reserved. Reprinted with permission.

Table 5–7. Examples of Outcomes from Systematic Reviews

Criteria	Yes	No
Did the review address a focused clinical question?		
Were tables used to show key features and to facilitate comparisons of studies?		
Were the criteria used to select articles for inclusion appropriate?		
Is it unlikely that important relevant studies were missed?		
Was the validity of the included studies appraised?		
Were assessments of the studies reproducible?		
Were the results similar from study to study?		
Are the results of a systematic review clear?		
Are the results precise?		
Can the results be applied to my client care?		
Were all clinically important criteria considered?		
Are the benefits worth the harms and costs?		
Were potential conflicts of interest disclosed?		

Sources: Adapted from *Systematic Review* (pp. 85–101), by K. Seers, In M. Dawes, P. Davies, A. Gray, J. Marx, K. Seers, and R. Snowball (Eds.), 1999, New York, NY: Churchill Livingstone; and "Making Sense of an Often Tangled Skein of Evidence," by the Editors, 2005, *Annals of Internal Medicine, 142*(12), pp. 1019–1020.

a biomedical model of health; of no relevance to real world; (4) must include statistical analysis (meta-analysis); (5) require experts; (6) can be done without experimental information/library support; and (7) substitute for good individual studies.

Systematic reviews about speech-language treatment have been criticized. Pring (2004) believes many researchers do not follow appropriate procedures for clinical outcomes research. In addition, many studies on which systematic reviews are based have methodological problems and often fail to adequately describe treatment, thereby making it impossible to evaluate or compare different types of treatment.

Garrett and Thomas (2006) responded to Pring's (2004) "Ask a silly question: Two decades of troublesome trials" by stating that systematic reviews using qualitative and/or statistical methods for combining studies can be completed within or across any phase of outcome research. Furthermore, systematic reviews can be informative because they help bring together what is, and what is not, known, and suggest treatments that may be beneficial or in need of further research.

Pring (2006) replied to Garrett and Thomas (2006) by stating that "systematic reviews are essential to evidence-based practice" (p. 208). Three advantages of systematic reviews were identified by Pring: (1) they can provide an overall effect size for treatment of a client group; (2) where different types of treatment have been provided, systematic reviews can compare the effect sizes to determine which treatment is more effective; and (3) the influence of experimental design on the overall effect size can be determined. Furthermore, methodological problems associated with systematic

reviews "serve as a further reminder that primary research must be both systematic in its development and rigorous in its procedures" (p. 110).

J. R. Johnston (2005) voiced concerns about the meta-analysis of treatment for children with developmental speech and language delay/disorder by Law, Garrett, and Nye (2004). These concerns were related to limitations in content, exclusion of practice sections, focus on very young children, and lack of sufficient attention to duration or methods of treatment. Law, Garrett, and Nye (2005) replied that "one person's narrowing is another person's strength" (p. 118). The concern about lack of information about treatment was valid. The age of the children included in the review was wider than J. R. Johnston (2005) suggested. The age of the children was in the birth to 16 year age range not just 2- to 3-year-olds.

The Cochrane Collection prepares, maintains, and disseminates systematic reviews. The Collection requires that systematic reviews address: Specific decisions points; objective; criteria for considering studies; types of studies; types of participants; types of intervention; types of outcome measures; search strategy; methods for selection of studies; awareness of methodological quality; date management; and data synthesis (Douglas, Brown, & Barry, 2004).

Difference Between Narrative and Systematic Reviews

There are major differences between a regular narrative review of the literature and a systematic review. Narrative reviews may lack the objectivity, rigor, and comprehensiveness of systematic reviews (Johnson, 2006). Systematic reviews use more specific search strategies and criteria for inclusion. These and other differences are compared in Table 5–8, systematic reviews are considered superior to narrative reviews for synthesizing research (Meline, 2006b).

Meta-Analysis

Meta-analysis is a systematic review in which a statistical summary is provided. It is a relatively recent approach to quantitative synthesis of previous studies which should not be confused with traditional reviews of the literature. In other words, meta-analysis is a statistical approach for combining studies about the same problem to determine the efficacy of a procedure or treatment (Haynes & Johnson, 2009; McMillan, 2005).

Steps in developing and completing a meta-analysis are listed in Table 5–9.

Table 5–9. Steps of a Meta-Analysis

- Selection of a research hypothesis
- Definition of eligibility criteria for inclusion and exclusion
- Development of a search strategy
- Identification of studies for inclusion
- Conversion of study statistic to common effect-size metric
- Complete summary effect and interpret its meaning

Table 5–8. Differences Between Narratives and Systematic Reviews

Feature	Narrative Review	Systematic Review
Question	Broad, general question	Focused or hypothesis to be tested
Sources and Search	Usually unspecified, risk for bias; do not usually attempt to locate all relevant literature	Comprehensive sources; specific search strategy
Selection	Usually unspecified risk for bias	Criterion-based selection, uniform application; limit selection bias
Appraisal	Variable; do not consider differences in study method or quality	Rigorous systematic critical appraisal; investigate potential biases and sources of heterogeneity
Synthesis	Qualitative	Quantitative
Inferences	Sometimes evidence-based; do not differentiate between sound and unsound studies	Usually evidenced-based; base conclusions on most methodologically sound studies

Sources: From "Systematically Reviewing the Evidence," by M. Law and I. Phillip, 2002. In M. Law (Ed.). *Evidence-Based Rehabilitation* (pp. 109–126). Thorofare, NJ: Slack Incorporated; "Systematic Reviews: Synthesis of Best Evidence for Clinical Decisions," by M. D. Cook, C. D. Murlow, and R. B. Haynes, 1997. *Annals of Internal Medicine, 126*(5), pp. 376–380; and "Systematic Reviews for Astronomy to Zoologoy: Myths and Misconceptions," by M. Petticrew, 2011. *British Medical Journal, 322*, pp. 98–101.

A preliminary step in meta-analysis is selection of a model of analysis. There are two analysis models: fixed effects and random effects. Fixed effects analysis is appropriate when most of the primary studies are obtained, and are reasonably homogeneous. Random effects analysis is appropriate when primary studies have random samples or are heterogeneous (Robey, 1999; Robey & Dalebout, 1998).

Meta-analysis can provide evidence, especially if it includes several randomized controlled trials (RCT), although it is influenced by the evidence available in the literature (Gloper et al., 2001). The highest evidence ratings are assigned to meta-analysis studies of RTCs (ASHA, 2004a). Thus, RTCs are considered the gold standard for evidence, but they are not infallible (Hartling et al., 2005).

Meta-analysis can provide information about treatment results. It included an average effect size that is considered clinically important and provides evidence that statistical power is adequate to detect and affect. Maxwell and Satake (2006) define *effect size* as "the degree to which the null hypothesis in false" (p. 511). That is, meta-analysis provides an average effect size to estimate whether a null hypothesis can be rejected, or the treatment has no influence on outcome. Maxwell and Satake (2006) developed a worksheet for meta-analysis review that is shown in Table 5–10. Another approach for reviewing meta-analysis is a series of questions, which are presented in Table 5–11. Critical review of meta-analysis reporting is important because of limitations associated with this type of analysis. Among these limitations are invalid primary studies, overemphasis on statistical significance, heterogeneous data, overestimation of treatment effectiveness, concern with whole populations

rather than individual's, and technical skill required for meta-analysis (Law & Philip, 2002;, Maxwell & Satake, 2006; Robey, 1999). Furthermore, meta-analysis may or may have specific criteria for selection of studies. The criteria for inclusion and evaluation of studies may not be as specific as the criteria should be. Therefore, meta-analysis reviews warrant critical appraisal.

Best-Evidence Systhesis

Best-evidence synthesis is an alternative to meta-analysis. It is a review of both qualitative and quantitative studies which are selected according to specific criteria (McMillan, 2004). Cook, Mulrow, and Haynes (1997) suggest that systematic reviews are synthesis of best-evidence for making clinical decisions. These are usually synthesis or experimental research, which is higher level research and excludes opinion(s).

Clinical Practice Guidelines

Most guidelines are a combination of clinician experience, expert opinion, and research evidence (Cook, Greengold, Elrod, & Weingarten, 1997). All practice guidelines are not equal. Some are based on expert opinion/consensus and/or evidence-based practice. The former are variable from high quality and credible to low quality, that is, biased and even deceptive and misleading, the latter are explicit statements that assist speech-language pathologist, audiologists and their clients to make informed decisions about appropriate care for specific speech-language-hearing problems.

Table 5–10. Meta-Analysis Review

Check one: ☐ Assessment article ☐ Intervention article

Reference:
_____
_____

Purpose Statement:
_____
_____

Number of Studies: _____

1	2	3	4	5

Seems inappropriate   Appropriate   Appropriate
No rationale   Limited rationale   Useful rationale

Comments: _____

Time Range for Inclusion: _____

1	2	3	4	5

Seems inappropriate   Appropriate   Appropriate
No rationale   Limited rationale   Useful rationale

Comments: _____

Types of Designs Included: Check all applicable:

☐ Large randomized controlled trials
☐ Small randomized controlled trials
☐ Repeated randomized single-case designs
☐ Non-randomized study with control group(s)
☐ Single-case design using alternating treatments or multiple baseline methods
☐ Case control study
☐ Case reports

1	2	3	4	5

Seems inappropriate   Appropriate   Appropriate
No rationale   Limited rationale   Useful rationale

Comments: _____

Criteria for Inclusion in Meta-Analysis:
_____

Comments: _____

Table 5–10. *continued*

Variables Studied:

Comments: _____

Main Points/Strategies Found to be Effective:

Comments: _____

Effect Size:

_____

Comments: _____

Interpretation of Results:

1	2	3	4	5
Interpretation beyond data		Some extension of interpretation beyond data		Data related tied to past research

Comments: _____

Credibility of Source:

1	2	3	4	5
Source unknown self-published/reported		Trade journal or edited publication		Peer-reviewed professional journal

Comments: _____

Source: Meta-analysis review. From *Research and Statistical Methods for Communication Sciences and Disorders (p. 485)*, by D. L. Maxwell and E. Satake, 2006, p. 485. Clifton Park, NY: Thomson Delmar Learning. Copyright 2006 Thomson Delmar Learning. Adapted with permission.

Table 5–11. Criteria for Meta-Analysis Studies

- Was the method for accumulating results from individual studies clear and appropriate?
- Were the methods for combining study effects appropriate?
- Were the data tested for heterogeneity and an appropriate statistic model utilized for the analysis?
- Where the data inspected for possible moderate variables?
- Were interpretation and conclusions consistent with the results?
- Were implications for future research discussed?

Source: From *Research in Communication Sciences and Disorders*, by T. Meline, 2006, Columbus, OH: Pearson Merrill. Reprinted with permission.

Furthermore, practice guidelines should be current, that is, developed, reviewed, or revised within the last 5 years (Johnson, 2006). Some practice guidelines may be outdated and need to be updated because of advances on clinical practice (Shojania, Sampson, Doucette, & Moher, 2007). ASHA's 25 evidence-based clinical practice guidelines were all published within the past three years. The majority of the 31 (78%) ANCDS (2011) evidence-based practice guidelines were published more than five years ago.

Determining when to develop guidelines should be considered carefully because of the amount of resources, skill, and time required (Slutsky, 2005). Criteria used to develop guidelines include:

- Potential to change outcomes or costs
- Availability of evidence on which to develop guidelines
- Topic clinically important
- Topic complex enough to initiate debate about recommendations
- Variation between actual and appropriate care
- No existing or relevant guidelines available to use
- Evidence available to support evidence-based development
- Recommendations acceptable to potential users
- Implementation of guidelines feasible.

Evidence-based guidelines are based on the best available evidence and professional judgment. Melnyk and Fineout-Overholt (2005) describe evidence-based practice guidelines as " . . . specific practice recommendations that are based on a methodologically rigorous review of

the best evidence on a specific topic" (p. 587). ASHA has also defined practice guidelines as part of its preferred practice patterns for speech-language pathology and audiology (ASHA, 2004b). These guidelines "define generally applicable characteristics of activities directed toward individual patients/clients and that addresses structural requisites of the practice, processed to be carried out, and expected outcomes (ASHA, 2004b).

There are three types of clinical practice guidelines based on evidence: traditional or narrative (TPG), systematic reviews (SR), and evidence based practice (Hargrove, Griffer, & Lund, 2008). Differences between these clinical practice guidelines are listed in Table 5–12.

There is a hierarchy of clinical practice guidelines with traditional-narrative reviews being the lowest rank (meeting the fewest criteria). Traditional reviews met only two of seven criteria. According to Hargrove, Griffer, and Lund (2008) evidence-based reviews differ " . . . from systematic reviews primarily in the quality of the evidence that is considered. Systematic reviews generally only consider only higher quality evidence, whereas evidence-based practice guidelines consider evidence from a variety of levels, including case studies and even expert opinions" (p. 290). This information is useful in making decisions about using and recommending clinical practice guidelines. The National Evidence-Based Center of ASHA (2011) uses the Appraisal of Guidelines for Research and Evaluation (AGREE) for evaluating and recommending systematic reviews. These reviews are highly recommended, recommended with reservations, or not recommended.

The Academy of Neurologic Communication Disorders and Sciences (ANCDS)

Table 5–12. Difference Between TCPs, SRs, and EBCPGs

Evidence Criteria	TCP	SR	EBCPG
Based on a comprehensive, methodical review of the literature	No	Yes	Yes
Based on the consensus of a panel of experts	No	Yes	Yes
Can include expert opinion	Yes	No	Yes
Identifies evidence that supports recommendations	No	Yes	Yes
Evaluates the quality of the literature used to support the recommendations	No	Yes	Yes
Expertise of the expert or group of experts is disclosed	No	Yes	Yes
Can include case studies, retrospective, nonrandomized research designs	Yes	No	Yes

Source: "Procedures for using clinical practice guidelines," by P. Hargrove and M. Griffer, 2008, *Language Speech, Hearing, and Services in Schools, 39,* 289–302.

as developed evidence-based practice guidelines (EBPG). These EBPGs focus on five areas: aphasia, acquired apraxia, cognitive dysarthria, and communication disorders related to traumatic brain injury and dementia.

Obviously there is a variation in reporting clinical practice guidelines. Sniffman and associates (2003) developed a standardized format for reporting clinical practice guidelines which is based on 15 factors.

Some practice guidelines do not meet the criteria for systematic review and are narrative rather than systematic. There may be limited information about the outcome measures used the literature search strategy or key words used, and no inclusion/exclusion criteria for the studies reviewed. Thus, it is important for speech-language pathologists and audiologists to critically appraise practice guidelines.

Finding appropriate guidelines depend on being able to critically evaluate the reliability of a guideline because guidelines do not always confirm the best practice (Slutsky, 2005). Criteria for evaluating guidelines include: validity; reliability and reproducibility; clinical applicability; clinical flexibility; clarity; documentation; development by a multidisciplinary program; and plans for review. Additional information about practice guidelines is provided in Chapter 13.

Summary

Narrative reviews in speech-language pathology and audiology are underutilized, whereas systematic reviews, including meta-analysis are underutilized. It is encouraging that in recent years there has been an increase in systematic reviews which is expected to continue because of the focus on evidence-based practice. A major evidence in evidence based practice and systematic reviews is formulation of the question. Two strategies were described: PICO and PESICO. Meta-analysis ranks very high in terms of the hierarchy of evidence considered in evidence-based practice. Organizing and reviewing evidence is challenging as the Editors (2005) of the *Annals of Internal Medicine* suggest as attempts at "making sense of an often tangled skein of evidence" (p. 1019).

DISCUSSION QUESTIONS

1. Outline the steps for performing and organizing a literature review.
2. Differentiate between a literature review chart and a concept matrix.
3. What are the differences between narrative and systematic reviews?
4. What are some common misconceptions about systematic reviews?
5. What are the major components of a systematic review?
6. How can systematic reviews be evaluated?
7. Define meta-analysis and discuss its use in speech-language pathology and audiology.
8. What are the steps in conducting a meta-analysis?
9. How can systematic reviews be evaluated?
10. How can meta-analysis be evaluated?
11. What is a best-evidence synthesis?
12. Explain the importance of practice guidelines.
13. How is practice guidelines developed?
14. Outline a hierarchy for clinical practice guidelines.
15. What is the difference between systematic review and an evidence based clinical practice guideline?
16. How can clinical practice guidelines be used for making clinical decisions?
17. Why should the use of clinical practice guidelines be encouraged?
18. What do clinicians not use clinical practice guidelines?
19. Describe PICO. Describe PESICO. What are the differences between PICO and PESICO?
20. What are the differences between clinical practice guidelines, systematic reviews, and evidence-based clinical practice guidelines?

References

Academy of Neurologic Communications Disorders and Sciences. (2011). *Evidence based practice documents.* Retrieved from http://www.ancds.org/index

American Psychological Association. (2010). *Publication manual for the American Psychological Association* (5th ed.). Washington, DC: Author.

Hearing Association. (1997). *Preferred practice patterns for the profession of audiology.* Rockville, MD: Author.

American Speech-Language-Hearing Association. (2004a). *Evidence-based practices in communication disorders: An introduction.* Retrieved from http://www.asha.org/members/deskref-journal/deskref/default

American Speech-Language-Hearing Association. (2004b). *Preferred practice patterns for the profession of speech-language pathology.* Rockville, MD: Author.

American Speech Language-Hearing Association. (2011). *Clinical practice guidelines.* Retrieved from http://www.asha.org/member/guidelines.aspt

Bannigan, K., Droogan, J., & Entwistle, V. (1997). Systematic reviews: What do they involve? *Nursing Times, 93*(18), 54–55.

Cook D. J., Mulrow, C. D., & Haynes, R. B. (1997). Systematic reviews: Synthesis of best evidence for clinical decisions. *Annals of Internal Medicine, 126*(5), 376–380.

Creswell, J. W. (2003). *Research design.* Thousand Oaks, CA: Sage.

DePoy, E., & Gitlin, L. N. (2011). *Introduction to research.* St. Louis, MO: Mosby.

Douglas, J., Brown, L., & Barry, S. (2004). The evidence base for the treatment of aphasia after stroke. In S. Riley, J. Douglas, & J. Oates (Eds.), *Evidence-based practice in speech pathology.* London, UK: Whurr.

Evidence-based practice tool available. (2006). *ASHA Leader, 11*(8), 19.

Garrett, Z., & Thomas, J. (2006). Systematic reviews and their application to research in speech and language therapy: A response to T. R. Pring's "Ask a silly question: Two decades of troublesome trials" (2004). *International Journal Language Communication Disorders, 41*(11), 95–105.

Golper, L. A., Wertz, R. T., Fratteli, C. M., Yorksten, K., Meyers, K., Katz, R., . . . Wambaugb, J. (2001). Evidence-based practice guidelines for the management of communication disorders in neurologically impaired individuals. *ANCDS Practice Guidelines,* pp. 1–12.

Hargrove, P., Gruffer, M., & Lund, B. (2008). Procedures for using clinical practice guidelines. *Language Speech and Hearing Services Schools, 39,* 289–302

Hartling, L., McAlister, F. A., Rowe, B. H., Ezekowitz, J., Frierson, C., & Kiassen, T. P. (2005). Challenges in systematic reviews of therapeutic devices and procedures. *Annals of Internal Medicine, 142*(12), 1100–1111.

Haynes, W. O., & Johnson, C. E. (2009). *Understanding research and evidence-based practice in communication disorders.* Boston, MA: Pearson.

Huang, X., Lin, J., & Dummer-Fushman, D. (2006). Evaluation of PICO as a knowledge representation for clinical questions. *AMJA Annual Symposium Proceedings,* p. 355–363.

Jewell, D. (2011). *Guide to evidence-based physical therapist practice.* Sudbury, MA: Jones and Bartlett.

Johnson, C. J. (2006). Getting started in evidence based practice for childhood speech language disorders, *American Journal of Speech-Language Pathology, 15,* 20–35.

Johnston, J. R. (2005). Re: Law, Garrett, & Nye (2004). The efficacy of treatment for children with developmental speech and language delay/disorder: A meta-analysis. *Journal of Speech, Language, and Hearing Research, 4*(5), 1114–1117.

Johnston, L. (2005). Critically appraising quantitative evidence. In B. M. Melnyk & E. Fineout Overholt (Eds.), *Evidence-based practice in nursing and health care* (pp. 79–126). Philadelphia, PA: Lippincott Williams & Wilkins.

LaRue, F. M., Draus, P. S., & Klem, M. (2009). A description of a Web-based educational tool for understanding the PICO framework in evidence-based practice. *Computer Information in Nursing, 27*, 44–49.

Law, J., Garnett, Z., & Nye, C. (2004). The efficacy of treatment for children with developmental speech and language delay/disorder. A meta-analysis. *Journal of Speech, Language, and Hearing Research, 47*(4), 924–943.

Law, J., Garnett, Z., & Nye, C. (2005). The specificity of a systematic review is the key to its value: A response to Johnson (2005). *Journal of Speech, Language, and Hearing Research, 48*(5), 1118–1120.

Law, M., & Philip, I. (2002). Systematically reviewing the evidence. In M. Law (Ed.), *Evidence based rehabilitation,* (pp. 109–126). Thorofare, NJ: Slack.

Marshall, J., Goldhart, J., & Roulstone, S. (2011). Application of systematic reviews speech and language therapy. *Intervention Journal Language and Communication Disorders, 46*, 261–272.

Maxwell, D. L., & Satake, E. (2006). *Research and statistical methods in communication sciences and disorders*. Clifton Park, NY: Thomsom-Delmar Learning.

McCauley, R. J., & Hergrove, R. (2004). A clinician's introduction to systematic reviews in communication disorders. *Contemporary Issues in Communication Sciences and Disorders, 31*, 173–181.

McMillan, J. H. (2004). *Educational research: Fundamentals for the consumer*. Boston, MA: Pearson.

McMillan, J. H., & Shumacher, S. (2010). *Research in education*. Boston, MA: Pearson.

Meline, T. (2006a). *Research in communication sciences and disorders*. Upper Saddle River, NJ. Pearson Merrill.

Meline, T. (2006b). Selecting studies for systematic review: Inclusion and exclusion criteria. *Contemporary Issues in Communication Sciences and Disorders, 33*, 21–27.

Melnyk, B. M., & Fineout-Overholt, E. (2005). *Evidence-based practice in nursing and health care*. Philadelphia, PA: Lippincott Williams & Wilkins.

Mertens, D. M. (2005). *Research and evaluation in education and psychology*. Thousand Oaks, CA: Sage.

Nursing Library and Information Resources. (n.d.). Retrieved from http://www.med.49.e.ed

Petticrew, M. (2001). Systematic reviews from astronomy to zoology: Myths and misconceptions. *British Medical Journal, 332*, 98–101.

Polit, D. F., & Beck, C. T. (2010). *Nursing research: Principles and methods*. Philadelphia, PA: J. B. Lippincott.

Portney, L. G., & Watkins, M. P. (2009). *Foundations of clinical research*. Upper Saddle River, NJ: Pearson.

Pring, T. (2004). Ask a silly question: Two decades of troublesome trials. *International Journal of Language Communication Disorders, 39*(3), 285–302.

Pring, T. (2006). Systematic reviews require a systematic approach to therapy research: A reply to Garrett and Thomas (2005). *International Journal of Language Communication Disorders, 41*(11), 107–110.

Richardson, W., Wilson, M., Nishikawa, J., & Hayward, R. (1995). The well-built clinical question: A key to evidence-based decisions. *ACP Journal Club, 123*, A112–A113.

Robey, R. R. (1994). The efficacy of treatment for aphasic persons: A meta-analysis. *Brain and Language, 47*, 582–608.

Robey, R. R. (1999). A meta-analysis of clinical outcomes in the treatment of aphasia. *Journal of Speech, Language, and Hearing Research, 41*(1), 172–187.

Robey, R. R., & Dalebout, S. D. (1998). A tutorial on conducting meta-analysis of clinical outcome research. *Journal of Speech, Language, and Hearing Research, 41*, 1227–1241.

Roy, N., Weinrich, B., Gray, S. D., Tanner, K., Stemple, J. C., & Sapineza, C. M. (2003). Three treatments for teachers with voice disorders: A randomized clinical trial.

Journal of Speech, Language, and Hearing Research, 46, 670–688.

Schlosser, R. W. (2000). Synthesis efficacy research in AAC. In R. W. Schlosser (Ed.), *The efficacy of augmentative and alternative communication* (pp. 230–259). New York, NY: Academic Press.

Schlosser, R, W., Kould, R., & Costello, J. (2007). Asking well-built questions for evidence based practice in augmentative and alternative communication in augmentative and alternative communication. *Journal of Communication Disorders, 40,* 225–238.

Seers, K. (1999). Systematic reviews. In M. Dawes, P. Davies, A. Gray, J. Marx, K. Seers, K., & R. Snowball (Eds.), *Evidence-based practice* (pp. 85–100). London, UK: Churchill, Livingstone.

Shojania, K. G., Simpson, M., Anscni, M. T., Doucette, S., & Moher, D (2007). How quickly do systematic reviews go over date? *Annals Internal Medicine, 147,* 224–233.

Slutsky, J. (2005). Using evidence-based practice guidelines: Tools for improving Practice. In B. M. Melnyk & E. Fineout-Overholt (Eds.), *Evidence-based practice in nursing and health care* (pp. 221–235). Philadelphia, PA: Lippincott Williams & Wilkins.

Sniffman, R. M., Shekelle, P., Overchag, M., Slutksy, J., & Grimshaw, R. (2003). Standardized reporting or clinical practice guidelines a proposal from the Conference on Guidelines Standardization. *Annals of Internal Medicine, 139,* 493–498.

The Editors. (2005). Making sense of an often tangled skein of evidence. *Annals of Internal Medicine, 142*(12), 1019–1020.

6

Measurement

LEARNING OBJECTIVES

Upon completion of this chapter the reader will be able to:

- Define nominal, ordinal, interval, and ratio levels of measurement
- Provide an example of each level of measurement
- Describe the differences in the levels of measurement
- Define validity and reliability
- Describe the various subtypes of validity and reliability
- Describe the importance of reliability and validity in research.

Scales of Measurement

One important phase of a research project is the measurement of the appropriate variables. Scales of measurement provide a means of assigning numbers to event or objects according to prescribed rules. Preparing numerical data according to these rules allows the application of statistical treatment. Four scales or levels of measurement are used to categorize data. They can be remembered by using the phrase, "No Oil In Rivers." They are in hierarchical order: *nominal, ordinal, interval,* and *ratio scales* (Table 6–1).

Nominal Level of Measurement

The nominal (lowest) level of measurement classifies an event or object into a category. Examples include gender, name, medical chart, number, individuals who do and do not stutter, individuals with and without a history of voice problems,

hearing sensitivity (normal or abnormal), etiology of hearing loss (conductive or sensorineural), and language development (normal or abnormal). A subject is measured at this level by assigning the individual to one of the categories. Some variables at the nominal level are naturally measured as numerics (e.g., medical chart number) whereas other variables are coded numerically (e.g., 1 = normal, 2 = abnormal). The numbers assigned denote differences and are not used mathematically for addition, subtraction, multiplication, or division. These functions would be meaningless at this level.

According to Portney and Watkins (2009), nominal categories are mutually exclusive. This means that no object or person can logically be assigned to more than one category. Use of the nominal data category also assumes that the rules for classifying a set of attributes are exhaustive; in other words, every subject can be accurately assigned to one category. Classifying blood type would follow these rules.

Table 6–1. Four Scales of Measurement Used to Categorize Data

Scale of Measurement	Definition	Example
Ratio	Equal intervals; true meaningful zero; possesses properties of all other scales	Age, IQ, weight; many personality and educational tests
Interval	Equal intervals; no meaningful zero; possesses properties of ordinal and nominal scale	Temperature
Ordinal	Ranked data; possesses properties of nominal scale	Heaviest-lightest Sweetest-sourest Tallest-shortest
Nominal	Named or counted data; classification of labeling	Color Label: male or female

Source: From *Research and Evaluation in Education and Psychology* (p. 304), by D. M. Mertens, 2005, Thousand Oaks, CA: Sage Publications. Reprinted by permission of Sage Publications, Inc.

Ordinal Level of Measurement

The ordinal level of measurement shows the position of one variable relative to another. The intervals between variables are not equal. Examples of variables at the ordinal level include college classification (i.e., freshmen, sophomore, junior, or senior), teaching ranks (i.e., instructor, assistant professor, associate professor, or professor), and severity of a disorder (i.e., mild, moderate, or severe). Examples of the ordinal categories for the variable, hearing sensitivity, include normal, mild, moderate, and severe. As with nominal level of measurement variables at the ordinal level are frequently coded numerically (e.g., 1 = freshman, 2 = sophomore, 3 = junior, and 4 = senior). However, mathematical or numeric operation (addition, subtraction, multiplication, division) remain meaningless with ordinal measures. Nonparametric statistical methods are used to examine ordinal data.

Interval Level of Measurement

Interval scales are used when there are equal intervals between values but no absolute zero. For numeric operation to yield meaningful results, it is necessary to have equal intervals between adjacent numerical values. For example, the difference between 3 and 5 should be the same as the difference between 23 and 25. In both the interval and ratio levels of measurement, there are constant differences in data entries. According to Portney and Watkins (2009), the interval scale does not allow for comparison of absolute magnitude of attribute because an absolute is not zero (like ordinal measurement).

Examples of variables at the interval include numerical ratings of vocal quality on a 5- or 7-point equal interval scale, numerical ratings reflecting attitudes of individuals who stutter based on 5-point Likert-type rating scales, standard or scaled scores on a language test, or IQ scores. Parametric statistics are used if the following criteria are met: (1) the subjects represent a "normal" population distribution; (2) the sample is sizable, usually more than 30; and (3) information is derived using the interval or ratio level of measurement (Ventry & Schiavetti, 1986). Thus, parametric statistical methods are used to examine equal interval data.

Ratio Level of Measurement

Ratio scales are interval scales with an absolute zero. In other words, it is assumed that the attribute being measured may not be present. This measure is more frequently appropriate for studies involving natural science than for studies in areas of social science. However, if the dependent variable is the frequency of events, such as frequency of moments of stuttering; has time measures, such as the latency period between seeing a printed word and saying it; involves a measure distance, such as measurement of the space constituting a velopharyngeal gap during phonation in patients with velopharyngeal incompetency; and so on, the ratio level may be appropriate. Height, weight, chronologic age, hearing level in decibels, and fundamental frequency of a complex wave are additional examples of variables that can be measured at the ratio level.

The differences between interval and ratio measurements are that multiples are meaningful at the ratio level (a 6-mm velopharyngeal gap is twice as large as a 3-mm gap), and the units of the variables measured at the ratio level can be changed by simple multiplication (i.e., feet are converted into inches by multiplying by 12). These properties do not hold true for measurements at the interval level. For example, a person with an IQ of 100 is not twice as intelligent as someone with an IQ of 50. All numbers at the ratio level of measurement have mathematical properties so parametric statistics are used to examine ratio interval data.

In summary, variables are treated as categorical (e.g., gender, age, disorder) or quantitative (e.g., height, weight, IQ, frequency of occurrence). It is important that categories for variables be classified so that each subject fits into only one category. Quantitative variables usually are measured in discrete units (e.g., frequency, pounds, milliseconds, and millimeters). These units must be carefully recorded as the data are collected.

Table 6–2 shows hypothetical data for fundamental frequency utilizing all types of measurements.

Validity of Measurement

When analyzing the accuracy of the results of a study, the investigator objectively attempts to answer questions of validity and reliability. When assessing the *validity* of a study, the primary question involves determining whether the information gathered actually contributes to answering the research question (Schiavetti, Metz, & Orlikoff 2011). For example, if the investigator identifies phonatory quality using a Visi-Pitch™ analysis with an inappropriate frequency range for some the subjects, perturbation data might be questioned. Portney and Watkins (2009) stated "validity implies that a measurement is relatively free from error; that is, a valid test is also reliable" (p. 79).

Hegde (1994) differentiates between the validity of the data defining the dependent variables and the validity of the experiment itself. Accuracy of the information about the phonation attributes of the subjects is an example of establishing the validity of data defining the dependent variable(s). The design of

Table 6–2. Hypothetical Data for Fundamental Frequency Utilizing All Types of Measurements

Subject	Ratio Measure	Interval Measure	Ordinal Measure	Nominal Measure
A	220	4	3	High
B	198	5	2	Medium
C	137	8	1	Low
D	235	3	4	High

Source: From *Foundations of Clinical Research: Application to Practice* (2nd ed., p. 56), by L. G. Portney and M. P. Watkins, 2000, Upper Saddle River, NJ: Pearson Education. Copyright 2000, Pearson Education, Inc. Adapted by permission.

a study, including control methods for observing, collecting, and recording data and control of the variables that might have an impact on the outcome of the study, contributes to the validity of the experiment itself. For example, consistent tracking of relevant phonatory habits and phonatory attributes of all subjects would contribute to the validity of the experiment.

Both internal and external validity are important to establish when analyzing the results of a research study. To establish *internal validity*, the experimenter determines if the experimental manipulation really made a difference (Kerlinger, 1973) by ensuring that extraneous factors that could influence the results are carefully controlled (Schiavetti & Metz, 2002). To establish internal validity, the design of a study should effectively rule out all variables that might affect the dependent variable so that it can be concluded that the independent variable was ultimately responsible for any change in the dependent variable (Doehring, 1988). Portney and Watkins (2000) cited several factors that affect internal validity. Some of these are the effectors of prior events, maturation, attrition, testing effects by repeated testing, instrumentation, statistical regression (regression toward the mean), compensatory rivalry, and resentful demoralization of respondents receiving less desirable treatments, In summary, internal validity involves answering the question of whether the experimental treatments actually made a difference in the study (Isaac & Michael, 1987).

For the voice study cited previously, internal validity could be established by demonstrating voice improvement using Visi-Pitch™ data and a comparison of pre-and post-experimental perceptual analyses of the quality of subjects' voices. Internal validity could be further established by reporting that: (1) the Visi-Pitch™ equipment was properly set and calibrated, (2) subjects with phonatory disorders related to pre-existing laryngeal conditions were not selected, (3) all perceptual judgments were made by the same speech-language pathologists whose perceptual judgments were calibrated to the same criteria in training sessions administered by the experimenter, (4) all subjects received the same training in identifying poor vocal habits and establishing good vocal habits, and (5) all received the same medical diagnosis at treatment.

External validity is the extent to which the results of a study satisfy representativeness or generalizability (Kerlinger, 1973) or can be generalized to the population as a whole (Schiavetti, Metz, & Orlikoff 2011). Practical clinical use of findings is determined by establishing external validity. The extent to which effects of independent variables on dependent variables apply to the natural setting must be determined to establish external validity (Doehring, 1988). Hegde (1994) cites effects of treatment during a study and knowledge of expected results by subjects as factors that may influence the external validity of a study. Isaac and Michael (1987) concluded that questions about external validity involving what populations, settings, treatment variables, and measurement variables to which an effect can be generalized may not be completely answerable. The researcher must attempt to control all variables as well as possible.

For the voice study, establishing external validity could be done by showing that: (1) the individuals selected for the study were typical in age, sex, and occupation to those generally reported in the literature as having chronic voice problems related to vocal abuse and/or inflammatory laryngeal conditions, (2) standard treatment information was given to all subjects about identification and reduction of vocal abuses, (3) typical medical management was used for the conditions diagnoses, and (4) establishing that the data provided by the Visi-Pitch™ and pre-and postperceptual analysis by examiners is typical of that collected by certified speech-language pathologists in varied clinical settings.

Three types of validity should be considered when using a test or questionnaire to measure an individual's knowledge or attitudes. These are content validity, criterion-related (including predictive and concurrent) validity, and construct validity. *Content validity* concerns whether the substance or content of a measure adequately represents the universe of content of the attribute being measured or how well the content of the attribute being measured or how well the content of a test reflects the subject matter from which conclusions will be drawn (Isaac & Michael, 1987; Kerlinger, 1973; Portney & Watkins, 2009). Kerlinger (1973) further explained that content validation is basically judgmental in that each item is judged for its pertinence or applicability to the property or characteristic being measured.

Schiavetti, Metz, and Orlikoff (2011) further described content validity as a subjective means of logically explaining and evaluating test items to determine how well they reflect the characteristics to be measured. Content validity is concerned with adequately assessing all the aspects of the behaviors to be measured.

For example, to assess IQ, the research usually assesses quantitative and verbal ability abilities because both have been shown to correlate with intelligence. For example, the content validity of a test of language development would be determined by identifying the important behaviors that reflect good or poor language performance, then determining whether the content of the test items reflects those behaviors or skills.

Schiavetti, Metz and Orlikoff (2011) define *criterion-related validity* as a test of whether a test (or measure) correlates with a known indicator (validating criterion) of the behavior (characteristic) being measured. Two types of criterion-related validity include concurrent and predictive validity (Kerlinger, 1973). Kerlinger (1973) further described concurrent criterion-related validity as involving the ability to check a currently administered measuring instrument against an outcome occurring now. Predictive criterion-related validity involves the ability to check a currently administered measuring instrument against a future outcome. For example, future achievement is predicted by aptitude tests (predictive) and present (concurrent) and future (predictive) achievement are predicted by achievement tests. Present and future ability to learn and solve problems are predicted by IQ tests (Kerlinger, 1973). Thus, it is difficult to separate the predictive and concurrent components of criterion-related validity.

Criterion-related validity involves a test's ability to predict current or future performance. This may involve using correlation measures to compare test scores with criteria known to identify the same skills as the proposed test (Isaac & Michael, 1987). In fact, criterion-related data may be collected concurrently with the test to ascertain whether the test involves criteria-related procedures (Isaac & Michael, 1987). The major difficulty in establishing criterion-related validity is determining whether criteria exist to predict a specific skill or performance such as teaching effectiveness. The question of what constitutes appropriate criteria to measure teaching effectiveness has proved a hotbed of controversy for many years.

Construct validity involves scientific inquiry by testing a hypothesized relationship and validating a test and the theory behind it (Kerlinger, 1973). By investigating the qualities a test measures, the degree to which the concepts or theory behind the test account for performance on the test may be determined (Isaac & Michael, 1987). Thus, construct validity is concerned with the extent to which a tester questionnaire measures what it is supposed to measure by reflecting the theory, behavior, or characteristic to be measured (Schiavetti & Metz, 2002). The scores on a test are correlated with other accepted measures of the same behavior. If subjects scores on a new test are strongly correlated with their scores on an established test, then construct validity has been established.

Reliability of Measurement

Reliability refers to the consistency of a rater or of a measurement. Several words have been used to define reliability: dependability, predictability, consistency, credibility, and stability. In research, reliability refers to the consistency or cor-

relation among repeated measures or observations. Reliability does not ensure accuracy or validity. Observations can be consistent without being accurate. For example, children's responses to audiometric screening in a noisy environment might very well be consistent but certainly would not be considered accurate or valid indicators of their hearing sensitivity.

Three types of reliability: intraexaminer (intrarater or intrajudge), interexaminer (interrater or interjudge), and test-retest reliability should be assessed when establishing the reliability of the results of a study. Strong *intraexaminer reliability* implies that in repeated observations of the same subject the same examiner gets similar results. Intraexaminer reliability is usually not difficult to establish. However, *interexaminers reliability* implies agreement among different observers measuring the same phenomenon. Interexaminer reliability is considered a crucial measure of objectivity and is a necessary element to subjecting a study to scientific review (Hegde, 2003). *Test-retest reliability* involves how well subjects perform on one set of measurements as compared to their performance on a second evaluation of the same measurements.

The relationship between validity and reliability is shown in Figure 6–1. A measurement may be very reliable, but not be very valid (Figure 6–1A). A measurement with random error is usually not considered either reliable or valid (Figure 6–1B). If a measurement has only a small amount of error, then it is possible to have relatively valid and reliable measurements (Figure 6–1C). If a measurement has no variance and is consistently reliable and valid, then the confidence in those measurements is high (Figure 6–1D).

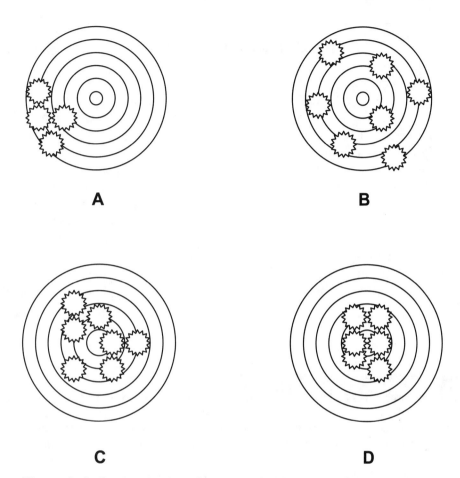

Figure 6–1. Representation of targets to illustrate the relationship between reliability and validity. **A.** Scores are highly reliable, but not valid, demonstrating systematic error. **B.** Scores are neither reliable nor valid, demonstrating random error. **C.** Reliability had improved but is still low; scores are somewhat valid. **D.** Scores are both reliable and valid. From *Foundations of Clinical Research: Application to Practice* (2nd ed., p. 80), by L. G. Portney and M. P. Watkins, 2000, Upper Saddle River, NJ: Pearson Education. Copyright 2000, Pearson Education, Inc. Adapted by permission.

Summary

Measurement of variables includes the control of factors which may influence reliability and validity. The level of measurement may be nominal, ordinal, interval, or ratio. It is important that the level of measurement used fit the study so appropriate analysis of the data can be used. It is important for all researchers to understand that validity and reliability are interrelated. Various types of factors may influence internal and external validity and different forms of reliability.

DISCUSSION QUESTIONS

1. What significance does the phrase, "No Oil In Rivers," have for measurement?

2. Describe nominal and ordinal levels of measurements. What are the major properties that distinguish these two levels of measurement?

3. Provide an example of interval level of measurement. Does it have an absolute zero?

4. Ratio level of measurement allows for what type of mathematical operations? Why is this advantageous?

5. Differentiate between content and construct validity? Provide an example of each.

6. What is reliability? How does reliability relate to validity?

7. Can a study have good reliability and poor validity? Give an example.

8. Differentiate between interjudge and intrajudge reliability? When might each of these be used during clinical research?

References

Doehring, D. G. (1988). *Research strategies in human communication disorders*. Boston, MA: College-Hill Press.

Hegde, M. N. (1994). *Clinical research in communicative disorders*. Austin, TX: Pro-Ed.

Hegde, M. N. (2003). *Clinical research in communicative disorders* (4th ed.). Austin, TX: Pro-Ed.

Isaac, S., & Michael, W. B. (1987). *Handbook in research and evaluation*. San Diego, CA: Edits Publishers.

Kay Pentax Inc. Visi-Pitch™. (2006). Retrieved from http://www.kaypentax.com

Kerlinger, F. N. (1973). *Foundations of behavioral research*. New York, NY: Holt, Rinehart & Winston.

Portney, L. G., & Watkins, M. P. (2009). *Foundation of clinical research: Applications to practice* (3rd ed.). Upper Saddle River, NJ: Prentice-Hall Health.

Schiavetti, N., Metz, D. E., & Orlikoff, R. F. (2011). *Evaluating research in speech pathology and audiology*. Boston, MA: Allyn & Bacon.

Ventry, I., & Schiavetti, N. (1986). *Evaluating research in speech pathology and audiology*. New York, NY: Macmillan.

7

Research Design and Strategy

LEARNING OBJECTIVES

Upon completion of this chapter the reader will be able to:

- Describe several group designs for between-subjects and within-subjects

- Discuss single-subject designs related to clinical practice

- Describe the basics of sequential clinical trials

- Describe the basics of the Statistical Package for Social Sciences

- Discuss the advantages and disadvantages of group, single-subject, and sequential clinical trials designs.

Introduction

All types of research have a strategy or design which permits statistical analysis of differences between and within groups of subjects (Doehring, 1988; Maxwell & Satake, 2006; Portney & Watkins, 2009). Several types of research were described in previous chapters. Research strategy and design refer to the plans for answering research questions and testing research hypotheses. Some authorities differentiate between these terms; others do not. The strategy or design of a study indicates the methods and procedures used in the investigation. There are essentially two types of research designs: group designs and single-subject-designs. *Group designs* include between-subject, within-subject designs, and mixed group designs. *Single-subject designs* include case studies, within-subject experimental designs, multiple baseline, and multiple treatment designs. Group research designs and single-subject designs are compared in Table 7–1.

Characteristics of a Good Design

Good research design may be described in terms of a number of characteristics. In order to understand that systematic changes are the result of the experiment being conducted involves the use of "the researcher's ability to manipulate and control variables and measurements, so that rival hypotheses are ruled out as a possible explanation for the observed response" (Portney & Watkins, 2000, p. 153). Essentially, there are two types of extraneous variables: (1) intrinsic and (2) extrinsic (Polit & Hungler, 1999; Portney & Watkins, 2000). *Intrinsic variables* are variables associated with subjects of an investigation such as age, gender, socioeconomic status, and marital status. There are a number of ways to reduce intrinsic variability such as randomization (each subject has an equal chance of being assigned to any group), homogeneity (choosing only subjects who have the same characteristics), blocking (building extraneous variables into the design by using them as independent variables), using the subject as his or her own control, and analysis of covariance (selecting a covariate and adjusting scores statistically to control for differences on the extraneous variable) (Portney & Watkins, 2009). *Extrinsic variables* are variables associated with the research situation or environment. The variables are related to the place and time the research was conducted and adherence or not to the research specification or protocols. The most effective method of controlling external factors is directly related to the consistency of conditions under which an investigation is performed, that is, the conditions under which data are collected should be as similar as possible for every subject.

The second characteristic of good research design is that it should be appropriate for the question(s) being asked. Third, the design should not result in data that are biased. A fourth characteristic of good research design is precision, which can be accomplished by the use of a well-described protocol. Research designs differ considerably in the sensitivity with which statistically significant results can be detected. A fifth characteristic is the power of the design or its ability to detect relationships among variables. According to Portney and Watkins (2000), the power

Table 7–1. Comparison of Group-Research Designs and Single-Subject Designs

Group Designs	Single-Subject Designs
Compare at least 2 groups from a target population	Compare within-subject performance for 1 subject or a small group of subjects.
Minimum number of subjects: 10	Minimum number: 1
Outcome measures collected infrequently; usually only pretest/post-test.	Performance repeatedly measured over a period corresponding to requirements of design.
Unnecessary to run subjects more than once under each experimental condition.	Necessary to run subject more than once under each experiment.
Little or no subject feedback; emphasis on outcome.	Subject feedback monitored; emphasis on process and outcome.
Inflexible; changes not permitted once intervention is introduced.	Flexible, permits addition or elimination.
Standardized measurement procedures and comparisons between subjects.	Measurement procedures flexible, individualized.
Generalization	Limited generalization.
Expensive	Inexpensive
Statistical procedures well developed.	Statistical procedures relatively new.
Relatively easy to control for order and sequence effects.	Difficult to control for order and sequence effects.

Sources: From "Clinically Relevant Designs for Rehabilitation Research: The Idiographic Model," by K. J. Ottenbacher, 1990, *American Journal of Physical Medicine and Rehabilitation, 69,* pp. 286–292; *Research Design and Evaluation in Speech-Language Pathology and Audiology,* by F. H. Silverman, 1993, Englewood Cliffs, NJ: Prentice-Hall; and "Group Designs in Clinical Research," by G. M. Siegelo and M. A. Young, 1987, *Journal of Speech and Hearing Disorders, 52*(3), pp. 194–199.

of a statistical test addresses the ability of a test to reject the null hypothesis, that is, "to document a real relationship between independent and dependent variables" (p. 164). The appropriateness of research designs must also be considered relative to the current state of the art. Portney and Watkins (2009) suggest that when important extraneous variables cannot be controlled, a descriptive or correlational design may be more appropriate.

Portney and Watkins (2000) identified six critical questions that should be considered when choosing a specific design. These include:

1. How many independent variables are being tested?
2. How many levels do each independent variable have, and are these levels experimental or control conditions?

3. How many groups of subjects are being tested?
4. How will subjects be selected, and how will they be assigned to groups?
5. How often will observation of responses be made?
6. What is the temporal sequence of interventions and measurements?

Group Designs

Group designs permit comparison of the average or typical performance of a group to other groups or other conditions (Warren, 1986). Several terms are used for this design: between-groups design, between-subjects designs, correlational design, pre-experimental design, quasiexperimental design, and true experimental design (Bordens & Abbott, 1988; Portney & Watkins, 2009). Hegde (1999) indicates that the basic method for implementing group designs is to initially have two or more comparable groups that represent the populations from which they were drawn (especially when the random procedure is used); at least one of the groups receives a treatment (experimental group); another group does not (control group).

Between-Subjects Designs

A classic design for exploring cause-and-effect relationships includes the pretest-posttest randomized control group (Patten, 2005). Figure 7–1 illustrates the classic design, which assumes that all groups are equal except that one received an experimental treatment and the other did not. Patten (2005) states that the advantage of using a pretest is that it will allow a researcher to determine how much each group has gained or changed, not just whether they are different at the end of the experiment.

If a researcher is concerned that a pretest might make subjects more sensitive to what is being studied, an alternative is to implement the posttest-only design (Portney & Watkins, 2009). A researcher would have used random assignment of subjects and the groups would be comparable. The posttest-only design is most successful when the groups are large so the probability of balancing interpersonal characteristics is increased (Portney & Watkins, 2009).

Multiple control group design is a variation of the single factor, multiple group design. This design uses multiple control groups because a single control group is inadequate for assessing the impact of each potentially confounding factor

Assign subjects at random to groups	**Group A:** (Experimental group)	Pretest	Experimental Treatment	Posttest
	Group B: (Control group)	Pretest	Control condition	Posttest

Figure 7–1. Classic design for cause-and-effect relationship. Adapted from *Understanding Research Methods* (5th ed.), by M. L. Patten, 2005, Glendale, CA: Pyrczak Publishing.

of the dependent variables. Multiple control groups can be included in both parametric and nonparametric designs (Bordens & Abbott, 1988; Portney & Watkins, 2009).

Factorial designs manipulate two or more independent variables; one group in the design accounts for each possible combination of the levels of the independent variables. A factorial design is usually described according to its dimensions so that a two-way or two-factor design has two independent variables and a three-way or three-factor design has three independent variables. These designs can be described as a 2 × 2 design, which would pair two independent variables with two different levels. For example, if a researcher utilized two independent variables (types of speech sample) for connected speech and single word articulation production and manipulated the environment (child's home and another sample in the clinic) this would be designated as a 2 × 2 factorial design Again, all subjects would be assigned to one of four groups receiving a combination of connected or single word articulation speech sample in a home or clinic setting. A factorial design has two or more independent variables which are manipulated simultaneously; it permits analysis of the *main effects* of the independent variables separately and the *interaction effects* of these variables. Each main effect is a single-factor experiment and the interaction addresses the question of the effect of one variable at different levels of the second variable (Portney & Watkins, 2009).

Multivariate designs involve two or more dependent variables, and provide information about the effect of the independent variable on each dependent variable and on a composite dependent variable formed from a weighted combination of the individual independent variables. In a multivariate design, Gutierrez-Clellen and Heinrichs-Ramos (1993) examined the referential cohesion of the narratives of Spanish-speaking children.

The validity of between-subjects experimental designs can be confounded or damaged by a variety of sources such as nonrandomization. randomization, experimenter bias, and poor planning and execution of experimental conditions. Confounding can be avoided by randomization, use of blinding, and careful planning and execution of a research protocol. *Double-blinding* is where neither the subjects nor the investigators are aware of the identity of the treatment groups until after data are collected (Portney & Watkins, 2000). *Single-blinding* of a study involves only the investigator(s) not knowing which treatment is used. It is often difficult to offer a placebo for studies involving rehabilitation procedures; therefore, single-blinding is more often used to try new or experimental procedures.

Within-Subjects Designs

In within-subjects designs, every subject in the experiment is exposed to all the experimental or treatment conditions. Fewer subjects are required for this design than for an equivalent between-subjects design. Sometimes referred to as a repeated measures design, within-subjects designs are a group of designs that incorporate the same basic structure, that is, using the same subjects in all conditions (Borden & Abbott, 1988; Patten, 2005; Portney & Watkins, 2009). Within-subjects designs are classified or described similarly to between-subject designs and include two treatments, single factor, multilevel, factorial, multiple control group, and multivariate designs.

The advantages of within-subjects designs include fewer subjects required, matching of subject factors, and power in detecting effects of dependent variables. Disadvantages include less power than equivalent between-subject designs if the dependent variable is only weakly related to subject differences, and possible carryover effects when exposure to one treatment influences behavior in a subsequent treatment. Carryover can be reduced by randomizing the order of presentation of levels of the independent variable. More frequently, counterbalancing is used in which individual subjects are exposed to the treatments in different orders. Utilizing treatment order as an independent variable makes it possible to determine whether carryover effects are present and, if so, their magnitude and direction. Despite the advantages of making treatment order an independent variable, there are disadvantages. The primary disadvantage is that every treatment order requires a separate group of subjects who must be tested under every treatment condition. This is expensive in terms of number of subjects and the time required testing them. Chapman, Sindberg, Bridge, Gigstead, and Hesketh (2006) utilized a repeated measure design when studying the effect of memory support and elicited production of new words by adolescents with Down syndrome.

Mixed-Group Designs

Mixed designs combine within-subjects and between-subjects designs and are used to investigate the effects of treatment for which carryover effects would be a problem while repeatedly sampling behavior across time or trials. Warren (1986) and Portney and Watkins (2009) consider mixed designs both descriptive and experimental. Three advantages of mixed designs are ease of implementation, generalizability of findings, and availability of statistical techniques. Frequent misinterpretation and overinterpretation of the results are the primary disadvantages. Altenberg and Ferrand's (2006) study about the attitudes of monolingual English, bilingual Cantonese-English, and bilingual Russian-English speakers toward individuals with voice disorders utilized a mixed experimental design.

The *nested design* is a variation of the mixed group design that combines within-subjects and between-subjects designs. It involves more than one task for each level of the independent variable. For example, assume that you were conducting an experiment on the ability to write diagnostic reports. The between-subjects factor might be difficulty (low, moderate, and high). Under each level of difficulty, two sets of diagnostic data would be included, with all subjects in each level of difficulty completing both sets of reports. By demonstrating the effect of item difficulty with different tasks, effects are not limited to a specific type of problem. This design is useful when subjects must be tested in groups rather than individually. It also has the advantage of increasing the generality of results (Bordens & Abbot, 1988; Portney & Watkins, 2009).

Clement and Wijner (1994), in a study of vowel contrasts, analyzed their data utilizing a "three way ANOVA, with factors subject group, vowel, and subject (nested under subject group)" (p. 86).

It is important to note that subjects are always nested under subject group. An example of a nested design, with speech-language pathologists nested within states, follows:

A group of six speech-language pathologists, two each from Louisiana, Oklahoma, and Texas, were discussing the treatment of patients with spasmodic dysphonia. The speech-language pathologists from Louisiana decided that Botox injections were the best means of treatment; therefore, their patients were injected with Botox, received no voice management, and were re-evaluated 3 months later to determine the amount of improvement. The speech-language pathologists from Oklahoma decided that voice management coupled with Botox injections were the best means of treatment; therefore, their subjects were injected, received voice management for 3 months, and then were reevaluated to determine the amount of improvement. The speech-language pathologists in Texas decided that voice management was the best means of treatment; therefore, their patients received voice management for 3 months and then were re-evaluated to determine amount of improvement. All data were then analyzed statistically.

Further information about nested designs may be found in Portney and Watkins (2009).

Advantages and Disadvantages of Group Designs

Advantages and disadvantages of group designs are summarized in Table 7–2 and discussed briefly here. Group designs have several advantages. Statistical procedures for determining reliability are available for group designs. Another advantage is that it is possible to con-

Table 7–2. Advantages and Disadvantages of Group Designs

Advantages	Disadvantages
Reliability of data	Assumption of homogeneity of group members
Availability of statistical procedures	
Generalization from sample to population	Subject attrition
	Availability of subjects
Established population characteristics	Typical subject may not be typical
Control order or sequence of effects	Generalizability of results
	Quantitative information
	Ethical considerations

Sources: From *Research Strategies in Human Communication Disorders*, by D. G. Doehring, 1988, Boston, MA: College-Hill Press; *Research Design and Evaluation in Speech-Language Pathology and Audiology* (4th ed.), by F. H. Silverman, 1998, Needham Heights, MA: Allyn & Bacon; *Language Intervention Strategies in Adult Aphasia* (pp. 66–80), by R. L. Warren, In R. Chapey (Ed.), 1986, Baltimore, MD: Williams & Wilkins; *Understanding Research Methods: An Overview of the Essentials* (5th ed.), by M. L. Patton, 2005, Glendale, CA: Pyrczak; and *Foundations of Clinical Research: Applications to Clinical Practice* (2nd ed.), by L. G. Portney, 2000, Upper Saddle River, NJ: Prentice-Hall Health.

trol order or sequence effects because a relatively large number of subjects permits randomization (Portney & Watkins, 2009; Silverman, 1998). Group designs also allow generalization of results from samples of subjects to the population as a whole (Doehring, 1988; Portney & Watkins, 2009). Another advantage is the ability to demonstrate causal relationships (Patten, 2005; Portney & Watkins, 2000).

Despite the advantages of group designs, there are several disadvantages. First, is the assumption of homogeneity of group members, that is, that all members of a group respond similarly to an experimental condition. Related to this is subject attrition which can affect results because loss of group members may disrupt group equivalency (Portney & Watkins, 2009; Warren, 1986). A second disadvantage is related to availability of subjects; in group designs more subjects may be required than are available (Silverman, 1998). Third, the typical subject may not be typical; in other words, the mean or average of the group may not accurately reflect differences in individual performance (Patten, 2005; Portney & Watkins, 2009; Silverman, 1998). Fourth, it may be difficult to generalize results because of the possibility of uncertain validity (Portney & Watkins, 2009; Silverman, 1998). Another disadvantage is related to limitations of quantitative information (Doehring, 1988). Last, there are ethical considerations about group designs because of concern about withholding treatment for research projects (Portney & Watkins, 2009; Warren, 1986).

Single-Subject Designs

Single-subject designs focus on the behavior of one or a few subjects. These designs are also referred to as applied behavioral analysis designs or behavioral analysis, idiographic designs, single-subject experimental designs, single-case designs, intrasubject replication designs, small N-approach, and within-subjects designs. The use of the term is confusing because it is also used to refer to a variety of group designs (Hegde, 1999). Cardon and Azuma (2011) describe the use of single-subject research designs for individuals with autistic spectrum disorders (ASD). These authors stated that individuals with ASD are a rather heterogeneous group to study; therefore, single-subject research designs may be very helpful when describing the impact of various types of clinical treatment.

It is misleading to consider any design that uses one or a few subjects as a single-subject design. Designs that use single subjects also can be classified as case studies or single-subject designs (Warren, 1986). Single-subject designs are experimental designs that attempt to establish cause-and-effect relations. According to Portney & Watkins (2000), "Single-subject designs are structured around two core elements that distinguish them from a case study or group studies; repeated measurement and design phases" (p. 224). Single-subject designs can be used to study comparison between several types of treatment or between treatment and no treatment (Portney & Watkins, 2000).

Bordens and Abbott (1988) described four characteristics of single-subject designs:

1. Individual subjects are observed intensely under each of several treatment conditions; these observations provide a baseline against which any future change induced by the independent variable can be evaluated.

2. All incidental variables that may affect the dependent variable are controlled as rigidly as possible.
3. Each subject is observed under all treatment conditions, and each treatment is repeated at least twice during the course of the experiment. This repetition of intrasubject replication shows the reliability of the findings. Subjects usually remain in each treatment of the experiment until the behavioral measure meets a stability criterion.
4. If more than one subject is used, the additional subjects are included to evaluate the generality of findings across subjects. This intersubject replication establishes whether the results obtained with one subject are similar or dissimilar to those obtained with other subjects. (p. 263)

There are many types of single-subject designs but two basic categories of single-subject designs known as baseline designs and discrete trials designs have been identified (Bordens & Abbott, 1988; Portney & Watkins, 2009). *Baseline designs* include designs that manipulate a single independent variable (single factor designs), those that manipulate two or more independent variables (multifactor designs), and those that measure several dependent variables (multiple baseline designs). In baseline designs the variable(s), also known as the target behavior, is measured prior to the experimental treatment of intervention. *Single factor designs* include a baseline condition (A) during which a baseline of subject performance is established and a treatment or intervention condition (B) in which the effect of the treatment or intervention is observed. There are several types of these designs include AB,

ABA, ABAB, ABAC, and BAB (Portney & Watkins, 2009; Silverman, 1998). These symbols are designed as follows:

A = baseline

B = first treatment or intervention

C = second treatment or intervention different from first.

Multifactor baseline designs include more than one independent variable and require that different combinations of the independent variable be tested across the study. The effects of the independent variables and their interactions can be assessed. A factorial design may be used or specific combinations may be evaluated (Portney & Watkins, 2000). These designs can be very time consuming because each treatment is evaluated at least twice for intrasubject replication.

Multiple baselines designs involve observation of different behaviors and establishing baselines for each. Thus, several behaviors are observed within the experimental context to provide multiple baselines. Treatment is considered effective if the level of each behavior changes after the treatment is applied to it.

In *single-subject discrete trial designs*, individual subjects receive each treatment condition of the experiment dozens of times. Each treatment or trial produces one data point for each dependent variable measured. Extraneous variables that could introduce unwanted variability in the dependent measure are rigidly controlled. If possible, the order of treatments is randomized or counterbalanced to control order effects. Intersubject replication is established by comparing the behavior of individual subjects undergoing the same treatment.

The advantages and disadvantages of single-subject designs are summarized in Table 7–3. Single-subject designs often are frequently used to determine treatment efficacy (Hegde, 1999; Portney & Watkins, 2009). These designs are economical in terms of time because single-subject research frequently can be conducted during regular clinical hours and during regularly scheduled treatment sessions (Gillam & Gillam, 2006). Furthermore, single-subject designs are similar in form to the design of therapy and are the best, if not the only, appropriate strategy to advance clinical knowledge and make use of evidence-based practice. Table 7–4 provides examples of studies using single-subject designs in ASHA journals between 2002 and 2006.

Sequential Clinical Trials

Group studies often require a fixed sample size prior to starting an experiment (Portney & Watkins, 2009). An alternative to group studies and single-subject designs includes sequential clinical trials (SCTs). Instead of waiting until the end of an experiment for data analysis, the SCT allows for analysis when each subject is tested and can be stopped at any point as the evidence is there to determine a significant difference between treatments (Portney & Watkins, 2009). An SCT can be used to compare two treatments such as an "old" or standard treatment to a "new" experimental treatment.

Once the parameters of the study have been adequately defined, then the first eligible subject can be enrolled. The patient is assigned to either the standard or experimental treatment by some randomization process. When the next eligible patient is enrolled, that patient is enrolled in a condition that is the opposite of the first patient.

Portney and Watkins (2000) stated that it is often "convenient to evaluate the relative effectiveness of two treatments by collecting a series of qualitative

Table 7–3. Advantages and Disadvantages of Single-Subject Designs

Advantages	Disadvantages
Control of error variance	Limited generalization
Establish causal relationships	Control of extraneous variables
Identify individual differences	Control of order and sequence effects
Flexibility	Limited availability of statistical procedures
Small number of subjects (as few as 1)	
Focus on actual behavioral outcomes	
Practical clinical application	
Can be done during scheduled treatments	
Economical	

Sources: From *Research Design and Methods*, by K. S. Bordens and B. B. Abbott, 1988, Mountain View, CA: Mayfield; *Research Design and Evaluation in Speech-Language Pathology* (4th ed.), by F. H. Silverman, 1988, Needham Heights, MA: Allyn & Bacon; and *Foundations of Clinical Research: Applications to Practice* (2nd ed.), by L. G. Portney and M. P. Watkins, 2000, Upper Saddle River, NJ: Prentice-Hall Health.

Table 7–4. Examples of Studies Using Single-Subject Designs in ASHA Journals between 2002–2006

Author(s)	Topic
Davidow, Bothe, & Bramlett (2006)	Stuttering treatment research and evaluation and assessment tool (STREAT)
Gillam & Gillam (2006)	Evidence-based decisions about child language intervention in schools
Inglehart (2004)	Speech perception by students with cochlear implants using sound-field systems in classrooms
Kay-Raining Bird, Chapman, & Schwartz (2004)	Fast mapping of words and story recall by individuals with Down syndrome
Kiran & Thompson (2003a & 2003b)	Semantic complexity in treatment of naming deficits in fluent aphasia
Lund & Light (2003)	Effectiveness of grammar instruction with AAC users
Marshall & Freed (2006)	Personalized cuing method
Weiss (2004)	Child language and stuttering
Woods & Wetherby (2003)	Early identification and intervention for infants and toddlers at risk for autism

preferences in favor of one or the other" (p. 205). The preference by the subject is defined on the "basis of clinically meaningful differences between two treatments" (p. 205).

There are four possible outcomes for classifying preference. First, both subjects could indicate "improvement." Second, both subjects could indicate "no improvement" with their treatment. Third, one subject could indicate "improvement" and the other subject could show "no improvement." Fourth, the situation could be reversed in which the first subject showed "no improvement" and the other subject showed "improvement." For further discussion about data collection and analysis, one should consult

Portney & Watkins (2009). Table 7–5 describes advantages and limitations for SCTs.

Technologic Applications and Research Designs

Whether using group or single-subject research designs, a researcher should make use of the technology available when conducting data analysis. Group designs usually involve more inferential statistics because a researcher is interested in making inferences from a sample to a population (Pyrczak, 2004). Descriptive statistics can be used with

Table 7–5. Advantages and Limitations for Sequential Clinical Trials (SCTs)

Advantages	Limitations
Fixed sample size not needed to start	Only compare 2 treatments
Can analyze data as subjects complete trials	Do not explore multiple or interaction effects
Subjects can be enrolled once eligible	Control extraneous variables only with randomization of pairs
Statistical technique can be done without computer	If a pair doesn't state preference those data are discarded
Holds much potential in rehabilitation research	Effects of treatment should be soon so time is limited

Source: From *Foundations of Clinical Research: Applications to Practice* (2nd ed.), by L. G. Portney and M. P. Watkins, 2000, Upper Saddle River, NJ: Prentice-Hall Health.

a variety of research designs (group, single-subject, SCTs) and would include information about, but not limited to, the mean, standard deviation, mode, median, and correlations.

One of the most often used statistical programs in behavioral and social sciences is the Statistical Package for Social Sciences® (SPSS) published by Prentice-Hall, a division of Pearson Education, Inc. available at http://www.prenhall.com. Student versions of SPSS are available that typically provide sufficient capacity for studies involving up to 50 variables and 1,500 data entries. Holcomb (2006) describes that SPSS can be used with a variety of levels of measurement in research including nominal, ordinal, interval, and ratio.

When utilizing SPSS it is important that a researcher understand there are many methods that can be used for the collection of data (e.g., pencil-paper, direct observation, etc.), but SPSS assists dur-ing the analysis of the data. Initially, all data must be entered into the SPSS program in which the researcher de-fines the variables to be entered and analyzed. After defining variables, the next step involves data input that follows the system developed within SPSS (Holcomb, 2006).

SPSS supports the researcher by saving data to a file that can be analyzed and graphically displayed in a variety of ways. This includes, but is not limited to, descriptive statistics, *t*-tests, ANOVA, linear regression, correlations, and multiple linear regressions (SPSS, 2006). There are useful tools to support a researcher when making decisions about statistical analysis in SPSS, including a tutorial program, statistics coach, and results coach.

A researcher must be mindful that SPSS, or any other statistical analysis program will only provide support in terms of the calculations and graphically displaying the information (which can be exported to text documents). It is still the responsibility of any researcher or team of researchers to determine which type of design to use, what statistical methods will help answer questions, and accurate interpretation.

Summary

Group research designs require the formation of two or more groups. Single-subject designs are based on individual subject's performance under different conditions. Although group designs are often used, they do not meet the practical needs of speech-language pathologists and audiologists to evaluate treatment. These designs were described as if they were mutually exclusive, but this is not so. Some studies use designs that generate both types of data. Different study designs have different strengths and weaknesses. It is important to remember that research designs that are appropriate today may not be in the future. Technology supports the analysis of data used with a variety of research designs, but still requires the researcher to make decisions regarding the appropriate application of the technology, data analysis, and interpretation.

DISCUSSION QUESTIONS

1. Distinguish between strategic planning and research design.
2. Distinguish between group and single-subject designs. What are the advantages and disadvantages of each?
3. When would a between-subjects design be appropriate? When would a within-subjects design be used?
4. Why might there be ethical concerns with certain types of research designs?
5. Why should single-subject designs be used by clinicians?
6. Are single-subject designs used by clinicians on a daily basis in some form? Explain your answer.
7. When would sequential clinical trials be used? Why are SCTs not frequently seen in rehabilitation literature?
8. What is SPSS? How would SPSS help a researcher? When doesn't SPSS help a researcher?
9. Explain to your faculty advisor that the graduate program needs to invest in SPSS.
10. Choose one of the single-subject designs listed in Table 7–4. Describe the statistical analysis that was used. What did you find interesting about it?

References

Altenberg, E. P., & Ferrand, C. T. (2006). Perception of individuals with voice disorders by monolingual English, bilingual Cantonese-English, and bilingual Russian-English women. *Journal of Speech, Language, and Hearing Research, 49,* 879–887.

Bordens, K. S., & Abbott, B. B. (1988). *Research designs and methods.* Mountain View, CA: Mayfield.

Cardon, T. A., & Azuma, T. (2011). Deciphering single-subject research design and autism spectrum disorders. *ASHA Leader.*

Chapman, R, S., Sindberg, H., Bridge, C., Gigstead, K., & Hesketh, L. (2006). Effect of memory support and elicited production on fast mapping of new words by adolescents with Down syndrome. *Journal of Speech, Language, and Hearing Research, 49,* 3–15.

Clement, C. J., & Wijner, F. (1994). Acquisition of vowel contrasts in Dutch. *Journal of Speech and Hearing Research, 37,* 83–89.

Davidow, J. H., Bothe, A. K., & Bramlett, R. E. (2006). The Stuttering Treatment Research Evaluation and Assessment Tool (STREAT): Evaluating research as part of evidence-based practice. *American Journal of Speech-Language Pathology, 15,* 126–141.

Doehring, D. G. (1988). *Research strategies in human communication disorders.* Boston, MA: College-Hill Press.

Gilliam, S. L., & Gilliam, R. B. (2006). Making evidence-based decisions about child language intervention in schools. *Language, Speech, and Hearing Services in Schools, 37,* 304–315.

Guitierrez-Clellen,V. P., & Heinrichs-Ramos, L. H. (1993). Cohesion in the narrative of Spanish-speaking children: A developmental study. *Journal of Speech and Hearing Research, 36*(3), 559–567.

Hegde, M. N. (1999). *Clinical research in communication disorders* (4th ed.). Austin, TX: Pro-Ed.

Holcomb, Z. C. (2006). *SPSS® basics: Techniques for a first course in statistics.* Glendale, CA: Pyrczak.

Inglehart, F. (2004). Speech perception by students with cochlear implants using soundfield systems in classrooms. *American Journal of Audiology, 13,* 62–72.

Kay-Raining Bird, E., Chapman, R. S., & Schwartz, S. E. (2004). Fast mapping of words and story recall by individuals with Down syndrome. *Journal of Speech, Language, and Hearing Research, 47,* 1286–1300.

Kiran, S., & Thompson, C. K. (2003a). The role of semantic complexity in treatment of naming deficits: Training semantic categories in fluent aphasia by controlling exemplar typicality. *Journal of Speech, Language, and Hearing Research, 46,* 608–622.

Kiran, S., & Thompson, C. K. (2003b). The role of semantic complexity in treatment of naming deficits: Training semantic categories in fluent aphasia by controlling exemplar typicality. *Journal of Speech, Language, and Hearing Research, 46,* 773–787.

Lund, S. K., & Light, J. (2003). The effectiveness of grammar instruction for individuals who use augmentative and alternative communication systems: A preliminary study. *Journal of Speech, Language, and Hearing Research, 46,* 1110–1123.

Marshall, R. C., & Freed, D. B. (2006). The personalized cueing method: From the laboratory to the clinic. *American Journal of Speech-Language Pathology, 15,* 103–111.

Maxwell, D. L., & Satake, E. (2006). *Research and statistical methods in communication sciences and disorders.* Clifton Park, NY: Thomson-Delmar Learning.

Ottenbacher, K. J. (1990). Clinically relevant research designs for rehabilitation research: The idiographic model. *American Journal of Physical Medicine and Rehabilitation, 69,* 286–292.

Patten, M. L. (2005). *Understand research methods: An overview of the essentials* (5th ed.). Glendale, CA: Pyrczak.

Polit, D. F., & Hungler, B. P. (1999). *Nursing research: Principles and methods* (6th ed.). New York, NY: Lippincott.

Portney, L. G., & Watkins, M. P. (2000). *Foundations of clinical research: Applications to clinical practice* (2nd ed.). Upper Saddle River, NJ: Prentice-Hall Health.

Portney, J. G. & Watkins, M. P. (2009). *Foundations of clinical research: Applications to clinical practices* (3rd ed.). Upper Saddle River, NJ: Pearson.

Pyrczak, F. (2004). *Success at statistics: A work text with humor.* Glendale, CA: Pyrczak.

Siegel, G. M., & Young, M. A. Group designs in clinical research. (1987). *Journal of Speech and Hearing Disorders, 52*(3), 194–199.

Silverman, F. H., (1993). *Research design and evaluation in speech-language pathology and audiology* (3rd ed.). Englewood Cliffs, NJ; Prentice-Hall.

Silverman, F. H. (1998). *Research design and evaluation in speech-language and audiology* (4th ed.) Needham Heights, MA: Allyn & Bacon.

Statistical Package for Social Sciences® (Version 14.0). (2006). Retrieved from http://www.prenhall.com

Warren, R. L. (1986). Research design: Considerations for the clinician. In R. Chapey (Ed.), *Language intervention strategies in adult aphasia* (pp. 66–79). Baltimore, MD: Williams & Wilkins.

Weiss, A. L. (2004). Epilogue: What child language research may contribute to the understanding and treatment of stuttering. *Language, Speech, and Hearing Services in Schools, 35,* 90–92.

Woods, J. J., & Wetherby, A. M. (2003). Early identification of and intervention for infants and toddlers who are at risk for autism spectrum disorder. *Language, Speech, and Hearing Services in Schools, 34,* 180–193.

8

Quantitative Research

LEARNING OBJECTIVES

Upon completion of this chapter the reader will be able to:

- Describe characteristics of quantitative research
- Identify various types of quantitative research
- Select an appropriate statistic
- Explain different methods of descriptive statistics
- Describe methods used for inferential statistics
- Apply special methods such as meta-analysis
- Evaluate quantitative research.

Research can be classified as either qualitative or quantitative. The latter involves investigation of phenomena that lend themselves to precise measurement and quantification, often under controlled conditions that can be subject to statistical analysis (Maxwell & Satake, 2006; Polit & Beck, 2010). This chapter describes various aspects of quantitative research including descriptive and inferential statistics.

Characteristics of Quantitative Research

Quantitative research is a type of research in which objective data are gathered and analyzed numerically (McMillan & Schumacher, 2010). The emphasis is on numbers, measurement, deductive logic, control, and experimentation. Characteristics of quantitative research are shown in Table 8–1 and Figure 8–1.

Advantages and Disdvantages of Quantitative Research

Historically, quantitative research has been the gold standard for research, that is, superior to other types of research. A major strength of quantitative research is its credibility, which is the extent to which

Table 8–1. Qualitative Versus Quantitative Research: Distinguishing Features

Characteristics	Quantitative	Qualitative
Purpose	Explain and predict	Describe and explain
	Conform and validate	Explore and interpret
	Test theory	Build theory
Process	Focused	Holistic
	Known variables	Unknown variables
	Established guidelines	Flexible guidelines
	Predetermined methods	Emerging methods
	Somewhat context free	Context bound
	Detached view	Personal view
Researcher's role	Detached	Observer or participant
Data collection	Statistical analysis	Search for themes and categories
	Stress objectivity	Acknowledgment of subjectivity and bias potential
	Deductive reasoning	Inductive reasoning
Communication of findings	Numbers	Words
	Statistics, aggregated data	Narrative, individual quotes
	Formal voice, scientific style	Personal voice, literary style

Sources: Practical Research Planning and Design, by P. D. Leedy & J. E. Ormrod, 2010, Boston, MA: Pearson; and *Research in Education*, by J. H. McMillan & S. Schumacher, 2010, Boston, MA: Pearson.

Associated terms or phrases	Positivist*
	Experimental
	Hard data
	Statistical
Key concepts	Variable
	Operationalized
	Controlled
	Reliable
	Statistically significant
	Replicated
	Hypothesized
Goals	Test theory
	Establish facts
	Show relationships
	Predict
	Statistically describe
Design	Structure
	Predetermined
	Formal
	Specific
Sample	Large
	Representative
	Random selection
	Control group
	Stratified
Data	Quantities
	Count
	Measures/instruments
	Numbers
	Statistics
Techniques or methods	Experiments
	Quasiexperiments
	Structured observations
	Structured interviews
	Surveys
Data analysis	Deduction
	Statistical

Figure 8–1. Characteristics of quantitative research. (*Positivist or post-positivism is based on the assumption that phenomena should be studied objectively; the goal is obtaining a single true reality, or at least reality within known probabilities.) Adapted from *Educational Research,* by J. H. McMillan, 2004, Boston, MA: Pearson.

the data and conclusions are believable and trustworthy. Other advantages are objectivity, standardization, replication, and limited bias. There is no uniform agreement about disadvantages. The disadvantages that have been identified are superficial/oversimplification, unrelated to the real world, too intense, focus on hard data, and unnatural environment (French, Reynolds, & Swain, 2000).

Quantitative Research Designs

There are major differences in credibility nonexperimental and experimental designs. Quantitative designs may be viewed on a continuum. True experimental designs are at one end of the continuum (highest), and nonexperimental studies are at the other end (lowest). *Five major categories of research* designs have been identified: nonexperimental; pre-experimental; quasiexperimental; and experimental (true experimental); and single subject.

Nonexperimental Designs

Nonexperimental or observational designs are the weakest of all designs because they do not involve randomization, manipulation, or use of control groups. Furthermore, casual relations cannot be established (Maxwell & Satake, 2006). This type of research includes descriptive research and correlational studies. The advantages of nonexperimental research are its: (1) appropriateness for studying problems not mendable to for experimental research, and (2) efficien-cies and effectiveness for studying a large amount of information about a problem. The disadvantages are the failure to describe casual relationships and faulty interpretation on selection of groups and self-selection.

Nonexperimental research includes descriptive and correlational studies (Polit & Beck, 2010). Descriptive studies provide descriptive information about population parameters and relationships among subjects. Correlational studies describe relationships among variables (DePoy & Gitlin, 2011).

Non experimental research is undertaken when: (1) a number of independent variables such as gender and height are not amenable to randomization; (2) some variables cannot be ethically manipulated; (3) there are practical constraints to manipulating variables; and (4) avoiding manipulation achieves a more realistic understanding (Polit & Beck, 2010). There are a variety of nonexperimental research designs, which are summarized in Table 8–2.

Pre-experimental Designs

Pre-experimental designs are sometimes referred to as pseudo experimental designs because they do not meet at least two of the three criteria for true experiments; randomization; manipulation; or control. Furthermore, pre-experimental studies are limited to describing outcomes because appropriate statistical analysis cannot be performed. Thus, the goal of such studies is to explore or describe phenomena rather than explain their causes. Currently, the use of pre-experimental designs is limited due to inadequate control of numerous extraneous variables.

Table 8–2. Nonexperimental Quantitative Research Designs

Name of Design	Description
Case Study	In-depth analysis of single individual, a few individuals, or an institution.
Case control	Retrospective comparison of case and a matched control.
Case series	Three or more cases in a case study.
Cohort	Focuses on specific subpopulation from which different samples are selected at different points in time.
Correlational	Study of interrelationships among variables on interest without any active intervention of inferring causality.
Descriptive	Summarizes status on phenomena, that is, characteristic and/or frequency with which certain phenomena occur.
Ex post facto	Presumed cause that occurred in the past. Also called causal comparison.
Retrospective	Begins with outcome and looks back in time for antecedent caused.
Prospective	Begins with examination of presumed causes and then goes forward in time for its effect.
Natural experiments	Comparison of groups in which one group is affected by a seemingly random event.
Path analysis	Uses correlation of several variables to study causal patterns
Causal comparison	Dependent variable already occurred so its relationship to other variables can only be studied. Also called ex post facto.
Structural equation modeling	Relatively new method, more powerful than path analysis for studying correlations to identify causal patterns.
Surveys	Focuses on obtaining information about activities, beliefs, preferences, attitudes, by direct questioning.
Cross-sectional survey	Survey given at one time.
Longitudinal survey	Same or similar subjects surveyed over time.

Sources: Research and Statistical Methods, by D. L. Maxwell and E. Satake, 2006, Clifton Park, NY: Thomson-Delmar Learning; *Educational Research*, by J. H. McMillan, 2005, Boston, MA: Pearson; and *Nursing Research: Principles and Methods*, by D. F. Polit and C. T. Beck, 2010, Philadelphia, PA: Lippincott Williams & Wilkins.

Maxwell and Satake (2006) noted that pre-experimental designs " . . . give the impression of constituting credible scientific studies but are characterized by numerous sources on invalidity" (p. 204). These designs were described as "fools gold" because of the " . . . misleading impressions of belonging to more rigorous and powerful kinds of experimental methodologies" (p. 203). Schiavetti and Metz (2002); Orlikof (2011) pointed out that these designs are weak in both internal and external validity.

There are *four types of pre-experimental designs:* single group pretest only; single group pretest-posttest; time series design; and nonequivalent groups posttest only. These designs are summarized in Figure 8–2.

The weakest of the pre-experimental designs is the *one-group postdesign,* which is also known as the single group posttest only or one-shot case study. This design involves study of the presumed effect of an independent variable in one group of subjects by administering a posttest after some treatment.

The *single or one group pretestposttest design* also known as a before-after design compares pretest and posttest data subsequent to treatment. There is inadequate control for internal and external validity because there is no control group.

The *time series design* involves repeated measures before and after treatment using the same instruments with the same or similar subjects over an extended period of time. McMillan (2005) believes this is " . . . a good design for frequently occurring measures of the dependent variable at regular intervals" (p. 218). There is some confusion about the classification of time series designs. This design is classified by some as pre-experimental (McMillan, 2005; Mertens

Nonequivalent Groups Posttest Only
$$X\ O_1$$
$$X\ O_2$$

⇓

Static Group Comparison
$$X\ O$$
$$X$$

⇓

Single Group Pretest-Posttest
$$O,\ X,\ O_2$$

⇓

Single Group Posttest Only
$$XO$$

Figure 8–2. Nonexperimental research designs from highest to lowest (O = observation; X = treatment). Adapted from *Educational Research*, by J. H. McMillan, 2004, Boston, MA: Pearson; and *Research and Statistical Methods*, by D. L. Maxwell and E. Satake, 2006, Clifton Park, NY: Thomson-Delmar Learning.

2005) and by others as quasiexperimental (DePoy & Gitlin, 2011; Maxwell & Satake, 2006; Meline, 2006; Polit & Beck, 2010). The next section on quasiexermintal designs provides further information about time service designs.

Nonequivalent groups' posttest-only design has a comparison control group both of whom are tested after treatment and not before treatment. Another type of pre-experimental design is the static group comparison in which the performance of two groups is compared. One group receives treatment and the other does not (Maxwell & Satake, 2004).

Quasiexperimental Designs

These designs are commonly used in speech-language pathology and audiology research (Maxwell & Satake, 2004; Meline, 2006). Quasiexperimental are sometimes referred to as nonrandomized. These designs are sometimes called controlled times without randomization. These designs are almost true experiments but not quite because of the lack of randomization and a control group, that is, subjects are not randomly assigned to groups. Quasi- or semiexperimental designs combine some of the characteristics of both experimental and nonexperimental research (Kumar, 1996). These designs are used when true experiments are impractical or impossible.

Quasiexperiments are not as powerful as true experiments in establishing relationships between treatments and outcomes (Polit & Beck, 2010).

The *nonequivalent group pretests posttest design* involves the use of two nonrandomized comparison groups both of whom are tested before and after treatment. The most serious threat to validity of this design is that subjects are not randomly assigned to these groups (DePoy & Gitlin, 2001). This design is similar to the nonequivalent groups posttest-only design and static group comparison except for the addition of a pretest (Maxwell & Satake, 2006; McMillan, 2005).

Another type of quasiexperimental research are *single time series designs,* which are sometimes referred to as interrupted time series designs. These designs involve repeated data collection over time for a single group (DePoy & Gitlin, 2011).

The advantage of this design over the nonequivalent comparison group design, which has single pretest and posttest measures, is the use of several pretest and posttest measures (Maxwell & Satake, 2006). This, however, could threaten validity because administration of several pretest and posttest measures could result in a greater degree of test sensitization. Another disadvantage is the lack of a control group.

Single-Subject Designs

Single-subject designs can be used to study one subject or a small number of subjects for an extended period of time before and after treatment. This design involves a variation of several group designs (repeated measures; time series). Single-subject designs are classified as quasiexperimental (Maxwell & Satake, 2006) or experimental (McMillan, 2005). They have been described as a special application of experimental research. These designs are described in more detail in Chapter 7.

True Experimental Designs

True experimental designs or randomized controlled trials (RCT) are considered by many as the *gold standard,* that is, the strongest of the research designs (Maxwell & Satake, 2006; Polit & Beck, 2010). Randomization also called random assignment is the selection of a sample of subjects so that each member of a population has an equal probability of being selected (Polit & Beck, 2010). Random assignment is randomization of subjects to experimental and control groups so that the groups are comparable at the onset of the experiment. Control is the process of holding constant confounding influences of the dependent variable under study. This usually means a control group of subjects who do not receive treatment. These designs can provide information about cause-and-effect relationships among independent and dependent variables.

A *true experimental design* is characterized by manipulation (treatment or intervention), randomizations or random assignment (equal chance of being represented), and control. If a research design does not meet these three criteria, it is probably a quasiexperimental design. There are several types of experimental designs. Some of the more common designs are summarized in Table 8–3. Additional information about experimental designs is available in Blessing and Forister (2012) and Isaac and Michael (1987), Leedy and Ormrod (2005), Schiavetti et al. (2011), and Vogt (2006).

Quantitative Analysis

Quantitative, or statistical analysis, is the organization and integration of quantitative data according to systematic mathematical rules and procedures. Statistical analysis is guided by and dependent on all previous steps of the research process including the research problem, study, design, number of study variables, sampling procedures, and number of subjects. Each of these steps should lead to the selection of appropriate statistical analysis (DePoy & Gitlin, 2011). Statistical analysis and statistic warrant definition. Statistical analysis is concerned with summarizing m = numerical data, assessing its reliability and validity, determining the nature and magnitude and relationships among sets of data, and makinggeneralizations from current to future events (Nicolosi, Harryman, & Kresheck, 2004). *Statistic* according to Maxwell and Satake (2006) "is a number derived by counting or measuring sample observations drawn from a population that is used in estimating a population parameter" (p. 529). DePoy and Gitlin (2011) described statistic as a "number derived from a mathematical procedure as part of the analytic process experimental type research" (p. 324).

Descriptive Statistics

Descriptive statistics are used to describe and synthesize data. Table 8–4 summarizes the different types of descriptive statistics. The most basic statistic is frequency distribution., which is a systematic arrangement of values from lowest to highest with a count of times each value was obtained.

Graphs can be used to display frequency or relative frequency of percentages. The most frequently used graphs are *histographs* (bar graphs) and *frequency polygons* (line graphs). Other graphs for displaying distributions include pie graphs and trend charts.

Pie charts are used to represent the proportion of data falling into certain categories in the form of a circle containing segments which are also called slices, sections, or wedges. These graphs are rueful in illustrating percentages in relation to each other and to the whole (Nicol & Pexman, 2003). They are also referred to as pie charts, pie diagrams, cake charts, circle graphs percentage graphs, or 100% graphs. An example of a

Table 8–3. Experimental Designs

Name of Design	Description
Between-subjects	Comparison of groups treated differently on some independent variable.
Counterbalance	Variation of experimental design in which more than one treatment is tested and the order of participation in each treatment is manipulated.
Factorial (ANOVA)	Any design in which more than one treatment factor is investigated.
Latin square	Repeated measures design in which presentation of conditions is counterbalanced so that each occurs in each sequential position of a block.
Parallel	Experiments that generally have at least two randomly assigned independent groups of participants, each of whom receive only one of the treatments (independent variables) under investigation.
Posttest only (after only)	Data collected from subjects only after treatment. Most basic of the experimental designs
Pretest-posttest (before-after)	Data collected from subjects both before and after treatment. Most commonly used true experimental design.
Randomized block	Involves two or more factors (independent variables), only one of which is experimentally manipulated.
Repeated measures (crossover)	One group of subjects is exposed to more than one condition or treatment in random order..
Randomized clinical trial (RCT)	Experimental test of a new treatment, involving random assignment to treatment groups; typically a large and diverse sample. Also known as a phase III clinical trial.
Solomon four group	Uses a before-after design for one pair of experimental and control groups, and after only design for a second pair.
Split plot	Uses both within-subject and between-subject design elements of statistical analysis of treatment effects.
Within-subjects	Comparison within same subjects under circumstances in which they were exposed to two or more treatment conditions.

Sources: *Introduction to Research*, by E. DePoy and L. N. Gitlin, 2011, Philadelphia, PA: Elsevier Mosby; *Nursing Research: Principles and Methods*, by D. F. Polit and C. T. Beck, 2010, Philadelphia, PA: Lippincott Williams & Wilkins; and *Research and Statistical Methods in Communication Sciences and Disorders*, by D. L. Maxwell and E. Satake, 2006, Clifton Park, NY: Thomson-Delmar Learning.

Table 8–4. Descriptive Statistics

Type of Analysis	Method	Description
Shape of distribution	Skewed	Asymmetric distribution
	Positively skewed	Asymmetric distribution tail points to right (positive) side because frequency of low scores greatly outnumber high scores
	Negatively skewed	Asymmetric distribution; tail points left (negative) side because frequency of high scores greatly outnumbers low scores
	Modality	Describes number of peaks, values with high frequencies.
	Unimodal	Distribution of values with one park (high frequency)
	Bimodal	Distribution of values with two peaks
	Multimodal	Distribution of values with more than one peak.
	Leptokurtic	Too peaked
	Platykurtic	Too flat
Central tendency	Mode	Value that occurs most frequently
	Median	Point in distribution where 50% above and 50% below; mid-score
	Mean	Arithmetic average
Variability	Range	Difference between lowest and highest score
	Interquartile range	Range of middle 50% of scores
	Semiquartile	Same as interquartile range
	Sum of squares	Difference between each score and the mean
	Variance	Mean of squares deviation from the mean
	Standard deviation	Square root of the variance; indicates average deviation of scores around the mean

continues

Table 8–4. *continued*

Type of Analysis	Method	Description
Bivariable	Contingency table	Two-dimensional table that illustrates frequencies of responses for two or more nominal or quantitative variables
	Correlation	Describes relationship between two or more variables
	Pearson's product Moment correlation	Uses interval or ratio data; yields a score between −1 and +1
	Spearman's rho	Uses ordinal data; yields a score between −1 and +1; preferable to product moment for numbers under 20 nonparametric equivalent of Pearson *r*
	Kendall's tau	Used with ordinal data; yields a score between −1 and +1; preferable to *rho* for numbers under 10
	Point biserial	To examine relationship between a nominal variable and an internal level measure; yields lower correlation than *r* and much lower than *r* big
	Phi coefficient	Describes the relationship between two dichotomous variables
	Terrachoric correlation coefficient	Used when both variables are artificial dichotomies
	Cramer's *V*	Describes relationship between nominal level data; used when contingency table to which it is applied is larger than 242
	Contingency coefficient	Two dichotomous variables on a nominal scale; closely related to chi square
	Multiple correlation	One single variable and some combination of two or more other variables
	Partial correlation	Two variables studied; influence of their or several other variables held constant. Also called first order–correlation

Sources: Foundation of Clinical Research, by L. G. Portney and M. B. Watkins, 2009, Upper Saddle River, NJ: Prentice-Hall Health; *Handbook in Research and Evaluation*, by S. Isaac and W. B. Michael, 1987, San Diego, CA: Edits Publishers; *Nursing Research: Principles and Methods*, by D. F. Polit and C. T. Beck, 2010, Philadelphia, PA: Lippincott Williams & Wilkins; *Reading Statistics and Research*, by S. W. Huck, 2004, Boston, MA: Pearson; and *Research and Statistical Methods*, by D. L. Maxwell and E. Satake, 2006, Clifton Park, NY: Thomson-Delmar Learning.

pie chart is in Figure 8–3. The pie to the right is an *exploded pie chart* that emphasizes the proportion of time devoted to research (Bordens & Abbott, 1988). The major advantage of pie charts that people typically think of is a circle encompassing 100%.

Trend charts also can be used to illustrate frequencies or percentages of change in a data set which is organized in a developmental or temporal order. A trend chart is shown in Figure 8–4.

Shapes of Distributions

Data can describe relative to its shape. Several shapes have been described and are illustrated in Figure 8–5 and defined in Table 8–4. Some distributions occur so frequently that they have special names. The *normal curve or normal distribution* is a symmetrical bell-shaped curve that has a concentration of scores in the middle of the distribution with fewer scores to the right and left sides of the distribution (Figure 8–6). An important characteristic of the normal curve is that predictable percentages of the population are within any given portion of the curve (Leedy & Ormrod, 2010). About two-thirds (68.2%) of the population fall within plus or minus one standard deviation of the mean, 96% fall within plus or minus two standard deviations of the mean, and 99% of the population fall within plus or minus three deviations of the mean.

Central Tendency

Measures of central tendency provide statistics that indicate an average or typical value of a set of scores. There are three measures of central tendency; *mode; median;* and *mean* which are described in Table 8–4.

Variables

Measures of variability or dispersion are the degree of dispersion or the difference among scores. These measures include: the *range; interquartile range; sum of squares; variance;* and the *standard deviation.* See Table 8–4 for definitions of these measures.

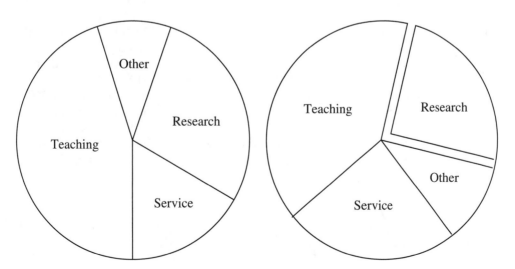

Figure 8–3. Pie chart and exploded pie chart.

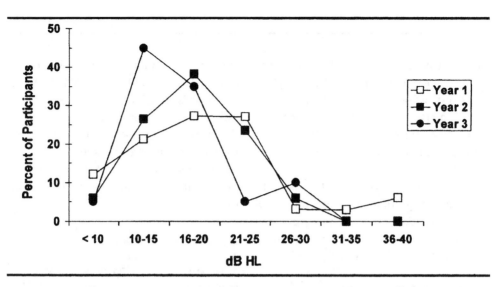

Figure 8–4. Trend chart showing distribution of average hearing levels for children with OME in years 1, 2, and 3. Data are presented according to hearing level (HL) categories in decibels (dB). Four-frequency (500, 1000, 2000, and 4000 Hz) average values displayed were derived by categorizing each participant's mean hearing levels across each study year. Reprinted by permission from "Effects of Otitis Media with Effusion on Hearing in the First 3 Years of Life," by J. S. Gravel and I. F. Wallace, 2000, *Journal of Speech, Language, and Hearing Research, 43*, p. 638. Copyright 2000 by American Speech-Language-Hearing Association. All rights reserved.

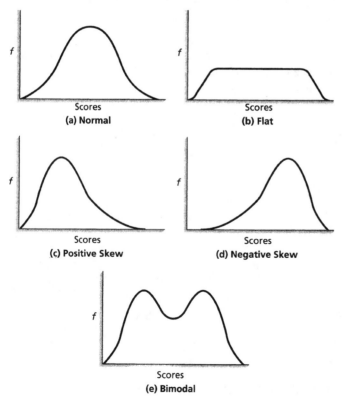

Figure 8–5. Frequency distributions. From *Educational Research: Fundamentals for the Consumer* (4th ed., p. 129), by J. H. McMillan, 2004, Boston, MA: Allyn & Bacon. Copyright 2004 by Pearson Education. Reprinted by permission of the publisher.

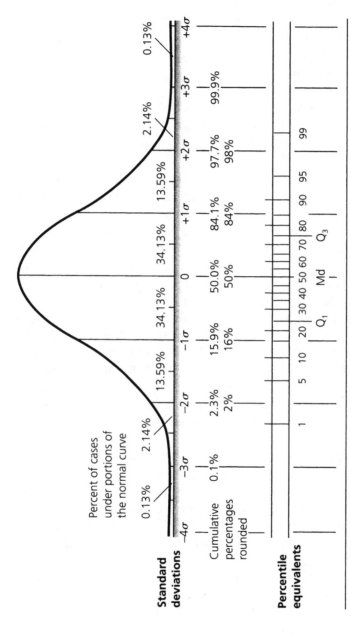

Figure 8–6. Normal distribution curve. From *Test Service Notebook #148.* Copyright 1980 by Harcourt Assessment, Inc. Reproduced with permission. All rights reserved.

Source: Seashore, H. G. (1980). Methods of expressing test scores. In *Test service notebook 148.* Courtesy of The Psychological Corporation.

Bivariate Descriptive Statistics

Bivariate descriptive statistics are a data reduction approach for describing relationships between two or more variables (DePoy & Gitlin, 2011). There are two methods: contingency tables and correlationalanalysis. A contingency table is a two-dimensional frequency distribution in which the frequencies of two nominal or ordinal level variables are cross-tabulated (Polit & Beck, 2010). Contingency tables are also used with nominal or ordinal data.

Correlation

Correlation is a statistical method for measuring the relationship between two or more quantitative variables for ordinal, interval, or nominal levels of measurement. This means that the value of one variable can be predicted by knowing the value of the other (McMillan, 2005). *Scatter plots* or diagrams can be used to graphically illustrate the relationship between tow variables. Scatter plots indicating correlation of variables are shown in Figure 8–7.

A *correlation coefficient* is a measure of the direction and strength of the relationship between variables usually ranging from 1.00 (perfect positive) through zero (no relationship) to −1.00 (perfect negative) relationships (Polit & Beck, 2010). The higher the value of the coefficient the stronger the relationship. Correlation coefficients between 0.10 and 0.30 are small or low relationships, 0.40 to 0.60 are moderate relationships and 0.70 and above are high relationships.

There are several types of correlation coefficients, as summarized in Table 8–4. The most frequently used correlation coefficient is the Pearson product moment correlation coefficient or Pearson's *r*.

There are several issues related to correlation: cause and effect, coefficient of determination, outliers, linearity, independence, and relationship strength. Correlation coefficients cannot be used to establish cause and effect. In other words, correlations should not be interpreted to imply a cause-and-effect relationship. A coefficient of determination is determined by squaring the raw correlation coefficient. This suggests that the raw correlation coefficient (the value of *r* not squared) exaggerated the relationship between variables.

Outliers are scores that are outside the range of most scores. Outliers can cause the size of a correlation coefficient to under or overestimate the strength of relationship between two variables.

A correlation coefficient is appropriate if the two variables have a linear relationship but not if there is a curvilinear relationship. A linear relationship requires that the path of data points be straight. If there is a curvilinear relationship the correlation coefficient will underestimate the strength of the relationship between the variables.

Correlation coefficients indicate the extent to which two measuring instruments are independent. Independence exists to the extent that *r* is close to zero, that is, high correlations suggest lack of independence whereas low correlations imply independence (Huck, 2004). There are no widely accepted criteria for describing the strength of relationship between two variables (correlation) (Portney & Watkins, 2009)

The relationship strength may be misinterpreted because of subjective interpretation for defining relationships as weak, moderate, or strong. Furthermore,

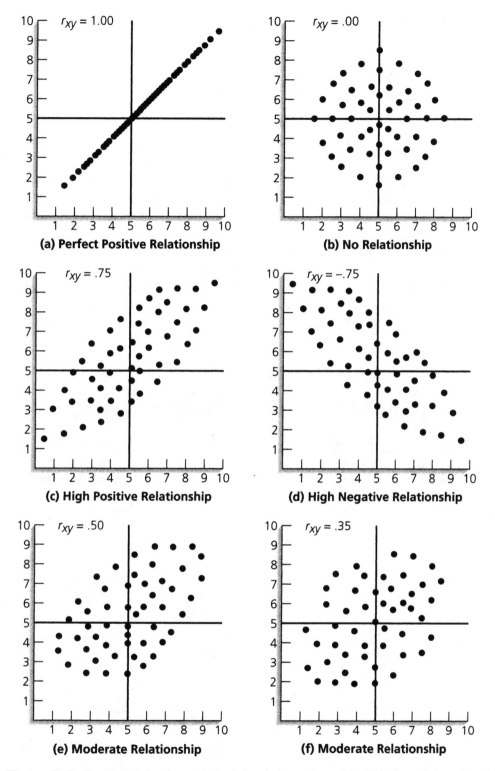

Figure 8–7. Scatter plots of correlations for various sizes (*N* = 50). From *Educational Research: Fundamentals for the Consumer* (4th ed., p. 135), by J. H. McMillan, 2004, Boston, MA: Allyn & Bacon. Copyright 2004 by Pearson Education. Reprinted by permission of the publisher.

there may be bias in selecting adjectives to describe results because of preconceived ideas about outcome.

Inferential Statistics

Inferential statistics are a type of statistics used to make inferences about whether relationships observed in a sample are likely to occur in the larger population, that is, infer characteristics about a population based on data from a sample. Inferential statistics are used to compare differences between groups (Mertens, 2005). Tables 8–5 and 8–6 provide descriptions of inferential statistical methods.

Statistical inference consists of two major approaches: estimating parameters and testing hypothesis. *Parameter estimation* is used to estimate a single parameter such as a mean. Estimates can take two forms: point estimates or intervals estimation. *Point estimation* is calculated by dividing the observed values from the sample by the size of the sample, that is, a single statistic to estimate the population parameter. Huck (2006) described point estimation as an educated guess on the basis of the sample data about the unknown value of the population.

Table 8–5. Summary of Statistical Methods

Level of Independent Measurement	Methods of Analyzing Relationships	Methods for Analyzing Differences	
		Related Samples	Samples
Nominal Test for Samples	Contingency	Cochran Q Test	Chi Square Independent (X^2)
Ordinal	Spearman Rank-Order Correlation Coefficient (*Rho*)	Two Samples Wilcoxon Matched Pairs Signed-Ranks Test (*T*)	Mann-Whitney U Test
ANOVA		More Than Two Samples Friedman Two-Way ANOVA	Kruskel-Wallis One-Way
Interval or Independent Ratio	Pearson Product-Moment Correlation Coefficient (*r*)	Two Samples *t*-test for correlated groups z-Ratio	*t*-Test for groups z-Ratio
	Multiple Regression Analysis	More Than Two Samples ANOVA (*F*) ANCOVA (*F*) MANOVA (*T², A, F*)	ANOVA (*F*) ANCOVA (*F*) MANOVA (*T², A, F*)

Source: Evaluating Research in Communication Disorders, by N. Schiavetti and D. E. Metz, 2002, Boston, MA: Allyn & Bacon. Reprinted with permission.

Table 8–6. Inferential Statistics

Parametric Statistics	
ANOVA	Comparison of three or more treatment groups or conditions or the simultaneous manipulation of two or more independent variables
ANCOVA	Used to compare two or more treatment groups while controlling effect of one or more extraneous variables (covariables)
Factor Analysis	Used to examine structure within a large set of variables and to determine underlying dimensions that exist within that set of variables
Pearson's *r*	Determine relationship between two variables
Structural equation models	Examines correlation among a number of variables to identify possible causal relationships. Includes methods such as path analysis and confirmatory analysis
t-test	Used for comparing two means. Also called student *t*-test
Nonparametric Statistics	
Chi square	Compares observed frequencies within categories to frequencies expected by change. Computed for nominal, ordinal, inferential, or ratio data
Fishers exact *t*-test	Used with small samples to test significance of difference in proportions
Kendall's tau	Measure of association or ordinal measuring
Kruskal-Wallis	Compares more than two independent groups representing levels of one independent variables; nonparametric counterpart of ANOVA
Mann-Whitney U test	Compares two independent groups; nonparametric counterpart of *t*-test
McNemar test	Used for nominal level measures to correlated samples: For Chi square test
Median test	Compares median values of two independent groups to determine if groups are from populations with different medians
Odds ratio	Estimate of relative risk by a case control study
Phi coefficient	Used to estimate relationship between two dichotomous variables
Spearman's rho	Correlation coefficient indicates magnitude of relationship between ordinal level measures
Wilcoxon signed rank test	Compares two correlated samples (repeated measures); nonparametric counterpart of *t*-test

Sources: Foundation of Clinical Research, by L. G. Portney and M. P. Witkins, 2009, Upper Saddle River, NJ: Prentice-Hall Health; and *Nursing Research: Principles and Methods*, by D. F. Polit and C. T. Beck, 2010, Philadelphia, PA: Lippincott Williams & Wilkins.

Internal estimation is a statistic that indicates the upper and lower limits of a range of values within which the parameter has a given probability of occurring, that is, the confidence intervals or the range of values within which a population parameter is estimated to lie. *Confidence intervals* are used to indicate the degree of confidence to which the data reflect the population's mean (Mertens, 2005). Confident limits are the upper and lower limits of the confidence level (Polit & Beck, 2010).

Huck (2004) provided four cautionary statements about point and intervals estimation. First, the second of two numbers separated by a plus and minus sign may or may not be the numerical value of the estimated standard error. Second, sample data permit estimation of the standard error, not definitive determination of the standard error. Third, the sample statistic will always be located between the upper and lower limits of the confidence interval but will not always be located halfway between the interval's end points. Fourth, estimation requires that the data used for inference come from a random sample.

Hypothesis Testing

Hypothesis testing is concerned with making objective decisions based on statistical analysis of differences between groups or relationships of values. The *null hypothesis* is a statement that there is no difference or no relationship between variables, that is, the statistical hypothesis (Portney & Watkins, 2009). Rejection of the null hypothesis lends support to the hypothesis whereas not rejecting the null hypothesis indicates that the observed difference is not due to chance. There are two types of errors in testing hypothesis: rejecting a true null hypothesis (Type I) or accepting a false null hypothesis (Type II). Conversely, there are two possible correct decisions: accepting a true null hypothesis and rejecting a false null hypothesis. Figure 8–8 summarizes these decisions.

A *Type I error* occurs if the null hypothesis is rejected when it is true, namely, that a relationship exists when it does not. A *Type II error* is when the null hypothesis is accepted when it is false, namely, that no relationship exists when it does (Polit & Beck, 2010).

Status of null hypothesis

	Null hypothesis is true	Null hypothesis is false
Accept null hypothesis	Correct decision	Type II error
Reject null hypothesis decision	Type I error	Correct decision

Figure 8–8. Hypothesis decisions. Reprinted with permission from *Evaluating Research in Communicative Disorders,* by N. Schiavetti and D. E. Metz, 2002, Boston, MA: Allyn & Bacon.

The risk of being wrong is rejecting the null hypothesis (Type I error) is called the *level of significance* or *limit of confidence* (Schiavetti et al, 2011). The level of significance is indicated with the small letter *p* (probability) or by the Greek letter alpha. The most frequently used levels of significance are 0.05 and 0.01. This means that the probability of making a Type I error is 0.05 (5 chances in 100) or 0.01 (I chance in 100). This means at the 0.01 level the null hypothesis would be rejected when it should have been accepted in only 1 out of 100 samples.

The level of significance is affected by three factors (McMillan, 2005). First, the differences between the groups being compared; the greater the difference, the smaller the *p* value. Second, is the degree of sampling and measurement error; the lower the error, the smaller the *p* value. Third, is the sample size; the *p* value will be smaller for a very large sample that is, if a small sample size is used.

One- and Two-Tailed Tests

A *one-tailed (directional) test* of statistical significance is one in which only values at one extreme (tail) of a distribution are considered in testing significance (Polit & Beck, 2004). A one-tailed test may be appropriate if there is a strong basis for a directional hypothesis which is a hypothesis that makes a specific prediction about the direction and nature of the relationship between two variables. The use of one-tailed tests is controversial because differences found with two tailed tests are more significant than those found with a one-tailed test (Schiavetti et al., 2002).

Two-tailed (nondirectional) tests are usually preferred. These tests involve both ends of the sampling distribution to determine improbable values (Polit & Beck, 2010). Two-tailed tests are more strict or credible than one-tailed tests, that is, a greater difference between groups may be significantly different when using a two-tailed test (Schiavetti et al., 2011). Conversely, a smaller difference may not be significant with a two-tailed test but may be significant with a one-tailed test.

Parametric and Nonparametric Statistics

Parametric (distribution bound) statistics involve: estimation of at least one parameter; the use of interval or ratio measures; normal distribution; and a fairly large sample. The sample has a central high point and is not seriously skewed, that is, leptokurtic (Leedy & Ormrod, 2005). Parametric statistics are more powerful (more sensitive to differences and relationships) than nonparametric statistics and are usually preferred.

Nonparametric statistics are sometimes called distribution-free statistics because they do not involve rigorous assumptions about the distribution. They are used most often with nominal or ordinal measures. Tables 8–5 and 8–6 list parametric and nonparametric statistical methods.

Between and Within-Subjects Tests

There are *between-subject tests* (test for independent groups) for comparing separate groups of subjects and *within-subject test* (test for dependent groups) for comparing a single group of subjects under different conditions or at different points in time (Polit & Beck, 2010).

Steps in Hypothesis Testing

The steps of hypothesis testing are basically the same starting with stating a hypothesis and ending with a decision about the hypothesis. Sequence of these steps is illustrated in Figure 8–9. These steps are described as follows:

1. *State the hypothesis.* The null hypothesis is a statement of no difference between or among groups. The alternative hypothesis is a hypothesis that is different from the one being tested and usually different from the null hypothesis (Polit & Beck, 2010).

2. *Select the test statistic.* The following factors are usually considered: type of groups (independent, dependent, repeated measures, matched groups, randomized blocks, or mixed groups); the number of independent and dependent variables; the scale of measurement; and whether parametric tests are appropriate. DePoy and Gitlin (2011) developed a series of seven questions to consider in selecting appropriate statistical tests. These questions are presented in Table 8–7.

3. *Establish level of significance.* The level of significance for accepting or rejecting the null hypothesis is established before analyzing the data. The level of significance is usually set at 0.05 or less.

4. *Choose sample size.* The sample size influences the power of a statistical test. A larger sample usually results in a more powerful test of the null hypothesis (Meline, 2005). Small samples are at greater

State hypothesis

⇩

Select test statistic

⇩

Establish level of significance

⇩

Choose sample size

⇩

Select one-tailed or two-tailed test

⇩

Compute test statistic

⇩

Calculate degrees of freedom

⇩

Obtain tabled value for statistical test

⇩

Compare test statistic with tabled value

⇩

Make decision about hypothesis
(Reject or fail to reject the null hypothesis)

Figure 8–9. Steps in hypothesis testing. From *Nursing Research: Principles and Methods*, by D. F. Polit and C.T. Beck, 2004, Philadelphia, PA: Lippincott Williams & Wilkins; and *Research in Communication Sciences and Disorders*, by T. Meline, 2006, Upper Saddle River, NJ: Pearson Education.

Table 8–7. Guidelines for Selecting s Statistical Test

1. What is the research question?
  • Is it about differences?
  • Is it about degrees of a relationship between variables?
  • Is it an attempt to predict group membership?
 	
2. How many variables are being tested, and what types of variables are they?
  • How many variables do you have?
  • How many independent and dependent variables are you testing?
  • Are variables continuous or discrete?
 	
3. What is the level of measurement? (Interval level can be used with parametric procedures.)
 	
4. What is the nature of the relationship between two or more variables being investigated?
 	
5. How many groups are being compared?
 	
6. What are the underlying assumptions about the distribution of a measurement in the population from which the sample was selected?
 	
7. What is the sample size?

Source: Introduction to Research, by E. DePoy and L. N. Gitlin, 2005, Philadelphia, PA: Elsevier. Reprinted with permission.

risk for a Type II error that is, accepting the null hypothesis when it is false.

5. *Select a one-or two-tailed test.* Usually a two-tailed test is selected.

6. *Compute test statistic.* Calculate a test statistic using a computational formula or a computer. The test statistic is a standard score such as z or t statistic (Meline, 2006). The test statistic is computed using the formula in Figure 8–10.

7. *Calculate degrees of freedom.* Degrees of freedom are the number of values within a distribution that are free to vary, given restrictions on the data; often *n-1* (Portney & Watkins, 2009).

8. *Obtain tabled value for the statistical tests.* All test statistics have theoretical distributions. By examining these distributions it can be determined whether obtained values of the test statistic are beyond the range of what is probable if the null hypothesis is true. A table is consulted for the appropriate test statistic to obtain the critical value corresponding to the degree of freedom and significance level (Polit & Beck, 2010).

9. *Compare the test statistic with the tabled value.* If the test statistic is smaller than the tabled value, the results are nonsignificant. If

$$\text{Test Statistic} = \frac{\text{(statistic)} - \text{(parameter)}}{\text{standard error of the statistic}}$$

Figure 8–10. Computation of the test statistic.

the computed value is larger, the results are statistically significant.

10. *Make decisions about the hypothesis.* The final step involves making a decision about rejecting or nor rejecting the null hypothesis. If the null hypothesis is rejected, the alternative hypothesis is supported but not proven (Meline, 2006).

Evaluating Inferential Statistics

McMillan (2005) suggested eight criteria for evaluating inferential statistics. These criteria were: (1) basic descriptive statistic are needed to evaluate the results of inferential statistics; (2) inferential analyses refer to statistical, not practical or clinical, significance; (3) inferential statistics do not indicate external validity; (4) inferential statistics do not indicate internal validity; (5) the results of inferential tests depend on the number of subjects; (6) appropriate statistical tests should be used; (7) the level of significance should be interpreted correctly; and (8) be cautious of statistical tests with small numbers of subjects in one or more groups or categories.

Multivariate Statistics

The preceding statistical procedures were univariate or bivariate because one or two dependent variables were analyzed. *Multivariable statistics* analyze all the dependent variables in a single proce-

dure; this is important in understanding the relationship between dependent variables (McMillan, 2005). Multivariate statistical procedures are being used more often in speech-language pathology and audiology research to study complex relationships among three or more dependent variables. Most outcomes in speech-language pathology and audiology are fundamentally multivariable regardless of whether or not the study is designed for multivariable statistics.

Commonly used multivariable statistical procedures are multiple regressions, analysis of covariables, discriminate analysis, and factor analysis. Multiple regressions analysis is the most widely used multivariable statistical procedure (Polit & Beck, 2010). These and other multivariable statistical procedures are summarized in Table 8–8. Multivariable analyses are usually done by computer because computations are complex.

Meta-Analysis

Meta-analysis statistically combines the results of two or more studies, that is, conclusions are made about other researchers' statistical analyses. It is a specialized quantitative synthesis of the results of existing research. The major advantages of meta-analysis are: (1) increased power by increasing sample size; (2) improved estimated of effect; (3) resolution of uncertainty about conflicting results; and (4) improved generalizability of findings.

Table 8–8. Multivariable Statistics

ANCOVA (analysis of covariables	Extension of ANOVA; used to compare the means of two or more groups
Canocial correlation	Analyzes relationship between two or more independent variables and two or more dependent variables
Discriminary analysis	Used to determine if a set of variables can predict group membership
Factor analysis	Procedure for reducing a large set of variables into a smaller set of variables with common characteristic or underlying dimensions
Hierarchical multiple regression	Prediction variables are entered into the equation in steps that are prespecified
Hoxelling's T^2	Extension of t-test: comparison of two groups
LIS-REL (linear structural relations analysis	Another approach to causal modeling; does not have as many assumptions and restrictions as path analysis; uses maximum likelihood estimation
Logistic regression	Based on maximum likelihood estimation; used to predict categorical dependent variables
MA-NOVA (multivariable analysis of variables)	Extension of ANOVA; used to test significance of differences between means of two or more groups on two or more dependent variables considered simultaneously
MA-NOVA (multivariable analysis of covariables)	Controls extraneous variables (covariables) when there are two or more dependent variables
MCA (multiple classification analysis)	Supplement to ANCOVA; provides information about adjusted means of groups on a dependent variables after removing effect of covariables
Multiple regression	Method for predicting a continuous dependent variable on basis of two or more independent variables
Multiple classification analysis	Variant of multiple regression and ANCOVA; yields group means by the dependent variables adjusted for effects or covariants
Multiple correlation coefficient	Summarizes degree of relationship between two or more independent variables and a dependent variable
Path analysis	Regression-based procedure for testing causal models
Simultaneous multiple regression	All predictor variables are entered into the equation simultaneously. Also called direct or standard multiple regression
Stepwise multiple regression	All prediction variables are entered into the regression equation at the same time
Survival analysis	Used when dependent variables represent a time interval between an initial event and a terminal event

Source: Nursing Research: Principles and Methods, by D. F. Polit and C. T. Beck, 2004, Philadelphia, PA: Lippincott Williams & Wilkins.

Effect size is an important concept in meta-analyses. The *effect size* is a standardized scale-free measure of the relative size of the effect if an intervention (Turner & Bernard, 2006). Effect sizes are interpreted in two ways: (1) common benchmarks of small, medium, and large; or (2) by comparing reported effect size to those reported in prior studies of a similar nature. Schuele and Justice (2006) believe that authors should both report an interpret effect size. It has practical, clinical implications for speech-language pathologists and audiologists who are interested in estimating the effects of treatment; there are several methods for determining effect size (Maxwell & Satake, 2006; Turner & Bernard, 2000). For further discussion about meta-analysis, see Chapter 5.

The statistics methods used in meta-analyses vary widely and depend, in part, on the research designs used in the studies being analyzed (Leedy & Ormrod, 2010). For example, correlated studies require different meta-analytic procedures that do experimental studies.

Summary

In this chapter, quantitative research was discussed relative to design and analysis. Quantitative research uses procedures for collection of data that can be subjected to statistical analysis. There are several types of qualitative research designs; nonexperimental; pre-experimental; quasiexperimental; single subject; and experimental. Major differences between these designs are related to control, manipulation, and intervention (treatment). Quantitative analysis can be classified as descriptive statistics, inferential statistics, multivariable statistics, and meta-analysis. Guidelines for evaluating quantitative were also described.

DISCUSSION QUESTIONS

1. Define quantitative research.
2. Why is quantitative considered to be the sole standard for research?
3. Why must one be cautious when interpreting results from a quasiexperiment?
4. Compare the between-subjects, within-subjects, and single-subject designs.
5. What are the strengths and limitations of single-subject design?
6. What are the major characteristics of single-subject design? How can it be used in speech-language pathology and audiology research?
7. Why is it important to graph data?
8. What factors would affect your decision about which measure of central tendency to choose?
9. Compare parametric and nonparametric statistics.
10. What is the difference between cross-sectional and longitudinal studies?

11. What are the advantages and disadvantages or quantitative research?
12. Why is it necessary to use descriptive statistics? Inferential statistics?
13. How is the null hypothesis used in inferential statistics?
14. What is the difference between Type I and Type II errors?
15. What is the difference between parametric and nonparametric statistics?
16. What are the major characteristics of quantitative research?
17. What are the major characteristics of qualitative research?
18. What is the difference between quantitative and qualitative research?
19. Why is randomization an important consideration in choosing a statistical test?
20. What can be done when the basic assumptions for parametric inferential statistics are not met?
21. How can quantitative research be evaluated?

References

Blessing, J. D., & Forister, J. G. (2012*). Introduction to research and medical literature for health professionals.* Boston, MA: Jones & Bartlett.

Bordens, K. S., & Abbot, B. B. (1988). *Research design and methods.* Mountain View, CA: Mayfield.

DePoy, E., & Gitlin, L. N. (2011). *Introduction to research.* Philadelphia, PA: Elsevier.

French, S., Reynolds, F., & Swain, J. (2001). *Practical research.* Boston, MA: Butterworth Heinemann.

Gravel, J. S., & Wallace, I. F. (2000). Effects of otitis media with effusion on hearing in the first 3 years of life. *Journal of Speech, Language, and Hearing Research, 43,* 631–644.

Harris, R. L. (1999). *Informative graphics.* New York, NY: Oxford University Press.

Haynes, W. O., & Johnson, C. E., (2008). *Understanding research and evidence-based practice.* Boston, MA: Pearson.

Huck, S. W. (2004). *Reading statistics and research.* Boston, MA: Pearson.

Isaac, S., & Michael, W. B. (1987). *Handbook in research and evaluation.* San Diego, CA: Edits Publishers.

Kumar, R. (1996). *Research methodology: A step by step guide for beginners.* Thousand Oaks, CA: Sage.

Leedy, P. D., & Ormrod, J. E. (2010). *Practical research.* Upper Saddle River, NJ: Pearson.

Leedy, P. D., & Ormrod, J. E. (2010). *Practical research: Planning and design.* Boston, MA: Pearson.

Maxwell, D. L., & Satake, E. (2006). *Research and statistics methods.* Clifton Park, NY: Thomson-Delmar Learning.

McMillan, J. H. (2005). *Educational research.* Boston, MA: Allyn & Bacon.

McMillan, J. H., & Schumacher, S. (2001). *Research in education.* Boston, MA: Pearson.

Meline, T. (2006). *Research in communication science and disorders.* Upper Saddle River, NJ: Pearson.

Mertens, D. M. (2005). *Research and evaluation in education and psychology.* Thousand Oaks, CA: Sage.

Nicol, A. M., & Pexman, P. M. (2003). *Displaying your findings.* Washington, DC: American Psychological Association.

Polit, D. F., & Beck, C. T. (2004). *Nursing research: Principles and methods*. Philadelphia, PA: Lippincott, Williams & Wilkins.

Polit, F., & Beck, C. T. (2010). *Nursing research: Principles and methods*. Philadelphia, PA: Lippincott Williams & Wilkins.

Portney, L. G., & Watkins, M. P. (2009). *Foundation of clinical research*. Upper Saddle River, NJ: Prentice-Hall.

Schiavetti, N., Orlikoff, R. T., & Meta, D. E. (2002). *Evaluating research in communicative disorders*. Boston, MA: Allyn & Bacon.

Schuele, C. M., & Justice, L. M. (2006). The importance of effect sizes in the interpretation of research. *ASHA Leader, 11*(10), 14–15, 26–27.

Turner, T. M., & Bernard, R. M. (2006, Spring). Calculating and synthesizing effect size. *Contemporary Issues in Communication Science Disorders, 33*, 42–55.

Vogt, W. P. (2006). *Quantitative research methods for professionals in English and other fields*. Boston, MA: Pearson Education.

9

Qualitative Research Methods

LEARNING OBJECTIVES

Upon completion of this chapter the reader will be able to:

- Describe qualitative research
- Compare advantages and disadvantages of qualitative research
- Explain qualitative research designs
- Understand sampling
- Describe methods for collecting qualitative data
- Analyze qualitative data
- Evaluate qualitative research

Qualitative research was defined by Damico and Simmons-Mackie (2003) as " . . . a variety of analytic procedures designed to systemically collect and describe authentic, contextualized social phenomena with the goal of interpretive adequacy" (p. 132). Qualitative research is non-numerical and takes place in naturally occurring situations in comparison with quantitative research which is numerical and focused on control and manipulation. It provides a detailed description of a specific program, practice, or setting (Mertens, 2005). Sometimes, qualitative research is referred to as naturalistic inquiry (DePoy & Gitlin, 2011).

Until recently, research in speech-language pathology and audiology was dominated by quantitative methods. This trend was apparent in both textbooks and scholarly journals. Although most studies continue to be quantitative, a greater number of qualitative studies have been published in the last few years. Damico and Simmons-Mackie (2003) identified several reasons for this trend: (1) increasing recognition of need to focus on complexity of communication and context in which it occurs; (2) concentration of consumer-based issues, that is, efficacy, clinical outcomes, and impact of services on quality of life; (3) response to social and economic conditions and trends; (4) social diversification; and (5) recognition of relationship between clinical practice and research. Table 9–1 includes some of the qualitative research published in speech-language pathology and audiology. Furthermore, qualitative research is an important component of evidence-based practice (EBP). The first stage of EBP frequently involves qualitative

Table 9–1. Examples of Qualitative Studies in Audiology and Speech-Language Pathology

Author(s)	Topic
Angell, Bailey, & Stoner (2008)	Dysphagia
Barr, McLeod, & Daniel (2008)	Speech impairment
Baylor, Burns, Eadie, Britton, & Yorkston (2011)	Communication disorders in adults
Borton, Mauze, & Lieu (2010)	Children; unilateral hearing loss
Fitzpatrick, Angus, Durieus-Smith, Graham, & Coyle (2008)	Children's hearing loss
Wafaa, Kaf, Barboa, Fisher, & Snavely (2011)	Interdisciplinary service
Logue-Kennedy, Lyons, Carroll, Byme, Dignan, & Hagan (2011)	Central auditory processing disorders
McCormack, McLeod, McAllister, & Harrison (2008)	Speech impairment
Moeller, Hoover, Peterson, & Stelmachowitz (2009)	Hearing aid use

methods (Johnson, 2006). The purpose of this chapter is to describe how qualitative research differs from quantitative research, advantages and disadvantages of qualitative research, data collection and analysis, and evaluation of qualitative research.

Characteristics of Qualitative Research

The primary characteristic of qualitative research is that it focuses on understanding real-life events or situations. Qualitative research is more concerned with subjective, narrative information and is typically obtained under less structured conditions than quantitative research (Portney & Watkins, 2009). Qualitative research involves insight into the participant's personal experiences, the possibility of unexpected findings, understanding if individual needs and requirements,

and continued development of the therapeutic relationship (French, Reynolds, & Swain, 2001).

Other characteristics of qualitative research have been described (Creswell, 2004, McMillan, 2005; McMillan & Schumacher, 2010; Polit & Brock, 2010). These characteristics include: natural setting; direct data collection; data narrative; process orientation; inductive analysis, participant view, variable role of researcher, flexibility, application, and ongoing data analysis.

To further describe qualitative research, differences between qualitative and quantitative research are listed in Table 9–2. Barbour and Barbour (2003) believe there are dangers in underemphasizing the differences between qualitative and quantitative research. Earlier, Barbour (2001) warned that "checklists can be useful in proofing qualitative research methods, but overzealous and uncritical use can be counterproductive" (p. 1115).

Table 9–2. Differences Between Qualitative and Quantitative Research

	Qualitative	Quantitative
Key Concepts	Meaning	Variable
	Understanding	Operationalized
	Social Construction	Controlled
	Context	Reliable
	Naturalistic	Valid
		Statistically significant
		Replicated
		Hypothesized
		Prediction
Goals	Grounded theory	Test theory
	Develop understanding	Establish facts
	Describe multiple realities	Show relationships
	Capture naturally occurring behavior	Predict
		Statistically describe

Table 9–2. *continued*

	Qualitative	Quantitative
Design	Evolving Flexible General	Structured Predetermined Formal Specific
Sample	Small Normal presentation Purposeful	Large Representative Random selection Control groups Stratified
Data	Verbal descriptions Field notes Observation Documents Photographs People's own words Narrative Subjective	Quantities Counts Measures/instruments Numbers Statistic Objective
Methods/techniques	Observation Participant observer Open-ended interviews Review of documents/articles	Experiment Quasiexperiments Structured observers Structured interviews Survey
Data analysis	Inductive Ongoing Study model, themes, concept	Deductive Statistical
Results	Valid	Reliable
Other characteristics associated with the approach	Naturalistic Field research Ethnographic Phenomenologic Anthropologic Ecologic Interpretive Constitutive Case study	Positivism Experimental Hard data Statistical

Source: Adapted from *Educational Research,* by J. H. McMillan, 2004, Boston, MA: Pearson.

Advantages and Disadvantages of Qualitative Research

Qualitative research has advantages and disadvantages, that is, strengths and weaknesses. The best research method is the one that is most appropriate, singly or combination, to the problem and will produce credible information. Polit and Beck (2010) believe that an understanding of human behavior, problems, and characteristics is best achieved by the use of both qualitative and quantitative data. Nonetheless, some researchers argue against qualitative research because they consider it to be unscientific and subjective (French, Reynolds, & Swain, 2001). Three reasons for considering qualitative research are: (1) induction is a problem; (2) verification; and (3) lack of casual explanation (Lum, 2002). The primary advantage of qualitative research is its focus on phenomena that occur in natural settings. In addition, qualitative research may bridge the gap between research and clinical practice and involve studying these phenomena in all their complexity (Maxwell & Satake, 2006). In addition, qualitative research and lead to hypothesis generation as well as development of theories (Polit & Beck, 2010).

Despite the advantages of qualitative research, there are limitations. First is credibility which is based primarily on validity and reliability (McMillan, 2005). Qualitative research has been described as subjective or based, not suitable for generalization or systematic comparisons (Seers, 2000). Other disadvantages of qualitative research are that it is usually extremely time consuming, and limited to fewer participants (Polit & Beck, 2010). Last, it is difficult to describe cause and effect relationship in qualitative research; in addition, qualitative research relies on literacy and verbal fluency. According to French, Reynolds, and Swain (2001), "respondents' accounts vary not only with their personal experience but to the extent that they differ in their facilitation with language" (p. 11).

Misconceptions About Qualitative Research

Qualitative research is not a modification of quantitative research (Morse, 2005). If these differences are not recognized, assumptions about both qualitative and quantitative research are erroneous. First, there is a clear relationship between qualitative and quantitative research. It would be difficult to understand qualitative strategies without understanding qualitative analytic processed and goals, which are contradictory to quantitative sampling and analysis. Second, knowing quantitative research helps one learn and/or understand qualitative research.

Understanding quantitative research helps to explain qualitative research but does not help one to do qualitative research. Third, quantitative researchers can learn qualitative research by doing it. This is an oversimplification. Furthermore, learning qualitative research by trial and error can be a slow and difficult process.

Qualitative Research Designs

The general principle of qualitative research design is: there are many different qualitative research designs. Tesch (1990) listed 46 different qualitative designs. Some are closely related; others are somewhat unrelated. Some qualitative research designs are relatively common. These include case studies, content analysis, ethnography, ground theory, and phenomenologic study. Other designs such as critical theory, heuristic, life history, and narrative are less common. These designs differ in several ways: purpose; focus; data collection, and analysis. Table 9–3 provides a summary of qualitative designs. There are a number of publications with detailed information about qualitative research (Crabtree & Miller, 1999; Finlay & Ballinger, 2006; Flick, 2006; Hammell & Carpenter, 2004; Polit & Beck, 2010; Sandelowski & Barroso, 2006).

Case Study

One of the most frequently used qualitative research designs is the case study. A case study is a retrospective research method involving detailed analysis of one or more individuals, groups, institutions, programs, or other entities (McMillan, 2005; Polit & Beck, 2010). A case study may be an expansion of an earlier case study.

Typically, a case study is a detailed qualitative analysis of a single entity and use of qualitative methods. Case studies however, may be quantitative and occasionally combine quantitative and qualitative methods (McMillan, 2005).

Case studies have several purposes. Among these purposes are: understanding unusual patients and conditions; providing examples of creative or innovative treatments; generating and testing theory; and providing implications for further research (Portney & Watkins, 2009).

There are several types of case studies. Each type of case study has a different focus. These types of case studies are historical, observational, life history, situational, multicase, and multicare (McMillan, 2005).

The format for reporting case studies varies. Typically, case studies begin with background information about the person or problem (Botavia, 2001).

The primary advantage of case study research is its detailed analysis of an entity or experience which can be done for a variety of purposes (Polit & Beck, 2010, Portney & Watkins 2009). There are also other advantages such as challenging an accepted method of treatment (Haynes & Johnson, 2009). Several disadvantages have been identified. Perhaps the most serious limitation is the relatively low level of evidence (Haynes & Johnson, 2009). Other disadvantages are biased sampling, small number; limited generalization, and difficulty summarizing data (Polit & Beck, 2004; Portney & Watkins, 2008).

In case studies, there is usually some degree of sampling bias. This bias can affect both analysis and results. There are several types of biased sampling: convenience sampling; typical (representative) case sampling; extreme (atypical) case sampling; and maximum (extreme) case sampling (McMillan, 2005).

Data Collection

A variety of methods for collecting qualitative data have been identified: open-ended questions, interviews, and observations. Furthermore, multiple methods are often used for any single study. These methods include self-reports, observation,

Table 9–3. Qualitative Research Designs

Design	Description
Biographical study	Detailed study of a person's like, or of some specific period of a person's life.
Case Study	Focus on specific objects as a case, that is, person, topic, and location. Believed to be related to one or more cases.
Content analysis	Refers to several methods for gathering and analyzing data from texts, that is, content or spoken and written materials, films, videotapes, photographs, and so forth.
Conversational analysis	Designed to study social interaction through detailed description of conversation
Critical theory	Designed to understand experiences for social change
Discourse analysis	Focus on studies of language use (spoken or written), beyond boundaries of an utterance or sentence. Commonly used in conjunction with conversational analysis
Ethnography	Description or interpretation of complex and contextually sensitive aspects of social life and culture in natural setting
Field study	Data collected in natural setting to understand practices, behaviors, beliefs, or group in real life
Focus group	Uses small group interviews about a specific topic or problem
Grounded theory	Develop theory from data collected in natural setting, that is, theory generated from qualitative research
Heuristic	Focus on personal and lived experience
Historical research	Collection and evaluation of data related to past or more contextualized and deeper understanding
Life history	Information about what has occurred throughout an individual's life. Sometimes referred to as oral history
Narrative analysis	Understand experiences or marginalized individuals
Naturalistic meta-analysis	Applies naturalistic methods to analysis of several studies
Participatory action	Generate knowledge to inform action
Phenomenology	Focus on understanding meaning of experiences

Sources: From *Introduction to Research*, by E. DePoy and L. N. Gitlin, 2005, St. Louis, MO: C. V. Mosby; "Qualitative Research and Speech-Language Pathology," by J. S. Damico and N. N. Simmons-Mackie, 2003, *American Journal Speech-Language Pathology*, *12*, 131–143; *Research and Statistical Methods in Communication Sciences and Disorders*, by D. L. Maxwell and E. Satake, 2006, Clifton Park, NY: Thomson-Delmar Learning; and *Practical Research*, by P. D. Leedy and J. E. Ormrod, 2005, Upper Saddle River, NJ: Pearson.

interview, focus groups, and analysis of documents or other materials (Law & Phillips, 2002). Self-reports and observation are the most frequently used types of data collection in qualitative research.

Data collection and analysis occurs in overlapping phases. There are five phases of data collection: (1) planning; (2) beginning data collection: (3) basic data collection; (4) closing data collection; and (5) completion. Phases 2 through 4 involve data collection. The last phase (5) focuses on data analysis including development of tables and figures (McMillan & Schumacher, 2010).

Self-Reports

Self-reports is a method of collecting data that involves a direct report of information by the person being studied (Polit & Beck, 2010). The major advantages of self-report are directness and versatility. Self-reports can be retrospective or prospective, that is, about activities or events occurring in the past or planned for the future. Despite these advantages, there are disadvantages, which are related to validity and accuracy of self-reports.

Observation

Observation is comprehensive because it is continuous and total (McMillan, 2005). Observations can vary in the degree of structure from totally unstructured to highly structured (French, Reynolds, & Swain, 2001). In *unstructured observation*, there is no attempt to manipulate the situation. Events are observed as they occur naturally and in the total situation. *Semistructured observation* is more concerned with some aspects of the situation than others. In *structured observation,* what to observe is decided in advance and there is an observational schedule. A single observation may involve all these methods of observation. Unstructured and semistructured observations tend to be time consuming and labor intensive. These methods are most frequently association with qualitative research.

There are several types of observational methods which are based on the degree of participation and involvement of the researcher, ranging from complete participation at one end to complete observer at the other end (McMillan, 2005). A *participant observer* is when the researcher is an active participant in the activity being studied, that is, the researcher participates as a member of the group and is not known as the researcher. According to Meline (2004), participant observation "is more demanding than direct observation because the researcher must acclimate to the situation and become an accepted member in the scene" (p. 79). A complete observer or *passive participant* is detached from the group being studied and is known as the researcher.

Participation of the researcher may be undisguised (overt) or disguised (covered). The researcher's role is known as active participation but not known in complete participation (Maxwell & Satake, 2006).

There are several steps for observational research: (1) select a research design; (2) determine the amount of the time for the study; (3) select the site; (4) gain entry; (5) initial observations; (6) review role; (7) detailed observation; and (8) exit field. The first step is contacting the gatekeeper who grants assess to the site and participants. Gaining entry to the field requires mapping the field, obtaining information about special, spatial, and temporal structures (McMillan & Schumacher, 2010; Polit & Beck, 2010).

Observational research is particularly well suited to speech-language pathology and audiology. Speech-language pathologists and audiologists are in an advantageous position to observe the behaviors and activities of clients and their families. Moreover, speech-language pathologists and audiologist by training may be very reliable observers. Many speech-language-hearing problems are well suited to observational approach.

There are, however, disadvantages including possible ethical consideration, distorted behavior of the person being observed if the observer is conspicuous, a high refusal rate, and observer bias (Polit & Beck, 2010). French and associates (2001) identified several ethical considerations related to the use of observers. Many groups such as the homeless and prisoners lack the power to complain about such intrusions. Researchers may witness behaviors that they find disturbing or with which they disapprove. There may be disapproval of covert methods of observation so that researchers must be prepared for criticism or even worse consequences. Creswell (2003) believes " . . . first and foremost the researcher has an obligation to respect the rights, needs, values, and desires of the informant(s)" (p. 201). Observation is vulnerable to observation has for a number of reasons (Polit & Beck, 2010). Among these reasons are: emotions, prejudices, attitudes, and values of observers; personal interest and commitment; preconceived ideas about what is to be observed; and inappropriate decisions about data collection.

Interviewing

Interviewing is the most common method of data collection in qualitative research (Llewellyn, 1996). The *interview* is a form of data collection in which questions are asked orally and participant's responses are recorded (Maxwell & Satake, 2006). Interviews are conducted either face-to-face, by telephone, or electronically. Some general guidelines for interviewing are provided in Table 9–4.

Additional information about interviewing can be found in French, Reynolds, and Swain (2001); Haynes and Pindzola (1998); Shipley and McAlfee (2009); and Stein-Rubin, and Adler (2012).

Interviews have both advantages and disadvantages. Advantages are related to rapport with the participants which can

Table 9–4. Guidelines for Conducting Qualitative Research

- Identify questions in advance
- Make interviews representative of the group
- Obtain written permission
- Establish and maintain rapport
- Focus on actual rather than abstract or hypothetical
- Do not put words in people's mouths
- Record responses verbatim
- Keep your reaction(s) to yourself
- Remember you are not necessarily obtaining the facts
- When conducting a focus group, consider group dynamics

Source: Adapted from *Practical Research*, by P. D. Leedy and J. E. Ormrod, 2005, Upper Saddle River, NJ: Pearson.

enhance motivation and results in obtaining information that might not otherwise be obtained: clarification of participants' questions; follow-up on leads or probing; use with many different types of persons (illiterate or too young to read or write); and higher return of results (McMillan, 2005). Face-to-face interviews also have additional advantages such as observation of nonverbal behavior, and a tendency to reduce no and unknown answers or neutral responses.

The major disadvantages of interviews are cost, time, small sample size, possible subjectivity, or the training and experience of the interviewer. It is important that questions not be leading or suggest a specific response (McMillan, 2005).

Interviews may be structured, semistructured, or unstructured. *Structured interviews* are often used in telephone interviews (Maxwell & Satake, 2006). Structured interviews have the advantage of efficient use of time and allowing some flexibility (Llewellyn, 1996). *Semistructured interviews* are predetermined but the participants are not predetermined. Rather, the questions are open-ended but specific, which permits individual responses. *Unstructured interviews* are sometimes referred to as informal conversation or in-depth interviews because they are open-ended and flexible. This type of interview is especially useful for understanding individual behavior over time. The disadvantages of unstructured interviews are the time involved and resources needed to analyze the data obtained.

Focus Groups

Focus groups are a method of interviewing a group of individuals about a specific topic or issue. The same format used for individual interviews is used for focus groups: structured, semistructured, or unstructured. The advantages of focus groups are that multiple responses can be obtained in a relatively short period of time, observation of interaction between focus group members, and some people feeling more comfortable talking in a group than alone (Leedy & Ormrod, 2010). Disadvantages are related to possible domination of the group by one or more members. Furthermore, if the facilitator of the focus group is not skilled in group processes and interviewing methods, this will adversely affect the responses of others (Law, 2002).

Document Analysis

Another method of collecting data for qualitative research is by reviewing documents (McMillan, 2005). Documents are written or printed materials such as case notes and files, autobiographies, biographies, diaries, newspaper, magazines, professional journals, essays, and official statistics. Nonprint materials can also be used for documentary analysis including pictures, videotapes, memorabilia, and films. Documents can be either primary or secondary sources. *Primary sources* are firsthand data. *Secondary sources* are secondhand documentation based on what is seen or heard by someone else, or a summary of primary information. Obviously, primary sources are more credible than secondary sources.

Documentation research has several advantages: it is relatively economic, largely unobtrusive, and larger amounts of existing data can be analyzed (French, Reynolds, & Swain, 2001). The disadvantages are that documentation research can be isolating, time consuming, and restricted to topics and issues that have been written or spoken about. Last, the credibility and authenticity of the documents may be questionable or the information may be incomplete or misleading.

Sampling

Sampling in qualitative research is very different from sampling qualitative research, which involves random samples (Law & Phillip, 2002). Participants are selected for a specific purpose in qualitative research, that is, purpose for sampling. Sampling in qualitative research is continued until sampling redundancy or theoretical saturation of the data is achieved (DiLollo & Walter, 2004). In other words, sampling is continued to the point at which no new information is obtained and redundancy is achieved (Polit & Beck, 2010). Types of qualitative samplings are convenience, snowball, and theoretical sampling (Polit & Beck, 2010). *Convenience, or accidental, sampling* is using the most readily available persons as participants. Also known as nominated, network, or chain sampling, *snowball sampling* is the selection of participants by nomination or referral from earlier participants. *Theoretical or purposeful sampling* is the selection of participants based on emerging findings as the study progresses so adequate representation of important themes is assured. Varieties of qualitative sampling methods have been identified by Patton (2001) and are described in Table 9–5.

Analyzing Qualitative Data

Qualitative data analysis is challenging for many reasons. Among the reasons are:

(1) there are no systematic roles for analyzing and presenting qualitative data; (2) the amount of work required to organize and analyze the data; and (3) reduction of the data for reporting (Polit & Beck, 2010).

There are a variety of methods of analyzing qualitative data ranging from objective and systematic to subjective and interpretive (Maxwell & Satake, 2006). Qualitative data analysis is based on the following principles: (1) analysis is conducted concurrently with data collection; (2) the analytic process is systematic; (3) the data are divided into segments during analysis; (4) comparison is the main strategy used for doing analysis; and (5) the goal is synthesis of the data into a higher level of conceptualization (Llewellyn, 1996). In addition, four cognitive processes are involved in qualitative analysis: (1) comprehension, the process of making sense of the data, which occurs primarily while in the field: (2) synthesis or sorting the data and putting the pieces together, which begins in the field but continues after the field work has been completed; (3) theorizing or a systematic sorting of the data; and (4) recontextuation which is the further development of theory. The latter is difficult to undertake before synthesis is completed.

The main types of qualitative data analysis are: quasistatistical; template; editions; and immersion. *Quasistatistical, or manifest, content analysis* begins with some preconceived ideas about the analysis which have been specified in the code book, and then uses these ideas (codes) to sort the data. This method lends itself to basic statistical analysis such as the frequency of occurrence of specific themes (Maxwell & Satake, 2006; Polit & Beck, 2010). *Template analysis* involves interpretation of the data on

Table 9–5. Qualitative Sampling Methods

Method	Description
Critical case sampling	Purposeful selection of participants who are especially important or illustrative
Extreme (Deviant) sampling	Purposeful selection of most extreme or unusual participants
Homogeneous samples	Deliberate selection of participants with limited variation
Intensity samples	Similar to extreme sampling; purposeful selection of intense, but not extreme participants
Maximum variation samples	Purposeful selection of participants with a wide range of variation
Samples confirming and disconfirming	Confirming—additional participants that fit conceptualization and offer enhanced reliability. Disconfirming—do not fit; do not offer new insights
Theory-based sampling	Selection on basis of potential representation of important theoretical constructs
Typical case sampling	Selection of participants who will illustrate or highlight what is typical or average

Source: From *Qualitative Research and Evaluation Methods*, by M. G. Patton, 2002, Thousand Oaks, CA: Sage Publications. Copyright 2001 by Sage Publications, Inc. Reprinted by permission of Sage Publications, Inc.

which categorization is used for coding, sorting, and organizing the data. The *immersion, or crystallization, method* involves total immersion in the problem. This method is considered to be an insider's perspective.

Criteria for Evaluation of Qualitative Research

Qualitative research requires different criteria for evaluation because of differences in design and data. Several authors have described criteria for evaluation of quali-

tative research (Creswell, 2003; French, Reynolds & Swain, 2001; Leedy & Ormrod, 2010; McMillan, 2005; Polit & Beck, 2010; Powers, 2005; Silverman, 2005; Trochim, 2001). A checklist for evaluation of qualitative research by McMillan, (2004) is presented in Table 9–6. Eleven similar standards for evaluating qualitative research were described more recently by McMillan and Schumacher (2010). Barbour and Barbour (2003) warn that an over rigorous application of checklists for evaluating qualitative research can be counterproductive.

Reliability and validity are the fundamental criteria for evaluating qualitative

Table 9–6. Criteria for Evaluating Qualitative Research

Criteria	Yes	No
Researcher's background, training, interest, possible bias clear	☐	☐
Concept and theoretical framework clear	☐	☐
Sampling method clear	☐	☐
Setting described	☐	☐
"Researchers and participants" involvement clear	☐	☐
Field notes provide detailed objective descriptions	☐	☐
Data analysis appropriate and described	☐	☐
Data analysis permits review and revision as new data emerge	☐	☐
Triangulation of data sources	☐	☐
Tables and figures easy to read and interpret	☐	☐
Sufficient data to support conclusions	☐	☐
Discrepant data explained	☐	☐
Discussion considered question and rationale	☐	☐
Implications for theory and/or practice	☐	☐

Sources: From *Educational Research*, by J. H. McMillan, 2004, Boston, MA: Pearson; and *Practical Research*, by P. D. Leedy and J. E. Ormrod, 2005, Upper Saddle River, NJ. Pearson.

research. These criteria have been identified by McMillan (2005):

1. The researcher's experience, interest, and potential biases should be clear.
2. The conceptual and theoretical background of the study should be clear.
3. The method of subject selection should be clear.
4. The degree of researcher involvement should be clear.
5. Fieldnotes should contain detailed information.
6. Researchers should be trained in qualitative data collection and analysis.
7. Credibility of the research should be considered.
8. Descriptions and interpretation should be separate.
9. Multiple methods of data collection should be used.

A study should be long enough to achieve the intensive involvement needed for qualitative research. Polit and Beck (2010) identified evaluation criteria based on validity, statistical conclusion, and internal and external assessment. Statistical inference is the process of inferring attributes about the population based on information from a sample using laws of probability. General guidelines for evaluating qualitative research were also described by Polit and Beck (2010).

Credibility, transferability, dependability, and conformability are used to evaluate the trustworthiness of qualitative data (Maxwell & Satake, 2006; Polit & Beck, 2010). *Credibility* is the extent to which data are believable and trustworthy, that is, confidence in the truth if the data. Several methods have been suggested for improving and documenting the credibility of qualitative research such as persistent observation, negative case analysis, peer debriefing, prolonged engagement, member checks, search for counterevidence, credibility of the researcher, and triangulation. *Triangulation* also known as crystallization refers to the use of multiple methods to improve the credibility of findings, or the truth. It may involve comparison of data from different sources or analysis to reduce or eliminate boas and errors (Maxwell & Satake, 2006; Meline, 2006; Polit & Beck, 2010). There are five major types of triangulation data: (1) data triangulation; (2) investigator triangulation; (3) theory triangulation; (4) method triangulation; and (5) analysis triangulation. *Dependability* is the qualitative equivalent to reliability of quantitative research, whereas conformability is the equivalent to objectivity (Mertens, 2005). *Transferability* is the extent to which findings from a qualitative study can be transferred to similar circumstances. *Conformability* refers to sharing findings with participants by informant checks or feedback sessions to confirm views of the person being studied. This maximizes accuracy of findings by minimizing bias.

Summary

There are a variety of qualitative research designs: case study; content analysis; ethnography; grounded theory; and phenomenologic study. The methods commonly used for data collection are observation and interviews.

Qualitative research is well suited to the interests of speech-language pathologists and audiologists. The increasing popularity of qualitative research in speech-language pathology and audiology is evident in the growing number of qualitative studies reported in the past few years. For example in 2003, *Language Speech and Hearing Services in Schools* had a special forum on qualitative studies; however, quantitative research continues to be the most frequent type of research. It should be remembered that both quantitative and qualitative research contribute to the knowledge base of the professions.

DISCUSSION QUESTIONS

1. Define and describe qualitative research.
2. What are the similarities between qualitative and quantitative research?
3. What are the reasons for the increase in qualitative research?
4. Compare qualitative and quantitative research.
5. What are the advantages and disadvantages to qualitative research?
6. List and briefly describe qualitative research designs.

7. How are data collected for qualitative research?
8. Explain observer participation and involvement.
9. What are the advantages and disadvantages of interviews?
10. What is the difference between structured and unstructured interviews?
11. How can focus groups be used to collect data?
12. Describe the advantages and disadvantages of focus groups.
13. How is document analysis used in qualitative research?
14. What are print documents? Nonprint documents?
15. What are the differences in sampling between qualitative and quantitative research?
16. Describe the different types of qualitative sampling.
17. Why is analysis of qualitative data challenging?
18. How can qualitative data be analyzed?
19. What are the criteria for evaluation of qualitative data?
20. What are the advantages and disadvantages of case study?
21. List and briefly describe the different types of case study.
22. Why are case studies high risk for bias?
23. What are the characteristics of qualitative research?
24. How can and why should qualitative research be explained?
25. Outline and describe steps for qualitative observation.

References

Angell, M., Bailey, R. L., & Stoner, J. (2008). Family perceptions of facilitators and inhibitors of effective school-based dysphagia management. *Language Speech and Hearing Services in Schools, 39,* 214–226.

Bailey, R. L., Parette, H. P., Stoner, J. B., Angell, M. E., & Carroll, K. (2006). Family members' perceptions of augmentative and alternative communication device use. *Language Speech and Hearing Services in Schools, 37,* 50–60.

Barbour, R. S. (2001). Checklist for improving rigor in qualitative research: A case of the tail wagging the dog? *British Medical Journal, 322,* 1115–1117.

Barbour, R. S., & Barbour, M. (2003). Evaluating and synthesizing qualitative research: The need to develop and distinctive approach. *Journal of Evaluating Clinical Practice, 9,* 179–186.

Barr, J., McLeod, S., & Daniel, G. (2008). Siblings of children with speech impairment: Cavalry on the hill. *Language Speech and Hearing Services in Schools, 39,* 21–32.

Baylor, C., Burns, M., Eadie, T., Britton, D., & Yorkston, K. (2011). A qualitative study of interference with communicative participation across communication disorders is adults. *American Journal of Audiology, 20,* 269–287.

Baylor, C. R., Yorkston, K. M., & Eadie, T. I. (2005). The consequences of spasmodic dysphonia on communication-related quality of life: A qualitative study of the insider's experience. *Journal of Communication Disorders, 38*(5), 395–419.

Borton, S. A., Mauze, E., & Lieu, J. E. (2010). Quality of life in children with unilateral hearing loss: A pilot study. *American Journal Audiology, 19,* 61–72.

Botavia, M. L. (2001). *Clinical research for health professionals*. Boston, MA: Butterworth-Heinemann.

Crabtree, B., & Miller, W. L. (1999). *Doing qualitative research*. Thousand Oaks, CA: Sage.

Creswell, J. W. (2004). *Research design*. Thousand Oaks, CA: Sage.

Culatta, B., Kouarski, D., Theadore, G., Franklin, A., & Timier, G. (2003). Quantitative and qualitative documentation of early literacy instruction. *American Journal of Speech-Language Pathology, 12*(2), 172–188.

Curenton, S. M., & Justice, L. M. (2004). African American and Caucasian preschoolers' use of decontextualizes language: Literate language features in oral narratives. *Language Speech Hearing Services in Schools, 35*, 240–253.

Damico, J. S., & Simons-Mackie, N. N. (2003. Qualitative research and speech-language pathology: A tutorial for the clinical realm. *American Journal of Speech-Language Pathology, 12*(2), 131–143.

DePoy, E., & Gitlin, L. N. (2011). *Introduction to research*. St. Louis, MO: Elsevier.

DiLollo, A., & Walter, J. (2004, June 8). Qualitative research in communication disorders. *ASHA Leader*, pp. 4–5, 16–17.

Dromey, C., & Bates, E. (2005) Speech interactions with linguistic, cognitive, and visumotor tasks. *Journal of Speech, Language, and Hearing Research, 45*, 295–305.

Farinella, K. A., Hixton, T. J., Hoit, J. D., Story, B. H., & Jones, P. A. (2006). Listener perception of respiratory-induced voice tremor. *American Journal of Speech-Language Pathology, 15*, 72–82.

Finlay, L., & Ballinger, C. (2006). *Qualitative research for allied health professionals*. Hoboken, NJ: John Wiley & Sons.

Fitzpatrick, E., Angus, D. Durieus-Smith, A., Graham, I. D., & Copyle, D. (2008). Parents' needs following identification of childhood hearing loss. *American Journal of Audiology, 17*, 387–349.

Flick, V. (2006). *An introduction to qualitative research*. Thousand Oaks, CA: Sage.

French, S., Reynolds, F., & Swain, J. (2001). *Practical research*. Woburn, MA: Butterworth-Heinemann.

Hammell, K. W., & Carpenter, A. (2004). *Qualitative research in evidence-based rehabilitation*. New York, NY: Churchill Livingstone.

Haynes, W. O., & Pindzola, R. H. (1998). *Diagnosis and evaluation in speech pathology*. Boston, MA: Allyn & Bacon.

Johnson, C. J. (2006). Getting started in evidence-based practice for childhood speech-language disorders. *American Journal of Speech-Language Pathology, 15*, 20–35.

Law, M. (2002). *Evidence-based rehabilitation*, Thorofare, NJ: Slack Incorporated.

Law, M., & Phillip, I. (2002). Systemically reviewing the evidence. In M. Law (Ed.), *Evidence-based rehabilitation* (pp. 97–108). Thorofare, NJ: Slack Incorporated.

Leedy, P. D., & Ormrod, J. E. (2010). *Practical research*. Upper Saddle River, NJ: Pearson.

Liiva, C. A., & Cleave, P. C. (2005). Roles of imitation and responsiveness in access and participation for children with specific language impairment. *Journal of Speech, Language, and Hearing Research, 48*, 868–883.

Llewellyn, G. (1996). Qualitative research. In F. Stein & S. K. Cutler (Eds.), *Clinical research in allied health and special education* (pp. 411–424). San Diego, CA: Singular.

Logue-Kennedy, M., Lyons, R., Carroll, C., Byrne, M., Dignan, E., & O'Hagan, L. (2011). Services for children with central auditory processing disorders in the republic of Ireland: Current and future service provision. *American Journal of Audiology, 20*, 9–18.

Lum, C. (2002). *Scientific thinking in speech and language therapy*. Mahwah, NJ: Lawrence Erlbaum Associates.

Maxwell, D. L., & Satake, E. (2006). *Research and statistics methods in communications* . Clifton Park, NY: Thomson-Delmar Learning.

McCormack, J., McLeod, S., McAlister, L., & Harrison, L. J. (2010). My speech problems, your listening problems, and my frustration: The experience of living with childhood speech impairment. *Language, Speech and Hearing Services in Schools, 41*, 379–392.

McMillan, J. H. (2005). *Educational research: Fundamentals for the consumer.* Boston, MA: Pearson.

McMillan, J. H., & Schumacher, S. (2001). *Research in education.* Boston, MA: Pearson.

McMillan, J. H., & Schumacher, S. (2010). *Research in education* (7th ed.). Boston, MA: Pearson.

Meline, T. (2004). *Research in communication science and disorders.* Columbus, OH. Pearson.

Mertens, D. M. (2005). *Research and evaluation in education and psychology.* Thousand Oaks, CA: Sage.

Moeller, M. P., Hoover, B., Peterson, B., & Stelacjowicz, P. (2009). Consistency of hearing aid use in infants with early identified hearing loss. *American Journal of Audiology, 18*, 14–23.

Morse, J. M. (2005). Qualitative research is not a modification of quantitative research. *Qualitative Health Research, 15*(8), 1003–1005.

Patton, M. G. (2001). *Qualitative research and evaluation methods.* Newbury Park, CA: Sage.

Polit, D. F., & Beck, C. J. (2010). *Essentials of nursing research:* Philadelphia, PA: Lippincott Williams & Wilkins.

Portney, L. G., & Watkins, M. P. (2009). *Foundation of clinical research.* Upper Saddle River, NJ: Prentice-Hall.

Powers, B. A. (2005). Critically apprising qualitative evidence. In B. M. Mellynk & E. Fineout-Overholt (Eds.), *Evidence-based practice in nursing and healthcare* (pp. 127-162). Philadelphia, PA: Lippincott, Williams & Wilkins.

Sandelowski, M., & Barroso, J. (2006). *Handbook for synthesizing qualitative research.* New York, NY: Springer.

Seer, K. (2000). Qualitative research. In M. Dawes, P. Davies, A. Gray. K. Seers, & R. Snowball (Eds.), *Evidence-based practice: A primer for health care professionals.* New York, NY: Churchill Livingstone.

Shipley, K. G., & McAfee, J. G. (2009). *Assessment on Speech-language Pathology.* Clinton Park, NY: Delmar Learning.

Silverman, D. (2005). *Doing qualitative research.* Thousand Oaks, CA: Sage.

Simmons-Mackie, N. N., & Damico, J. S. (2003). Contributions of qualitative research to the knowledge base of oral communication. *American Journal of Speech-Language Pathology, 12*(2), 144–154.

Stein-Rubin, C., & Adler, R. T. (2012). Counseling and the diagnostic interview for the speech-language pathologist. In C. Stein-Rubin & R. Fabus (Eds.), *A guide to clinical assessment and professional report writing in speech-language pathology.* Clifton Park, NY: Delmar.

Tesch, R. (1990). *Qualitative research. Analysis types and software tools.* New York, NY: Falmer Press.

Trochim, W. M. (2001). *The research methods knowledge base.* Cincinnati, OH: Atomic Dos.

Wafaa, A., Kaf, L. S., Barboa, B., Fisher, J., & Snave, L. (2011). Effect of interdisciplinary service learning experience for audiology and speech-language pathology: Students working with adults with dementia. *American Journal of Audiology, 20*, S241–S249.

10

Multimethod Research

Upon completion of this chapter the reader will be able to:

- Describe the sequences for combining qualitative and quantitative research
- Understand designs for multimethod research
- Acknowledge advantages and disadvantages of multimethod research
- Evaluate multimethod research.

Multimethod or mixed research combines quantitative and qualitative research methods. It uses the best of both methods. According to Creswell and Clark (2007) "the use of quantitative and qualitative approaches in combination provides a better understanding of research problems than either approach alone" (p. 5). Speech-language pathologists and audiologists should understand multimethod research because most clinical research combines quantitative and qualitative research methods.

Characteristics of Multimethod Research

Multimethod research is a growing trend that resulted from discussions and controversies about quantitative and qualitative research. Multimethod or mixed research combines both quantitative (outcome) and qualitative (process) feature collection, and analysis in the design, data collection, and analysis (McMillan, 2005, Mertens, 2005). The steps in multimethod research from determining the feasibility of the study through data collection to reporting the results are shown in Figure 10–1. Similar steps have been described by Creswell 2009; McMillan, 2005; and McMillan and Schumacher, 2010.

A number of publications describe methods for combining research (Creswell, 2009 Mertens, 2005; Polit & Beck, 2010; Tashakkori & Teddlie, 1998). The *Handbook of Mixed Methods in Social and Behavioral Research* (Tashakkori & Teddlie, 2003) and *Designing and Conducting Mixed Methods Research* (Creswell & Clark, 2007) are comprehensive publications about issues related to combining quantitative and qualitative research. Among the issues discussed are controversies about the use of mixed methods; mixed method designs and analysis, multidisciplinary application, collaborative research, and teaching mixed methods research. There are also journals reporting and advocating mixed method research such as Field Notes (Alta Mara Press, 1988).

Despite the increasing popularity of mixed method research, there is considerable debate (Adamson, Gooberman-Hill, Woolhead, & Donovan, 2004). These two methods of research are different and the results may be reported separately. Also, it may be difficult to combine quantitative and qualitative methods because of technical problems or conflicts between theoretical perspectives about research (Morgan, 1998).

Until recently, research in speech-language pathology and audiology has been dominated by quantitative studies. However, qualitative studies gained considerable attention during recent years. Another trend is the blending of quantitative and qualitative data. Multimethod studies are now published in a greater number of speech-language pathology and audiology journals.

Advantages and Disadvantages of Multimethod Research

There are both advantages and disadvantages in multimethod research. The major advantage is that by combining qualitative and quantitative methods the weaknesses of one may be reduced or avoided, that is, there's the potential for one to offset the other's weaknesses (Polit & Beck, 2010).

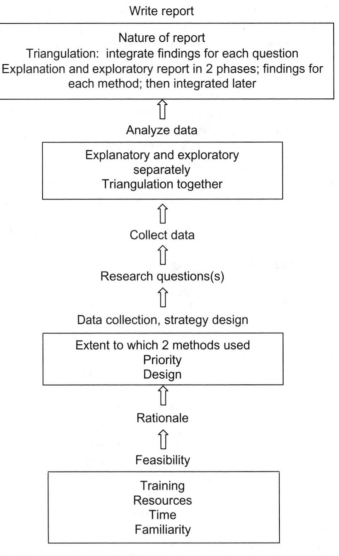

Figure 10–1. Steps in conducting multimethod research. Adapted from *Educational Research*, by J. H. McMillan, 2004, Upper Saddle River, NJ: Merrill/Prentice-Hall.

There are other advantages to multimethod research such as: (1) providing comprehensive data analysis both objective (quantitative) and subjective (qualitative); (2) permitting study of both process and outcome; (3) allowing for different types of research questions; (4) compensating for use of a single type of research method; and (5) enhancing credibility of findings (Abusabha, & Welfel, 2003; McMillan & Schumacher, 2010). In addition, multimethod approach may lead to theoretical insight that might be possible without combining methods.

Different methods are more appropriate for different phases of research, that is, qualitative methods are appropriate for exploration of hypothesis generation, and quantification is needed later for verification. Multiple and complementary types of data can improve the validity of results. When there are conflicting findings, careful review of the discrepancies between qualitative and quantitative data can provide new insights and enhance theoretical understanding.

There also disadvantages and limitations in combining qualitative and quantitative research. Depoy and Gitlin (2011) believe mixed-method research should not be viewed with skepticism and as nontraditional because of its inconsistency. Polit and Beck (2010) identified five limitations: (1) cost; (2) biases; (3) research training; (4) analytic challenges; and (5) publication biases. First, multimethod research is usually expensive. Second, there are extreme preferences; some prefer quantitative research whereas others prefer qualitative research. Third, training can be a challenge because multimethod research requires knowledge and understanding of both qualitative and quantitative research. Furthermore, many training programs offer training in only one method or the other, but not both. Fourth, there are analytic challenges related to combining numeric (quantitative) and narrative (qualitative) data, and resolving and interpreting inconsistent or contradictory results. In addition, writing the report and formatted conclusions can be challenging (McMillan & Schumacher, 2010). Fifth, are publication biases. Some journals prefer qualitative research; however, typically more journals prefer quantitative research. There is also the possibility of a mismatch or bias between the theoretical perspectives or reviewers and authors, that is, quantitative researchers serving as reviewers for qual-

itative research (Belgrave, Zabolotsky, & Guadagno, 1998). According to Meline (2006), "it is somewhat popular to indicate that research has both components, even though one of the two methods is only used superficially" (p. 288). Other issues identified by Tashakkori and Teddlie (1998) are related to overreliance on one method alone and the need for an alternative to mixed methods designs. The former involves going beyond mixing at the method level only, that is, mixing qualitative and quantitative methods throughout several phases of a study and more accurately reflects the research process. The latter suggests that mixed studies go beyond the mixing of methods to include combining other stages of the research cycle. Related to the disadvantages are several myths and misunderstandings that Creswell and Clark (2007) identified. The more common myths are: (1) multimethod research is just qualitative research; (2) it is a method that has always been used; and (3) multimethod research is universally accepted. Acceptance ranges from minimal to major/most. (Table 10–1).

Sequencing

Typically multimethod research is sequential. Figure 10–2 illustrates sequences for combining qualitative and quantitative research. An explanatory design may be the most common type of mixed-methods research. Quantitative data are collected first, and qualitative data are collected in the second phase, that is, qualitative follows quantitative. Another type of mixed methods research is an explanatory design in which qualitative data are collected first and then followed

Table 10–1. Checklist of Designing a Mixed Method Study

Is the basic definition of mixed methods research provided?	Yes	No
Does the reader have a sense for the potential use of a mixed methods strategy?	Yes	No
Are the criteria identified for choosing a mixed methods strategy?	Yes	No
Is the strategy identified, and its criteria for selection given?	Yes	No
Is a visual model presented that illustrates the research?	Yes	No
Is the proper notation used in presenting the visual model?	Yes	No
Are the procedures for data collection and analysis mentioned as they relate to the model?	Yes	No
Are the sampling strategies for both quantitative and qualitative data collection mentioned? Do they relate to the strategy?	Yes	No
Are specific data analysis procedures indicated? Do they relate to the strategy?	Yes	No
Are the procedures for validating both the quantitative and qualitative data discussed?	Yes	No
Is the narrative structure mentioned, and does it relate to the type of mixed methods strategy being used?	Yes	No

Source: From *Research Design*, by J. W. Creswell, 2009, Thousand Oaks, CA: Sage Publications. Copyright 2003 Sage Publications. Reprinted with permission.

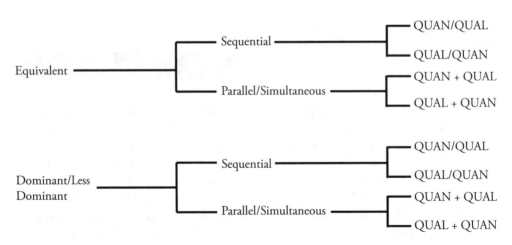

Figure 10–2. *Mixed Methodology*, by A. Tashakkori and C. Teddlie, 1998, Thousand Oaks, CA: Sage Publications. Copyright 2003 Sage Publications. Reprinted with permission.

by a quantitative phase, that is, quantitative follows qualitative. The other type of multimethod study is the triangulation design in which both qualitative and quantitative data are collected simultaneously (McMillan, 2005). Mixed methods research can also be described relative to the stage in which the methods occur (Tashakkori & Teddlie, 1998).

In equal status (equivalent) mixed methods designs, both quantitative and qualitative methods are used about equally. Dominant—less dominant mixed methods designs refers to studies in which one method is dominant and a small part of the study evolves from the other method. Qualitative and quantitative data are collected and analyzed simultaneously in parallel/simultaneous mixed methods designs.

Research Designs

The choice of research methods is frequently associated with a specific theoretical orientation (Adamson et al., 2004). There are, however, specific criteria for selection of appropriate mixed method designs (Creswell, 2009). These criteria are related to: (1) implementation for data collection (concurrent or sequential); (2) priority or equal weight given to quantitative or qualitative approach; (3) phase of research in which the two methods are combed; and (4) identification of theoretical orientation is used in the study.

A checklist of questions may help in designing a mixed methods study. Such a checklist is presented in Table 10–2. There are two major categories of designs in multimethod research: component and

integrated. The latter are more appropriate for theory building and tests than the former (Polit & Beck, 2010). In component designs, the quantitative and qualitative methods are implemented as different components and remain different during data collection and analysis. There are three types of component designs: (1) triangulated; (2) complementary; and (3) expansive. In *triangulated designs*, both quantitative and qualitative methods are used to study the same entity or concept with a focus on convergence (similarities) and increased validity. *Complementary design* is the result of the dominant research method being enhances or clarified by results from the findings of the other type of research. The *expansion design* involves using different methods for different components.

In addition to sequential and integrated designs for combining quantitative and qualitative methods, Meline (2006) described two other designs: parallel and coordinated substudies. *Parallel designs* involve qualitative methods such as case studies, focused ethnographic observation, multiple linked in-depth interviews, or some combination of time in combination with other methods. *Coordinated substudies* are qualitative studies which are part of a larger program project or long term study.

Combining qualitative and quantitative methods can result in several possible outcomes (Brannen, 2005). Among the possible outcomes are: (1) corroboration, the same results from both methods; (2) elaboration, qualitative data analysis explains how the quantitative findings may apply; (3) complementary, the results differ but when combined they provide insights, and; (4) contradiction, the findings conflict.

Table 10–2. Levels of Acceptance for Mixed Methods Studies

Major Acceptance	
_____	Special issue of a journal focusing on the use of mixed methods in the profession
_____	Publication of mixed methods studies in top professional journals
_____	Course on mixed methods research as part of graduate training programs
Moderate Acceptance	
_____	Leaders in the profession advocate for use of mixed methods research
_____	Workshops on mixed methods research forums dedicated to the profession
_____	Funding agencies supporting mixed methods research
_____	Methodological discussions of mixed methods in journals devoted to the profession
Minimal Acceptance	
_____	Awareness within the profession of qualitative research
_____	Publication of actual mixed methods studies in professional journals
_____	Graduate students using mixed methods in dissertation research
_____	Discussions in journals about need for mixed methods
_____	Mixed methods research discussed at professional conferences

Source: From *Designing and Conducting Mixed Methods Research*, J. W. Creswell and V. L. R. Clark, 2007, Thousand Oaks, CA: Sage Publications. Copyright 2007 by Sage Publications, Inc. Reprinted by permission of Sage Publications, Inc.

Moffatt, White, Mackintosh, and Howel (2006) described strategies for explaining and integrating data when mixed methods conflict. The strategies for explaining contradictory data include: (1) treating the methods as fundamentally different; (2) explaining the methodological rigor of each component; (3) exploring the data set comparability; (4) collecting additional data and making further comparisons; (5) exploring whether the intervention under study worked as expected, and (6) exploring whether the outcomes of the quantitative and qualitative parts match.

Data Analysis

Data analysis occurs quantitatively (descriptive and inferential statistics), and qualitatively (descriptive and thematic text or image analysis). Four strategies for data analysis described by Creswell (2003) were: (1) data transformation; (2) exploration of articles; (3) instrument development; and (4) examination of multiple levels.

Evaluating Multimethod Research

Questions for evaluating multimethods research were described by Creswell and Clark (2007). These questions reflect relatively general standards such as basic knowledge of multimethod research, rigor of the research, and advanced knowl-edge of specific designs. The questions are: (1) is the study a multimethod study; (2) does the study show rigorous multi-method research; (3) does the study include advanced multimethod features consistent with multimethod design; and (4) does the study show sensitivity of some of the challenges of using the design.

The questions in Table 10–3 may be used to analyze methods research. These questions refer to issues related to quality which would be referred to as credibility or trustworthiness in qualitative terms or validity in quantitative research. Mertens (2005) also described questions for ana-lyzing mixed methods research that are in Table 10–3. The questions require nar-rative answers.

Table 10–3. Questions for Analyzing Mixed Methods Research

- What are the purposes and questions that justify the use of a mixed-methods design?
- Has the researcher matched the purposes and questions to appropriate methods?
- To what extent has the researcher adhered to the criteria that define quality for the quantitative portion of the study?
- To what extent has the researcher adhered to the criteria that define quality for the qualitative portion of the study?
- How has the researcher addressed the tension between potentially conflicting demands of paradigms in the design and implementation of the study?
- Has the researcher appropriately acknowledged the limitation associated with data that were collected to supplement the main data collection of the study?
- How has the researcher integrated the results from the mixed methods? If necessary, how has the researcher explained conflicting findings that resulted from different methods?
- What evidence is there that the researcher developed the design to be responsive to the practical and cultural needs of specific subgroups on the basis of such dimensions as disability, culture, language reading levels, gender, class, and race or ethnicity?

Source: From *Research and Evaluation in Education and Psychology*, by D. M. Mertens, 2005, Thousand Oaks, CA: Sage Publications. Copyright 2005 by Sage Publications, Inc. Reprinted by permission of Sage Publications, Inc.

Summary

Combining qualitative and quantitative data collection and analysis has several advantages. Despite the advantages, there are also several barriers. However, reducing these barriers is worth the time and effort. Furthermore, most quantitative research contains some qualification and vice versa. More widespread use of mixed methods research may enhance the overall quality of the evidence-base in speech-language pathology and audiology. Most clinical activities combine quantitative and qualitative research, that is, are multimethod research.

DISCUSSION QUESTIONS

1. What is multimethods research?
2. What are its characteristics?
3. Why should speech-language pathologists and audiologist understand multimethod research?
4. Describe the major categories of multimethods research.
5. What are the advantages and disadvantages of multimethods research?
6. Identify the different types of component designs.
7. How can contradictory data be explained?
8. How are integrated designs classified?
9. What are the different types of mixed methods designs?
10. Why should a mixed method design be used?
11. What are the advantages and disadvantages of mixed methods research?
12. What are the strengths and weaknesses of mixed methods research?
13. What are the main design options for mixed methods research?
14. Explain the advantages and disadvantages of multimethod research.
15. Do the advantages of multimethod research outweigh the disadvantages? Why?
16. How can multimethod research be evaluated?

References

Abusabha, R., & Welfel, M. (2003). Qualitative vs. quantitative methods: Two opposites that make a perfect model. *Journal of the American Dietetic Association, 103*(5), 566–569.

Adamson, J., Gooberman-Hill, R., Woolhead, G., & Donovan, J. (2004). Questerviews: Using questionnaires in qualitative interviews as a method of integrating qualitative and quantitative health services research. *Journal of Health Services Research Policy, 9*(3), 139–145.

Alta Maria Press. (1988). *Field notes.* Thousand Oaks, CA: Author.

Belgrave, L. L., Zablotsky, D., & Guadagno, M. A. (1998). How do we talk to each other? Writing qualitative research for quantitative readers. *Qualitative Health Research, 12*(10), 1427–1439.

Brannen, J. (2005). Mixed methods: The entry of qualitative and quantitative approaches into the research process. *International Journal of Social Research Methodology, 8*(3), 173–184.

Creswell, J. W. (2009). *Research design.* Thousand Oaks, CA: Sage.

Creswell, J. W., & Clark, V. L. R. (2007). *Designing and conducting mixed methods research.* Thousand Oaks, CA: Sage.

Depoy, E., & Gitlin, L. N. (2011). *Introduction to research.* St Louis, MO: Elsevier.

McMillan, J. H. (2005). *Educational research.* Boston, MA: Pearson.

McMillan, J. H., & Schumacher, S. (2010). *Research in education.* Boston, MA: Pearson.

Meline, T. (2006). *Research in communication science and disorders.* Columbus, OH. Pearson.

Mertens, D. M. (2005). *Research and evaluation in education and psychology.* Thousand Oaks, CA: Sage.

Moffatt, S., White, M., Mackintosh, J., & Howel, D. (2006). Using quantitative and qualitative data in health services research: What happens when mixed method findings conflict? *BMC Health Services Research, 6*(28). Retrieved May 8, 2006, from http://www.biomedcentral.com/1472-6963/6/28

Morgan, D. I. (1998). Practical strategies for combining qualitative and quantitative methods: Applications to health research. *Qualitative Health Research, 8*(3), 362–376.

Polit, D. F., & Beck, C. J. (2010). *Nursing research: Principles and methods.* Philadelphia, PA: Lippincott Williams & Wilkins.

Tashakkori, A., & Teddlie, C. (2003). *Handbook of mixed methods in social and behavioral research.* Thousand Oaks, CA: Sage.

Turkstra, L. S. (2005). Looking while listening and speaking. Eye-to-face gaze in adolescents with and without traumatic brain injury. *Journal of Speech Language and Hearing Research, 48,* 1429–1441.

11

Reporting and Disseminating Research

LEARNING OBJECTIVES

Upon completion of this chapter the reader will be able to:

- Identify reasons for reporting research
- Correct misconceptions about research reporting
- Avoid misconceptions about research reports
- Effectively manage time for reporting research
- Maintain a research log
- Develop a schedule for reporting research
- Use appropriate professional writing style
- Request permission for copyright materials
- Understand rewriting and revision
- Translate research reports into manuscript
- Identify different types of research reports
- Select a journal to submit a manuscript
- Evaluate and review reports.

Reporting and disseminating research studies are essential to the advancement of science in speech-language pathology and audiology. Students and practicing professionals are often not prepared to write and publish research reports. What distinguishes the unpublished from the published is a matter of attitude, training, and perseverance. First is a positive attitude of confidence and determination that suggests, "I can and I will publish." Second is the probability that those who do not publish do not know how to publish. Throughout schooling, students have had to write and have been graded on writing, but have not been taught how to write for publication. Irwin, Pannbacker, and Kallail (1992) suggest that "university faculty should instruct students about the process of publishing in a journal" (p. 122). Third, an unpublished paper is often one that someone gave up on. Fourth, many people think they have good writing skills but a few do; good writers edit and rewrite, again, and again (Henson, 1993).

The purpose of this chapter is to: (1) describe common myths about research reports: (2) identify reasons for reporting the results of research: (3) managing time to report research; (4) describe the organization and style of research reports; (5) explain research reports at professional meetings; (6) classify and describe visual supplements; and (7) explain submission and review of research reports.

Reasons for Reporting Research

There are numerous reasons for reporting research including ethical responsibility, improving clinical service, academic survival, and personal and group recognition. Hegde (2003b) believes "dissemination or research findings are an ethical responsibility." (p. 560). According to the ASHA Code of Ethics (ASHA, 2010), speech-language pathologists and audiologists have ethical responsibilities related to "dissemination of research findings and scholarly activities" (p. 3). In *A History of the American Speech and Hearing Association 1925–1958,* Paden (1970) stated, "one of the chief reasons for the existence of a profession or learned society is the sharing of knowledge on the field among its members" (p. 21). ASHA provides many opportunities for disseminating research including its scholarly journals, teleseminars, and annual meetings.

Reporting research is fundamental to the advancement of diagnosis and treatment of speech, language, and hearing problems. Silverman (1998) pointed out that if clinical speech-language pathologists and audiologists do not formally disseminate clinical outcome research the potential to help persons with speech-language-hearing problems is restricted to their caseload and those of colleagues with whom they communicate.

Academic survival is related to understanding "publish or perish." Publication has a significant impact on academic survival and promotion, tenure, and merit salary raises (Anderson, 1992; Boyes et al., 1984; Holcomb & Roush, 1988; Schilling, 2005; Sininger, March, Walden, & Wilber, 2003). Publishing makes a difference to speech-language pathologists and audiologists employed in colleges or universities. Those who are promoted have published more than those who have not been promoted. For these reasons, there is tremendous pressure to publish among academicians (Luey, 1987). Academic survival (graduation) of students is also related to completing a thesis or dissertation requirement (Cone & Foster, 2006; Davis & Parker, 1979; Rudestam & Newton, 2001; Sternberg, 1981). There are also several other reasons for reporting, which are listed in Table 11–1.

Table 11–1. Reason for Reporting Research

Ethical responsibility
Advancement of clinical practice
Academic survival; promotion, tenure
Graduation requirement (theses or dissertation)
Stimulate further research
Peer approval
Personal sense of achievement
Evidence of intellectual effort
Entry to professional networks
Quality indicator of group/program/ institution

These reasons are institutional as well as individual.

Reasons for not reporting research also warrant consideration. Two of the most frequently cited reasons are lack of time and negative attitudes (Bennett & Taylor, 2003; Meline, 2005). Time management for reporting research is discussed in the next section. Some speech-language pathologists and audiologist do not report research because of the fear of rejection, revisions, or self-censorship (Meline, 2005). In recent years, ASHA journals rejected between 39 and 66% of the manuscripts that were submitted (Table 11–2). Moreover, one or more revisions were usually required before any manuscript was accepted for publication (ASHA, 2000). Avoiding peer review may also be seen as a related response. Reports based on opinion and testimonials lack significant credibility and are not accepted for publication in peer-reviewed journals. Therefore, peer review is avoided and such reports are presently directed toward the public and others (Finn, Both, & Bramlett, 2005).

Table 11–2. Acceptance and Rejection Rates for ASHA Journals

Journal	Accept		Reject		Total
	#	%	#	%	#
American Journal of Audiology	58	63	37	39	95
American Journal of Speech-Language Pathology	81	35	158	66	230
Language, Speech and Hearing Services in Schools	106	42	148	58	256
Journal of Speech-Language-Hearing Research					
Speech	___	50	___	50	___
Language	___	42	___	58	___
Hearing	___	48	___	52	___

Myths and Facts About Research Reports

Despite attempts to debunk the myths surrounding research reports, there continue to be several common misconceptions, which Sternberg (1993) identified in his book, *The Psychologist's Companion: A Guide to Scientific Writing for Students and Researchers*. These myths are described in Table 11–3. Identification and understanding of these myths should facilitate more accurate and realistic concepts about reporting research.

Time Management for Reporting Research

Most productive researchers have no more free time or no fewer commitments than those who do not do research. Instead, those who do research simply make the time to do it. It is a matter of prioritizing and managing time. Productive researchers frequently have to rearrange both personal and professional priorities to complete projects (Sternberg, 1981). Like anything else, with practice comes efficiency. The traditional approach to writing requires time for warm-up and reflection, large blocks of time, and uninterrupted working conditions. Another approach preferred by many involves writing in brief spurts (i.e., writing in brief daily sessions) (Boice, 1989).

Silverman (1999) indicated that research need not be excessively time consuming. There is a relationship between unproductive researchers and maladaptive delays of "busyness" and binging (Boice, 1989). Busyness involves keeping busy with less important tasks as a way to avoid high priority tasks. Binging is spending most time on a less important activity. Those who are too busy cannot get everything done, whereas bingers are likely to overprepare for classes.

According to Leedy and Ormrod (2010), the first step in the development of a reasonable writing schedule and sticking to it. Additionally, suggestions are identification of small accomplishable goals within the project; set reasonable dates for completing each goal; reward yourself each time you meet a goal; seek regular feedback; and build time into the schedule for at least two or three rewrites.

From the beginning, a target date should be set for completion of the research report. A personal deadline should pre-empt some time before the actual deadline. The research report should be organized so that it can be completed. If delayed by unavoidable influences, it is necessary to work twice as hard the next day or week, or to work over the weekend to stay on schedule. Robertson (2004) described strategies for managing time that may be helpful such as setting personal goals, using a master list, organizing work space, and being proactive.

It is helpful to develop a timetable of activities required to plan, write, and submit a research report (DePoy & Gitlin, 2011; Polit & Beck, 2010). Table 11–4 provides a list of activities and a schedule for completing a research report. Several activities overlap and some w involve little time; others are more time consuming. The identification and scheduling of tasks to complete the report should facilitate completion of the report within a reasonable period of time. In developing a schedule, several factors should be considered: available resources such as technology support and personnel will influence the amount of time required.

Table 11–3. Research Reports: Myths and Facts

Myth:	Clinicians are not researchers.
Facts:	Clinicians should be researchers.
Myth:	Writing the research report is the most routine, least creative aspect of research, requiring much time bit little creativity.
Facts:	Writing the research report requires both time and creativity.
Myth:	The important consideration is what is said rather than how it is said.
Facts:	How it is said (professional writing style) is an important consideration.
Myth:	Longer papers are better, more papers also better.
Facts:	Concise papers are better, quality of papers is more important that quantitative of papers.
Myth:	The main purpose of a research paper is presentation of facts, whether newly established (experimental research) or established (literature review, tutorials).
Facts:	Research papers have several purposes: analysis/synthesis of past and current research, drawing conclusions, and providing suggestions for future research.
Myth:	The difference between scientific writing and advertising is that the purpose of the former is to inform and the latter is to persuade.
Facts:	Scientific writing and advertising may both inform and persuade.
Myth:	An acceptable way to gain acceptance of a theory is to refute another theory.
Facts:	An acceptable way to gain acceptance of a theory is to provide credible evidence.
Myth:	Negative results which fail to support a hypothesis are as valuable as positive results that so not support the hypothesis.
Facts:	Both negative and positive results can improve knowledge and understanding.
Myth:	Logical development of ideas in a research paper reflects historical development of ideas.
Facts:	Logical development of ideas in a research paper may not reflect the historical background.

Table 11–4. Steps and Schedule of Writing a Research Report

Steps	Schedule
Prewriting/planning stage	
Review requirement for submitting report	
Obtain permission(s) to use previously published material(s)	
Decide on authorship and order of authors	
Determine level of evidence relevant to topic	
Assemble materials needed to write report	
Writing first draft	
Title page	
Abstract	
Key words	
Introduction (background)	
Statement of problem (purpose)	
Method	
Results	
Discussion	
Conclusions	
Author contributions	
Contact information	
References (all references cited both in text and list)	
Tables and figures	
Documentation of informed consent	
Documentation of IRB approval	
Resources and environment	
Review and revision	
Revise first draft and subsequent revisions	
Editing	
Review and revise the last complete draft	
Final editing and proofreading	
Prepare final report	
Submit manuscript and cover letter	
Assemble report copies and accompanying materials	

Source: Reprinted from *Writing and Publishing in Medicine*, by E. J. Huth, 1999, Baltimore, MD: Lippincott Williams & Wilkins. Copyright 1999, with permission from Elsevier.

Other activities that will take time include securing necessary permission and holding meetings or communicating with co-authors.

Efficient use of computer technology can increase productivity because of its speed and accuracy. Computers are used for a variety of research tasks: searching the literature, sampling, recording observations, and qualitative and quantitative data analysis (Maxwell & Satake, 2006; McMillan, 2004; Polit & Beck, 2010).

In addition, some types of research are less time consuming than others (Hegde, 2003b; Maxwell & Satake, 2006; Meline 2006). Single-subject research designs require less time because clinical service can be integrated with experimental evaluation. Use of single-subject designs can provide answers to many clinically relevant questions. As Connell and McReynolds (1988) concluded, "individual contact with a client over an extended time interval is the basic requirement for implementation of single-subject experimental designs" (p. 1062). This also helps dispel the myth that there is a division between clinical and research activities.

Procrastination

Related to time management is procrastination or needless delay in beginning or completing a research project. Procrastination may include discomfort, anxiety, busyness, or binging (Boice, 1989). It may reflect a fear of failure or success. And/or reflect a need to rebel. Carter-Scott (1989) refers to procrastination as the *manana syndrome* and describes it as "the precise behavior which keeps you from meeting deadlines, doing what you say you will do, and reinforcing the fact that you're not up to the challenges" (p. 21). Several strategies have been described to reduce procrastination such as cognitive-behavioral orientation, reprogramming negative attitudes, prioritization, contingency management, procrastination support groups, and time slots. Roth (1989) suggested maintaining a research log or journal from the beginning to the end of a research project, including the completed research report and submission of the report for presentation and/or publication Table 11–5. This information can also be used to determine authorship contributions.

Table 11–5. Research Log Example

Date	Time	Entry
Date of entry	Record time; stop and start	Specify what was done.
3/18/06	10:00–11:45 AM	Computer references search; located articles of interest; requested interlibrary load for journal articles not available.
3/19/06	1:00–2:30 PM	Reviewed articles.
3/21/06	9:30–11:00 AM	Drafted outline and working title.

Several professional journals request that authors disclose their contributions (AMA 2006; Bates et al., 2004). The log can also be used to verify supervision.

Format of Research Reports

Research reports contain most, if not all, of the sections listed in Table 11–6. Further description of selected parts of research follows in this section: abstracts, key words, author contributions and tables and figures. Sometimes the results and discussion sections are combined. The format of research is fairly consistent across different types of reports such as thesis, dissertations journal articles, and papers for professional meetings (Polit & Beck, 2010). Extensive discussions of the format for written reports can be found in the *Publication Manual of the American Psychological Association (2010),* the *American Medical Association Manual of Style* AMA, (2007), Schiavetti, Metz, and Orlikoff (2010), and Silverman (1998).

Table 11–6. Format for Research Report

Title page	Title, name of authors, and institutional affiliation
Abstract	Summary including methods, results, implications
Key words	Short list of words for indexing
Introduction	Untitled; begins body of paper; review of relevant literature, theoretical foundations and rationale, purpose/ research questions or hypothesis
Method	Design of study, subjects, sampling techniques, controls, equipment or test materials, experimental procedures, rationale for choice of statistics
Results	Summary and evaluation of relevant data, tables, and figures
Discussion	Comparison of findings to previous research, limitations, implications for clinical practice, and future research
Author information	Contains information
Author contributions	Disclose of contributions to report
Acknowledgments	Recognition of support from individuals and/or organizations
References	All cited sources of information
Tables and figures	Visual presentation of information
Appendix	Contains information that cannot be integrated in text; usually contains unpublished information

Abstracts

An abstract is a brief comprehensive summary of a report (APA, 2010). The *abstract* may be the most important part of a report because it may be the only part that many people read. Most professional journals use structured abstracts because they provide more detailed and consistent information. In addition, structured abstracts make literature searches easier (Editors, 2004).

There are two types of structured abstracts. The first is for original reports and the second is for review or tutorial reports. The primary information for these abstracts is summarized in Table 11–7. No information should be reported in the abstract that does not appear in the text of the paper (AMA, 2006).

ASHA journals use modified abstract which includes the following sections: purpose; method; results; and conclusions. The *Annals of Internal Medicine* (Editors, 2004) added a section on Limitations located immediately before Conclusions. The Limitation section reduced the risk of overgeneralization, overinterpre-

Table 11–7. Information Required for Structured Abstract

Original Reporting

1. Objective: exact question(s) addressed by the report
2. Design: the basic design of the study
3. Setting: the location and level of clinical care
4. Patients or participants: the manner of selection and number of patients or participants who entered and completed the study
5. Interventions: the exact treatment or intervention, if any
6. Main outcome measures: the primary study outcome measure as planned before data collection began
7. Results: the key findings
8. Conclusions: key conclusions including direct clinical applications

Review

1. Purpose: the primary objective of the review paper
2. Data sources: a succinct summary of data sources
3. Study selection: the number of studies selected for review and how they were selected.
4. Data extraction: rules for abstracting data and dhow they were applied
5. Results of data synthesis: the method of data synthesis and key results
6. Conclusions: key conclusions, including potential applications and research needs.

Source: Adapted from "More Informative Abstracts Revisited," by R. B. Haynes, C. D. Mulrow, E. J. Huth, D. G. Altman, and M. J. Gardner, 1996, *Cleft Palate Craniofacial Journal, 33*(1), pp. 1–9.

tation, or overexplaining the evidence. It also helps readers understand how one report differs from another on the same topic.

Key Words (Indexing Terms)

Most journals include a list of key words or indexing terms that represent content of the report including words in the title or abstract. They are placed on the abstract page following the abstract. These words assist in locating research reports in computer databases such as Medline and CINAHL (Depoy & Gitlin, 2011, McMillan, 2005; Silverman, 1998). MEDLINE is the database most commonly used in health care and is one of the largest in the world. CINAHL (Cumulative Index to Nursing and Allied Health Literature) focuses on publications from the allied health professions.

Author Contributions

Several professional journals require that authors disclose their contributions to a report. Each author specifies their contributions which are published before the acknowledgement section. Some examples are as follows:

Study concept and design

Acquisition of data

Analysis and interpretation of data

Drafting of the manuscript

Critical revision of the manuscript for important intellectual content

Statistical analysis

Obtaining funding

Administrative, technical, or material support

Study supervision.

All authors of a group should have full access to all of the data in the report and be responsible for integrity and accuracy of the report.

Tables and Figures

A wide variety of tables and figures have been described that are used to present complex information in a concise, visual format. Table and figures should not be used when results can be easily expressed in the test of a report (Nichol & Pexman, 1999). Tables generally present exact numerical values, and the data are arranged in an orderly display of columns and rows (APA, 2010). A figure is any kind of graphic illustration other than a table.

Harris (1999) defined and illustrated more than 400 tables and figures. Among the most frequently used figures are pie charts, bar graphs, scatter plots and curves (DePoy & Gitlin, 2011). Less frequently used figures are concept maps and V-diagrams. Curves refer to any line on a figure used to represent a set or series of data (Harris, 1999).

Computer software is available for preparation of tables and figures. Among the available programs are IBM SPSS, Microsoft Excel, Adobe Photoshop, Adobe Illustrator, PowerPoint, and Corel Draw.

Tables and figures should be clear enough to stand alone without explanation in the text (Bless & Forister, 2012). General guidelines for tables and figures are listed in Tables 11–8 and 11–9.

Table 11–8. Guidelines for Preparing Tables

- Select a clear and specific table
- Number tables consecutively
- Use subheadings for columns and rows
- Only include information related to the title
- Do not explain table in text it should stand alone
- Use consistent format that confirms to publisher's guidelines. Refer to instructions to Authors.
- Avoid excessive lines. Usually vertical lines are not needed
- Use appropriate units of measure

Source: From *Research and Medical Literature*, by J. D. Blessing and J. G. Forister, 2012, Burlington, MA: Jones and Bartlett.

Table 11–9. Guidelines for Preparing Figures

- Labeling table as a figure not a table
- Select appropriate type of figure based on data, statistical analysis and readability
- Title should be self-explanatory
- Refer to figure in text; number consecutively
- Check spelling and plotting of data
- Review publisher's guidelines for overall size, resolution and specification: See instruction for authors
- Include legends if necessary, define abbreviations
- Update permission from copyright holder

Source: From *Research and Medical Literature*, by J. D. Blessing and J. G. Forister, 2012, Burlington, MA: Jones and Bartlett.

Diagrams and Maps

There are several reasons for using diagrams and maps to display research data. Among the reasons are: (1) simplify complex information; (2) summarize or enhance certain findings; (3) illustrate complicated results; (4) demonstrate trends or redundancies in research (Nichol & Pexman, 2003).

According to the APA (2010) Manual, both diagrams and maps are types of figures. The main types of diagrams are graphs and charts. The former are described as "typically displaying the relationship between two quantitative indices, or between a continuous quantitative variable" and the later are "generally displays of quantitative information such as the flow of subjects through a process (APA, 2010, p. 150). Maps usually present spatial information (APA, 2010).

Diagrams and maps are often created by using available computer programs such as Microsoft Word and Microsoft Excel. There are a variety of diagrams and maps for displaying information. A V-diagram consists of 12 elements and is provided in Figure 11–1. Information Graphics by Harris (1999) is a comprehensive

CONCEPTUAL/THEORETICAL
(Thinking)

FOCUS/RESEARCH:

QUESTION

METHODOLOGICAL
(Doing)

WORLD VIEW:

The general belief system motivating and guiding the inquiry.

PHILOSOPHY:

The beliefs about the nature of knowledge and knowing guiding the inquiry.

THEORY:

The general principles guiding the inquiry that explain *why* events or objects exhibit what is observed.

PRINCIPLES:

Statements of relationships between concepts that explain *how* events or objects can be expected to appear or behave.

CONSTRUCTS:

Ideas showing specific relationships between concepts, without direct origin in events or objects.

CONCEPTS:

Perceived regularity in events or objects (or records of events or events or objects) designated by a label.

VALUE CLAIMS:

Statements based on knowledge claims declare the worth or value of the inquiry.

KNOWLEDGE CLAIMS:

Statements that answer the focus or research question(s) and are reasonable interpretations of the transformed records (or data) obtained.

TRANSFORMATIONS:

Tables, graphs, concept maps, statistics, or other forms of organization of records made.

RECORDS:

The observations made and recorded from the events/objects studied.

EVENTS AND/OR OBJECTS:

Description of the events(s) and/or object(s) to be studied in order to answer the focus/research question.

Figure 11–1. V-diagram (Adapted from *The Art of Educating with V Diagrams*, by D. B. Gowin and M. C. Alvarez, 2005, New York, NY: Cambridge).

448 page illustrated reference book. Yau (2011) has step by step guidelines for graphics from start to finish. These guidelines are for visualizing patterns over time, proportions relationship differences, and spatial relationships.

The following guidelines for diagrams and maps have been described by Nichol and Pexman (2003):

■ Must be referred to in test
■ Information should be as simple as possible
■ Only relevant information should be included;
■ Labels should be consistent; and
■ Use of color should be avoided because most print information is black and white.

General guidelines for evaluating diagrams and maps have been described by Nichol and Paxman (2003). These criteria are: text diagrams and maps use a simple format; font size in diagrams and maps do not vary by more than four fonts; captions are typed double spaced on a separate page; lines are thick enough to be clear after reduction; similar diagrams or maps within the same manuscript should have a similar appearance; and diagrams and maps are referred to in the text using the same number(s) as in the caption(s). Detailed strategies for evaluating V-diagrams and concept maps have been developed by Gowin and Alvarez (2005).

Writing Styles

Although there are different types of research reports, the style should be similar, that is, simple and clear as pos-sible. Clear writing is concise, not wordy or redundant. Research reports are of limited value if they are not understandable. Several guides for writing style are available (American Medical Association Manual of Style, 1998; American Psychological Association, 2010; Chicago Manual of Style, 2008; Hegde, 2010, Modern Language Association of America, 2003; Strunk & White, 1979; Turabian, 1995). The style should be consistent with the requirements of the university for theses, or dissertations, or of the journal to which the report is submitted.

APA Format

All publications of the America-Speech-Language-Hearing Association (ASHA) follow the style of the American Psychologal Association that is in the *Publication Manual of the American Psychological Association* (2010a). A training supplement to the APA publication manual (APA, 2010b) is available.

The *APA Manual* (2010a) provides information about content and organization of research reports as well as rules for citing references and organizing a reference list. The Manual also includes guidelines about punctuation, spelling, capitalization, headings, quotations, numbers, tables, and figures.

References

All parts of every reference should be checked against the original publication. Every reference cited in the text should be listed; conversely, every reference listed should be cited in the text.

Mistakes in referencing are too common. These mistakes are usually related to plagiarism, use of secondary sources, and not reading the source. Plagiarism is sometimes unintentional, that is, the author did not intend to plagiarize (DePoy & Gitlin, 2011). To avoid this potentially devastating mistake one should be aware of the standards for referencing. All work written by another person, even if not directly quoted, must be cited. The use of secondary sources is not acceptable, that is, only primary sources should be cited. Another common error is the use of citations that have not been read.

Personal Pronouns

The use of personal pronouns such as "I," "my," "you," and "we" should be avoided in research reports because of the appearance of subjectivity. However, several journals are beginning to break with this tradition (Polit & Beck, 2010).

Avoid Bias

Research reports should be objective and free from bias about gender, individuals, and groups (APA, 2010a; Hegde, 2010). APA (2010a) has specific guidelines to reduce bias in language: (1) describe at the appropriate level of specificity; (2) be sensitive to labels; and (3) acknowledge participation.

Racism and sexism are probably most common. Racist expressions should be avoided in describing participants and discussing results. Hegde (2003) advises that "if it is necessary to identify participants as belonging to a particular ethnic or cultural group, terms that are nonevaluative should be used. The best practice is to select the terms the group use to refer to themselves" (p. 479). Expressions

such as culturally deprived or disadvantaged are also biased and imply that one culture is the standard against which other cultures are evaluated.

Sexism in language has a long history and may not be easily recognized. It is inherently discriminatory and suggests an unjustified bias against an individual or a group, usually women, but sometimes men (Schneider & Soto, 1989). Sexist language should be avoided in speaking and writing. There is nothing more out of contact with reality than believing women are not equal to men. One of the most misused personal pronouns is *he*, which is frequently used to refer to someone of unidentified gender, such as a child, client, customer, or student (Hedge, 2003b). Indiscriminate use of personal pronouns may suggest that all authors, bankers, deans, department heads, doctors, editors, executives, fire fighters, lawyers, police officers, presidents, or professors are male. The noun *man* is often inappropriately used in ways that also implies sexism. For example, *chairman* of a department or organization. Chair*person* or simply *chair* is appropriate. Apparently, there is some truth in Barzun's (1986) statement that "sex is a source of chaos in language generally, as it is in life" (p. 37).

In 1979, the ASHA Committee on Equality of Sexes adopted the American Psychological Association Guidelines for Unbiased Language. These guidelines provide specific suggestions and examples for gender-free writing. ASHA (1993) also provided guidelines for gender equality in language usage which include "being specific about gender when inclusion of this information is relevant and avoids generalization which may lead to stereotyping" (p. 42). Other useful references are *The Handbook of*

Nonsexist Writing by Miller and Swift (1988), *The Nonsexist Communicator* by Sorrels (1983), and *The Elements of Nonsexist Usage* by Drummond (1990).

"Person first" language should be used to describe individuals with disabilities, that is, put the person first, not the disability. According to APA (2010a) "the guiding principle for nonhandicapping language is to maintain the integrity of individuals as human beings" (p. 76). Table 11–10 provides a list of person first phrases and those which should avoided. Folkins (1992) described five principles for the language used to describe individuals with disabilities. These principles are: (1) person first language; (2) disability versus handicap; (3) everyone likes to think of themselves as normal; (4) avoid terms that project unnecessary negative connotations; and (5) do not overdo it.

There are other words which are misused. Huth (1990) described some words as dehumanizing, for example, case and patient or client. Case is an episode or example of illness, injury, or disease. Patient or client is the person cared for by the speech-language pathologist or audiologist. Patients or clients are cared for, not cases. Another misused word is subject or participant. The term participants should be used because it acknowledges that participants have an active role in research studies (APA, 2010a).

Permissions

The legal reason for seeking appropriate permission when using previously published materials is related to copyright law (APA, 2010a; Huth, 1999). Most publications are copyrighted; legal ownership is vested to the copyright holder. Permission for reproduction of published material must be obtained from the copyright holder or the writer and publisher are at risk for legal action because of copyright infringement for unauthorized use of published materials. When in doubt about the need for permission, it is probably better to request it. Permission should be sought well in advance. Figure 11–2 provides an example of a letter requesting permission to use copy-

Table 11–10. Person First Language

Preferred	Avoid
Children with cleft palate	Cleft palate children
Persons who stutter	Stutterers
Adults with aphasia	Aphasic adults
The lawyer who has dyslexia	The dyslexic lawyer
The client with hearing impairment	The hearing-impaired client

Source: Adapted from *The Language Used to Describe Individuals with Disabilities,* by J. Folkins. Available from http://www.asha.org/about/publications/journal-abstracts/submission/person_first.htm#one. Copyright 1992 by the American Speech-Language-Hearing Association. All rights reserved.

righted material. Most publishers have form letters or online forms for requesting permission to use copyrighted mate- rial. Additional information about permission is available elsewhere (APA, 2010a; Huth, 1999).

I am preparing a manuscript:

_____
(title of book)

_____
(author/editor of book)

to be published in _____(approx. date) by

_____
(publisher's name and address)

I would like to include in it the material specified below:

Author:
Title:
Date:
Figure or table number(s):

I request permission to reprint the specified material in this book and in future revisions and editions thereof, for possible licensing and distribution throughout the world in all languages. If you do not control these rights in their entirety, would you please let me know where else to write. Proper acknowledgment of title, author, publisher, city, and copyright date (for journals; author, article title, journal name, volume, first page of article, and year) will be given. If the permission of the author is also required, please supply a current address. For your convenience, you may simply sign the release form below. A copy of this request is enclosed for your files.

Thank you,
Author_____   My return address is (please print)
                (please print)   _____
Date_____   _____
                                    _____

PERMISSION GRANTED:

_____   _____
Signature   Date

Figure 11–2. Request for permission. From *Singular Manual of Textbook Preparation*, by M. N. Hedge, 1991, San Diego, CA: Singular Publishing Group. Reproduced with permission fro copyright holder M. N. Hedge.

Rewriting and Revising

Rewriting and revision are an important part of writing because authors are usually asked to make revisions (Portney & Watkins (2009). For most, even those who are experienced writers—writing is hard work. The first or rough draft should not be the final draft. Even experienced writers revise manuscripts several times. Often, the final draft is much different from the first or original draft (Hegde, 2003). Editing and rewriting are the steps to good writing. These steps are listed in Table 11–11.

Rewriting is not easy for several reasons. Self-editing is difficult because it requires critical evaluation of one's own writing (Hegde, 2003b). Rewriting requires very focused attention to details and usually reorganization of the paper (Meline, 2006). Lack of time may also prevent revision of a paper. Another problem is related to co-authors who may not be able to respond with suggestions

Table 11–11. Steps in Writing and Revising Reports

Write first draft
Hold first draft 1–2 weeks, then revise
Second draft
Distribute copies to co-authors and to colleagues willing to critically review
Read draft, make notes on needed revisions
Get written recommendations for revisions from co-authors and colleagues
Third draft same sequences as second
Later drafts
Continue reading to co-authors
Concentrate on content and structure
When satisfied with content, revise style
Review and revise large elements first
Paragraph lengths
External and internal sequence of paragraphs
Consider sentences: length; variety
Elements of sentences: clarify and phrasing; modifying word choices
Read the revised text to identify and correct "overlooked flaws"

Source: Reprinted from *Writing and Publishing in Medicine,* by E. J. Huth, 1999, Baltimore, MD: Lippincott Williams & Wilkins. Copyright 1999, with permission from Elsevier.

for revision(s) (Huth, 1999). Rewriting and revising increased the likelihood of acceptance although it is no guarantee.

Some writers revise content, structure, and style of a paper at the same time; others revise content and structure first and then style. The content of a paper is more likely to determine whether it is accepted for publications than style. Writing style includes paragraph length and structure, paragraph linkage, sentence variety and word choices. Further detailed information about writing style is available in Huth's (1999) Writing *and Publishing in Medicine: The Publication Manual of the American Psychological Association (*2010a), and the *American Medical Association Manual of Style* (AMA, 1998). Strategies for improving writing styles are: writing from an outline; putting the first draft aside for a week or two before revising; and having colleagues critically review the draft (APA, 2010a; Huth, 1999).

Translating Research Reports to Published Papers

Most research presented at professional meetings (platform presentations and poster presentations) is not subsequently published in peer-reviewed journals. There are two reasons for this failure to complete a full manuscript and submit it to a peer-reviewed journal. First, research accepted for presentation at a professional meeting might not stand up under peer review because it is flawed. Second, preparing a manuscript can be overwhelming especially for beginning presenters.

Many of the reasons for a manuscript rejection can be avoided. Therefore, it is useful to be aware of reasons for rejecting manuscripts. Among the reasons are: inappropriate or incomplete statistics; overgeneralization of results; inappropriate or substandard instrumentation; sample too small or biased; writing style flaws; insufficient problem statement; inaccurate or inconsistent data; and inadequate tables or figures (Pierson, 2004).

Types of Research Reports

The organization and style of research reports is fairly consistent across different types of reports, although there is some variation. This section describes the major types of research reports: journal articles, these and dissertations, textbooks, and presentation at professional meetings. Other types of research reports, systematic reviews, and reports to funding agencies are described elsewhere in Chapters 5 and 14, respectively.

Journal Articles

Publication in a journal ensures wide circulation of research findings. Research reports are often substituted for publication after presentation at a professional meeting or they may be reduced reports of research findings from these and dissertations. Many manuscripts are now submitted online. Manuscripts submitted to ASHA are submitted online via ASHA manuscript central, online manuscript submission and review center at http://mc.manuscriptcentral.com/asha. When submitting a manuscript, it must include a cover letter requesting that the manuscript be considered for publication. The following information should be included in the cover letter:

- Request that the manuscript be considered for publication
- Verification that all authors have made contributions that justify authorship
- Affirms compliance with ethical considerations for protection of human and animal subjects in research
- Copy of permission granted to reproduce or adapt any copyright material
- Verification that the manuscript has not been previously published in the same, or essentially the same, form
- Notice that the manuscript is not currently under review elsewhere
- Disclosure of any real or potential conflicts of interest
- Author's professional address, telephone and fax numbers, E-mail address.

An example of a cover letter is shown in Figure 11–3.

Manuscripts submitted for publication in peer-review journals are reviewed and evaluated by peers who are experts in the subject area. Non-peer-reviewed journals do not require a critical review of manuscripts by peers with relevant expertise. There is a greater likelihood that the former contribute to the scientific knowledge base in speech-language pathology and audiology and have clinical relevance and credibility.

Journals in speech-language pathology and audiology publish several types of articles, which are described in the next section. ASHA journals provide descriptions of types of articles, at the end of each issue. Additional information about types of articles is also available in the *American Medical Association Manual of Style* (Iverson et al., 1993), *AMA Information for Authors* (2006), and the *Publication of the American Psychological Association* (APA, 2010a).

Selecting a Journal

Selecting a journal to submit a manuscript to is important and should be an early step in planning a paper. Steps in publishing a paper and possible outcomes are shown in Figure 11–4. In addition to ASHA journals, there are several other journals that publish information about speech-language pathology and audiology. Maxwell and Satake (1999) and Huth (1999) suggested the following questions be considered in selecting a journal:

1. Is the topic of the proposed paper within the scope of the journal?
2. Is the topic reported in the journal frequently or only rarely?
3. Would the journal be the best match of readers with that topic?
4. What formats does the journal accept?
5. Does the journal publish an "information for authors" page or issue similar information on-line?

Information relevant to these questions can usually be found on a journal's information-for-authors page in the journal or at its Web site. Huth (1999) suggests if one is uncertain about selecting the right journal "then write or call the journal's editor" (p. 16). This should probably be avoided because many editors of journals do not encourage such questions because the information is usually avail-

John Jones, PhD

Editor, Language and Speech Journal

9120 Miracle Road

Greenville, LA 54681

Dear Dr. Jones:

I am submitting this manuscript, "Happy days in Speech and Language," for publication consideration in the Language and speech Journal. The manuscript complies with ethical and authorship guidelines:

— Each authors' contributions are appropriate for authorship

— All of the authors have agreed to the order of authorship

— No copyrighted material is to be reproduced in the material

— The manuscript is not currently under review elsewhere

— Disclosure about previous public presentations elsewhere: the paper was presented in part as a poster session at the annual meeting of the American Speech Language Hearing Association

— There is no real or potential conflict of interest

I have assumed responsibility for keeping the co-authors informed about the status of the manuscript through the editorial review process, the content of the reviews, and any revisions.

Thank you for your time and effort on our behalf. I look forward to hearing from you.

Sincerely,

J. B. Smith

Senior Speech-Language Pathologist

Figure 11–3. Sample letter for submitting a manuscript.

able elsewhere, that is, in the instructions for authors.

It also may be helpful to consider the quality of the journals. This can be based on citation analysis which is an examination of the frequency and patterns of citations of print materials. Citation analysis reflects the quality of journals in print. The Impact Factor is also used as an indicator of quality. It is the number of times a report is cited in a given year divided by the total number of reports published. Higher values suggest greater credibility and greater and higher impact. There has

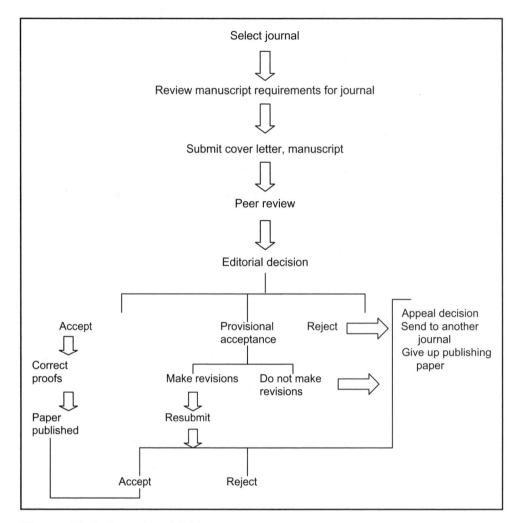

Figure 11–4. Steps in publishing a paper.

been criticism about the impact factor relative to its use to evaluate individuals rather than journals and distribute research funds (Hirschbok, 2011; Schute & Svec, 2007).

Black (2001) reported that the most important journals in communication disorders were:

Journal of Speech, Language, and Hearing Research

Journal of the Acoustical Society of America

Brain and Language

Journal of Fluency Disorders

Ear and Hearing

Language, Speech and Hearing Services in Schools

Journal of Communication Disorders.

Categories of Reports in ASHA Journals

ASHA publishers original research reports, reviews, and tutorials, special forums, letters to the editor, and general other categories of articles in their journals, namely, *American Academy of Audiology, American Journal of Speech-Language Pathology, Journal of Speech-Language and Hearing Research,* and *Language, Speech and Hearing Services in Schools.* Topics include subjects related to communication sciences and to the clinical practice of speech-language pathology and audiology.

Research reports are based on data, descriptive, ethnographic, or experimental studies. They also include case studies, which follow case study designs and require information about the reliability of the data reported. Reviews and tutorials are reports of interest to speech-language pathologists and audiologists that cover recent literature, clinical implications, and the need for further research. Special forums focus on a specific topic. Letters to the editor provide readers an opportunity to respond to recently published papers. Conversely, the author(s) of the report is given the opportunity to respond to a letter to the editor.

Theses and Dissertations

Some master's programs and most doctoral programs in speech-language pathology and audiology require completion of a written thesis (masters) or dissertation (doctoral). Theses and dissertations usually document a research project. Most universities have a required format for theses and dissertations. Examples of typical formats can be found in the *APA Manual* (2010a); Cone and Foster (2006); Davis (1997); and Polit and Beck, 2010). A written research proposal, or prospectus, is a prerequisite for approval of either a thesis or dissertation (Maxwell & Satake, 2006). Prior

to writing a prospectus, an advisor and a committee with relevant expertise are selected. A prospectus is important because it is as an action plan for the proposed research and may prevent future criticisms of the research by committee members. The content of theses and dissertations is often appropriate for publication but the format and content usually requires extensive revisions (ASHA, 2000). The format of theses and dissertations is similar to a book. The content is very detailed, and more comprehensive than required for publication. In other words, the length must be reduced for publication. Some suggestions for reducing length are: narrow the focus to a specific topic; be specific in reporting the results; avoid problems common to beginning authors; omit information that is not appropriate for journal articles; and be selective in the use of references. The only requirement for publication is that enough information is provided to replicate the study.

The best time to publish data from a thesis or dissertation is when the information is "fresh" (Davis, 1999). It is easier to prepare a manuscript while the data are new because it becomes increasingly difficult to so as time passes. Furthermore, the impact of the research will be limited if not submitted for publication. For these reasons, some advisory committees suggest that the thesis or dissertation be in the format of a journal article or articles.

Textbooks

There are five types of publishers for textbooks: professional associations; trade publishers; university-affiliated centers; university presses, and vanity presses. Publishers differ in the review process, types of manuscripts published, marketing strategies, and contractual arrangements with authors (Luey, 1987).

Some professional associations, including ASHA, publish books. ASHA's first book was published in 1954 (Paden, 1970). The Association's most recent book, *Business Matters: A Guide for Speech-Language Pathologists*, was published in 2004 (Gloper & Brown).

There are two types of trade publishers: (1) general trade publishers who target nonfiction of interest to the general public and (2) specialized or professional publishers who focus on specific professional groups. Frequently, universities publish books in their specialty areas, although these publications are sometimes limited to research sponsored by the university. University presses are the primary outlet for book-length scholarly reports. They vary greatly in size; some publish hundreds of books a year, others publish fewer than one a year. Some university presses publish on a variety of subjects; others focus on a few areas. Vanity or subsidy publishers charge money to publish; in other words, if the author pays, the vanity press publishes the book. Obviously, there is no peer review. Therefore, publications by a vanity press carry no prestige and no merit for academic promotion or tenure.

The primary issue in selecting a publisher is whether they publish information about issues related to speech-language pathology and audiology. A book proposal or manuscript submitted to a publisher should be in proper form for the publisher. The author should obtain guidelines for preparing proposals and manuscripts from the publisher to which they plan to submit their manuscript.

University presses and trade houses usually base their publishing decisions on the opinions of reviewers. When a publisher receives a manuscript, it is read by an editor to determine if it is appropriate for the publisher and to assess the quality of the writing. A manuscript may be rejected on the basis of the editor's reading or it may be sent out to reviewer's or referees. Publishers often request that reviewers complete questionnaires similar to the forms used for evaluating research reports. A manuscript may be accepted with revisions, or rejected.

Presentations at Professional Meetings

ASHA, AAA, state speech-language-hearing associations, and other professional organizations have meetings at which research is presented, either through oral reports or poster presentations. Presentation at a professional meeting is often linked with publication of similar information in a journal article. That is, oral reports or poster presentation may precede development of a manuscript for publication. Organizing and planning a presentation for a professional meeting and preparing a manuscript are smellier up to a point.

Presentations of research at professional meetings have several advantages: (1) there is usually less time between completion of the research and dissemination of the findings; (2) one receives immediate feedback; (3) it is interactive, that is, interaction between the author and audience; and (4) it allows networking with others who have similar interests and possible future research (Maxwell & Satake, 2006; Polit & Beck, 2010). Presentations at professional meetings are less valued as scholarly products. Table 11–12 provides a comparison about oral reports and poster presentations. Submitting a presentation for a meeting is somewhat simpler than for submitting a manuscript

Table 11–12. Comparison of Oral Reports and Poster Presentation

Characteristic	Oral Reports	Poster Presentations
Materials	Slides, computer, notes	Poster, Velcro
Subject	Justify objectives, refer to literature, support; methods and results	Justify objectives; refer to literature, support methods and results
Preparation	Formal speech to adhere to time limits	Answers to expected questions
	Prepare early; practice, review, revise	Prepare early, construct posters, review, revise
Style	More formal; contact one to many	Relatively informal; contact one to one or one to a few
	Speaker standing, audience seated	Both speaker and audience standing
Moderator	Moderator introduces, buffer audience, keep time	No moderator, direct control, no buffer
Time	Limited	Flexible
Audience	Captive, not likely to leave	Free, only interested stay
Discussion	Declamation from speaker with short questions	Chiefly questions and answer or conversational discussion
Handouts	Possible	Helpful

Source: Adapted from *Scientific Papers and Presentations,* by M. Davis, 1997, New York, NY: Academic Press.

to a journal. ASHA requires electronic submissions through the ASHA Web site. Some states organizations also require electronic submission, although others continue to use main-in submission.

Usually, the professional organization announces a "Call for Papers" on its Web site or written materials (newsletter, journals) about 6 to 9 months before the meeting. The announcement includes instructions/requirements and deadlines for submission. If the submission is accepted, the author is required to appear at the meeting to make the presentation.

Regardless of the type of proposed presentation, it must meet certain criteria to be accepted. ASHA's program committee selects proposals based on the following criteria: strength of theoretical rationale; originality of research; strength of research design; credibility of data; integration of findings; and overall clarity.

Oral Reports

Oral reports usually last between 10 and 15 minutes and are followed by a question-and-answer period. These presentations frequently use slides and occasionally handouts. Organization of oral reports is similar to that of a journal article (Silverman, 1998). However, there are differences related to length: less detailed because of limited time; style: less formal and more redundant; and language: less formal and more conversational.

General characteristics of an oral report are presented in Table 11–12. Additional guidelines include do not "wing it" or read the paper and, whenever possible, use appropriate visual supplements present complex information (APA 2010a). In addition, the skilled presenter: (1) captures the audience's attention at the very beginning; (2) clearly states the objectives of the presentation; (3) concentrates on concepts, not confusing details; (4) presents important concepts in different ways; (5) uses slides or less complexity than published table and figures; and (6) prepares for a question and answer period.

A first time presenter is usually more anxious that an experience presenter. Also to be considered is the size of the audience, typically as the larger the audience the greater the anxiety. Presenters should also be aware of other factors that affect oral presentations. These factors include:

- quality of the presenter's speech and manner;
- physical or nonverbal aspects the presenter (appearance, eye contact, facial expression, gesture enthusiasm, dress, grooming).
- confidence and poise;
- knowledge of information related to effective presentations, (Goldfarb & Serpanos, 2009).

Poster Presentations

Poster sessions have become a major format for presenting research at professional meeting. A poster session at a professional conference consists of several simultaneous visual displays of research studies. Attendees circulate around the posters during the session (Polit & Beck, 2011). Poster presentation may be formal or open. In formal poster presentations the author presents an overview of the poster with a moderator who guides discussion about each poster in a symposium format. The author is present at an open session to answer attendee's questions. Most organizations have specific instructions for poster presentations. Generally, the title is at the top followed by author(s) and affiliation. The introduction is in the upper left corner and the conclusions in the right lower corner. Traditional posters have the advantage of permitting simultaneous sessions within the same time period. Poster presentations allow participants to select information of interest, receive substantial information within a short period of time, and avoid posters dealing with topics of less interest to them. For some presentations, poster presentations are less threatening (Maxwell & Satake, 2006). Traditional poster presentations also have disadvantages. First, preparing posters requires more effort and expense than preparing for an oral report. Second, posters, like wedding dresses, are often not used subsequently. Third, a presentation can be seriously disadvantaged if placed in an awkward, crowded location or in poor lighting conditions (Simmonds, 1984). It might be best, if possible, to check the room in advance when doing a poster presentation (Deep & Sussman, 1990). Problems identified early may be resolved. An example involves placing posters on a crowded stage, which was inaccessible to participants in wheelchairs or on crutches. Fourth, posters at times can be difficult to transport (Bordens & Abbott, 1988).

In recent years more poster presentations have been electronic. The primary differences between traditional and electronic poster presentations are related to the presence of an author and attendees. These and other differences are compared in Table 11–13.

General guidelines for posters according to Bless and Forister (2011) are:

■ Keep the poster simple.
■ Include only enough information to support the conclusions.
■ Use tables and figures; less text is better.

Templates are available for preparing posters as well as computer generated programs such as Power Point, Microsoft Excel, and Statistical Programs for the Social Sciences (SPSS). Leedy and Ormrod (2010) provided detailed descriptions of Microsoft Excel and SPSS. Nichol and Pexman (2003) provided guidelines for the content and style of posters. Considerations related to content were to consider the main point, key points of information for attendees, crucial details, methodology, the most important results, and realistic conclusions. Style was related to available space: one large poster or a poster consisting of small panels.

Visual Supplements

Visual supplements are essential to oral presentations and posters. A visual supplement is any illustration used to clarify and analyze information in written or reports and oral presentations. The most common visual supplements are tables and figures which were discussed earlier in the chapter under the section on Format of Research Reports. Handouts may be used to supplement oral reports and poster presentations. They should include the title of the report, the authors 'name and affiliation, and where and when presented. PowerPoint slides or a mini poster are frequently used as handouts. It is recommended that handouts for oral reports be distributed prior to the

Table 11–13. Characteristics of Traditional and Electronic Poster Presentations

	Traditional	Electronic
Access	Live	Remote
Audience	Restricted	Widespread
Schedule	Fixed	Flexible
Frequency	Nonrepeatable	Repeatable
CEUs	Inconsistent	Consistent
Duplication	Impossible	Possible
Author and audience	Present	Not present
Access	Direct	Indirect or direct

presentation, not while the presentation is occurring. Instead of, or in addition to handouts, some presenters distribute diskettes containing information about the presentation (Nichol & Pexman, 2003). However, this can be expensive.

Guidelines for visual supplements are listed in Table 11–14. Criteria for visuals are: simplicity, legibility, unity, quality, and feasibility. Visuals should be cohesive and uniform with other visual supplements and with the written or spoken words. Production and presentation of visual supplements should be possible with available materials, facilities, and time (Davis, 1997). The *Publication Manual of the American Psychological Association* (2010a) provides extensive guidelines about traditional tables and figures.

Table 11–14. Guidelines for Visual Supplements

- Make them simple

- Make the images or letters large enough to be seen clearly

- Make a trial run long enough before the presentation to permit you to revise the visual aids if needed

- Coordinate the visual aids with the oral report or written text so that the audience is not distracted and the visual aid is relevant to the oral report or text

- Prior to a presentation that uses visual aids, be sure that any needed equipment is available and operational

---

Source: Adapted from *Scientific Papers and Presentations*, by M. Davis, 1997, San Diego, CA: Academic Press.

Evaluating and Reviewing Research Reports

Research reports should be read critically; just because a report has been published does not ensure its quality. The published research varies in both quality and value. Peer-reviewed journals ensure that reports "have received scrutiny by experts, and it maximizes the likelihood that serious errors of fact, reasoning, or method will be detected and eliminated" (ASHA, 2000). Another consideration is the impact factor which indicates how many times a journal's paper is cited in other journals (Huth, 1999). Some journals provide this information at the end of reports.

Readers are responsible for critically reviewing research reports and deciding their value. Critically evaluating and reviewing research reports is a skill that requires knowledge and experience. The most important considerations are scientific relevance, soundness of methodology, and the author(s). Several guidelines for evaluating research reports are available (APA, 2010a), Hegde, 2010; Polit & Beck, 2010; Schiavetti, Metz, & Orlikoff,, 2010; Silverman, 1998). These guidelines can also be used to evaluate oral reports and poster presentations.

Evidence-based practice uses specific criteria to evaluate the quality of evidence. The criteria differ according to whether the evidence is related to decisions about diagnosis or treatment (ASHA, 2005).

These guidelines can also be used to evaluate oral presentation and posters. There are also guidelines with specific focus such as the type of research, qualitative, or quantitative (McMillan, 2004; Leedy & Ormrod, 2010), clinical services, diagnosis or treatment (ASHA, 2005), and level of evidence (Haynes & Johnson, 2009; Jewell, 2011; Mc Mullern & Schumacher, 2009).

- Dollaghan (2007) developed brief summaries of evidence for a variety of topics:
- CATE—Critical Appraisal of Treatment Evidence
- CADE—Critical Appraisal of Diagnostic Evidence
- CASM—Critical Appraisal of Systemic Review or Meta-Analysis
- CAPE—Checklist for Appraising Patient/Practice Evidence
- CAPP—Checklist for Appraising Patient Preferences

Answer to questions can be used for evaluating reports (Bless & Forister, 2012). These questions are listed in Table 11–15.

CATs

Two methods have been suggested for brief critical reevaluations of the literature. Critically Appraised Topics (CATS) and Evidence-Based Communication Assessment and Intervention (EBCAI) structure appraisal abstracts.

A CAT is a brief summary of clinical quality and appraisal of the evidence that typically begins with a clinical bottom line that is a recommendation about use and application (Polit & Beck, 2010). There are several templates for CATs available online. CATS have two distinguishing characteristics: (1) based on specific clinical questions and developed by using the PICO format; and (2) inclusion of the bottom line or conclusions about the value

Table 11–15. Questions to Ask and Answer About Research

- What is the source of the report?
- Was the publication peer-reviewed?
- Who are the authors and their affiliations?
- What was the main subject of the study?
- What was the problem(s) investigated?
- What was the purpose or rationale for the study?
- Who or what constituted the sample or populations?
- What was the design?
- What statistical analyses were used?
- Are the results clear?
- Did the results answer the identified question(s)?
- Are the conclusions consistent with the design and analysis?
- Are the results consistent or contradictory with the results of similar studies?
- What do the results mean relative to clinical practice, and patients?
- Can the results be applied to your research or clinical practice?

Source: From *Research and Medical Literature*, by J. D. Blessing and J. G. Forister, 2012, Burlington, MA: Jones and Bartlett.

of the findings. The major advantage of CATs is the potential to improve patient care. Other advantages include a standard format, specific/focused questions, brevity, and possible reducing the amount of time for critical review. Disadvantages are short-term use as new evidence becomes available, limited access to the literature, based on only one or two studies, and variable skills and methods of analysis (EBCAI) structured appraisal abstracts can be used to evaluate evidence (Lackey & Ogletree, 2012). These abstracts are published in the peer-review journal, Evidence-Based Communication Assessment and Intervention. EBCAI abstracts can be used to evaluate credibility and determine the potential for application to clinical practice.

Summary

There are several reasons for reporting research. Among these reasons are ethical responsibility to contribute and disseminate professional information an indicator of, institutional quality, as well as recognition and academic survival.

It is difficult to report research without effective time management. Research is frequently not reported because of failure to make time to write and revise reports. There are, however, several strategies that can facilitate managing time for reporting research.

Research is incomplete until the reports have been disseminated at a professional meeting, as a written report, or both. The form and content of oral and written research reports are similar although there are differences primarily in manner of presentation and length. Written reports are usually longer. There are different types of written reports: journal articles; theses and dissertations; and textbooks. Evaluating and reviewing research reports is an important professional responsibility. Critical review and evaluation of research reports are an integral part of evidence-based practice which emphasizes the application and use of research evidence to make clinical decisions.

DISCUSSION QUESTIONS

1. What distinguished the unpublished from the published writer?
2. What are the reasons for reporting research?
3. Define "publish or perish."
4. Why is research not reported?
5. Explain the myths about research reports.
6. Why and how can these myths be eliminated?
7. How can time management facilitate research productivity?
8. What is the difference between "busyness" and binging?
9. Why should a timetable be developed and implemented for reporting research?
10. How can computer technology be used to increase research productivity?
11. Why do single-subject research designs require less time?
12. Describe procrastination.
13. How can procrastination affect research?

14. How can procrastination be avoided or reduced?
15. How can a research log be used to determine order of authorship?
16. List and briefly describe the major sections of research reports.
17. What is a structured abstract?
18. Compare structured abstracts for original and review of tutorial reports?
19. Why are key words important?
20. Why do professional journals require the authors disclose their contributions to a report?
21. What is the difference between tables and figures?
22. Why are tables and figures valuable to research reports?
23. What is meant by writing style?
24. How is writing style developed?
25. What is APA format?
26. Why are mistakes in referencing so common?
27. How can mistakes in referencing be eliminated or reduced?
28. What is biased language? How can it be avoided?
29. What is person first language?
30. When and why should one request permission to use previously published materials?
31. What are the steps in rewriting and revising a report?
32. What are rewriting and revising challenging?
33. List and briefly describe the types of research reports.
34. What is a cover letter? What information is included in a cover letter?

35. Define peer review. Why is peer review important?
36. How does one select an appropriate journal to submit a manuscript?
37. What types of articles are published in ASHA journals?
38. Briefly describe the different types of textbook publishers.
39. What is a vanity press? What are the limitations?
40. What are the advantages and disadvantages of presenting research at professional meetings?
41. What is a "call for papers"?
42. What are the advantages and disadvantages of poster presentations?
43. What are the differences between traditional and evidence-based poster presentations?
44. How can visual supplements be used in written reports and oral presentations?
45. Why should published research reports be evaluated and reviewed?
46. How can research reports be reviewed?
47. Which ASHA journal has the highest rate of acceptance for manuscripts submitted? The lowest? What are the implications?
48. What are the guidelines for tables and figures? Why is it important to be familiar with these guidelines?
49. What are the advantages and disadvantages of presenting research findings at professional meetings?

50. What are the major components of a V-diagram?
51. What information should be included in a cover letter when submitting a manuscript?
52. What factors can affect presentation of research findings at professional meetings?
53. What are the advantages and disadvantages of presenting research findings at professional meetings?
54. What are CATs? What are the different types of CATs?
55. How can research be evaluated?
56. Why should research be evaluated?
57. What factors influence poster presentation?
58. Compare traditional and electronic poster presentation? Which would have the most advantages? Why?

References

American Medical Association. (2006). Instructions for authors. *Journal of the American Medical Association, 295*(1), 103–111.

American Medical Association. (2007). *American Medical Association manual of style.* New York, NY: Oxford University Press.

American Psychological Association. (2010a). *Publication manual of the American Psychological Association.* Washington, DC: Author.

American Psychological Association. (2010b). *Mastering APA style.* Washington, DC: Author.

American Speech-Language-Hearing Association. (1979). Guidelines for nonsexist language in journals of ASHA. *ASHA, 21,* 973–977.

American Speech-Language-Hearing Association. (1993). Guide for gender equality: language usage. *ASHA, 35*(10), 42–46.

American Speech-Language-Hearing Association. (2000). Code of ethics. *ASHA Supplement, 23,* 13–15.

American Speech-Language-Hearing Association. (2004). *Evidence-based practice in communications disorders. An introduction.* Retrieved from http://www.asha.org/member/deskredf-journals/deskref/default

American Speech-Language-Hearing Association. (2005, June 1). Examples of levels-of evidence hierarchies. *ASHA Leader.*

American Speech-Language-Hearing Association. (2010). *Code of ethics.* Retrieved from http://www.asha.org

Anderson, M. (1992). *Imposters in the temple.* New York, NY: Simon & Schuster.

Barzun, J. (1986). *Writing, editing, and publishing.* Chicago, IL, University of Chicago Press.

Bates, T., Anie, A., & Marusic, A. (2004). Authorship criteria and disclosure contributions. *Journal of the American Medical Association, 292,* 86–88.

Bennett, D. M., & Taylor, D.M. (2003). Unethical practices in authorship of scientific papers. *Emergency Medicine, 15*(3), 263–270.

Betz, C. L., Smith, K., Melynk, B. M., & Rickey, T. (2005). Disseminating evidence. In B. M. Melynk & E. Fineout-Overholt (Eds.), *Evidence-based practice in nursing and healthcare* (pp. 361–433). Philadelphia, PA: Lippincott Williams & Wilkins.

Black, S. (2001). Using citation analysis to pursue a core collection of journals in communication disorders. *Library Resources and Technical Services, 45*(1), 3–9.

Bless, J. D., & Forister, J. G. (2011). *Research and Medical Literature.* Burlington, MA: Jones and Bartlett.

Boice, R. (1989). Procrastination, busyness, and binging. *Behavioral Research therapy, 27*(6), 605–611.

Bordens, K. S., & Abbott, B. B. (1988). *Research designs and methods.* Mountain View, CA: Mayfield.

Boyes, W., Happel, J., & Hogen, T. (1984). Publish or perish: Fact or fiction. *Journal of Economics Education, 15*(2), 136–141.

Carter-Scott, C. (1989). *Negaholics.* New York, NY: Fawcett Crest.

Chicago manual of style. (2001). Chicago, IL: University of Chicago Press.

Cone, J. D., & Foster, S. L. (2006). *Dissertations and theses from start to finish.* Washington, DC: American Psychological Association.

Connell, P., & McReynolds, L. (1988). A clinical science approach to treatment. In N. J. Lass, L. McReynolds, J. Northern, & D. Yoder (Eds.), *Handbook of speech-language pathology and audiology* (pp. 1058–1073). Philadelphia, PA: B. C. Decker.

Davis, G. B., & Parker, C. A. (1979). *Writing the doctoral dissertation.* New York, NY: Barron's Educational Services.

Davis, M. (1997). *Scientific papers and presentations.* San Diego, CA: Academic Press.

Deep, S., & Sussman, L. (1990). *Smart moves.* Reading, MA: Addison-Wesley.

DePoy, E., & Gitlin, L. N. (2011). *Introduction to research.* St. Louis, MO: C. V. Mosby.

Drummond, V. (1990). *The elements of nonsexist language usage.* New York, NY: Prentice-Hall.

Editors. (2004). Addressing the limitations of structured abstracts. *Annals of Internal Medicine, 140*(6), 480–481.

Finn, P., Bothe, A. K. & Bramlett, R. E. (2005) Science and pseudoscience in communication disorders: Criteria and application.

American Journal of Speech-Language Pathology, 14(3), 172–186.

Folkins, J. (1992). *The language used to describe individuals with disabilities.* Retrieved from http://www.asha.org/publication/

Goldfarb, R. & Serpanos, Y. C. (2009). *Professional writing in speech-language pathology and audiology.* San Diego, CA: Plural.

Golper, L. A., & Brown, J. E. (2004). *Business matters: A guide for speech-language pathologist.* Rockville, MD: American Speech-Language-Hearing Association.

Gowin, D. B., & Alvarez, M. C. (2005). *The art of educating with V diagrams.* New York, NY: Cambridge University Press.

Gustafson, M. (1981). Poster presentations more than a poster on a board. *Journal of Continuing Education in Nursing, 12*(1), 28–30.

Guyatt, G., & Rennie, D. (2002). *Users' guides to the medical literature.* Chicago, IL: American Medical Association.

Harris, R. L. (1999). *Informative graphics,* New York, NY: Oxford University Press.

Haynes, R. B., Mulrow, C. D., Huth, E. J., Altman, D. G., & Gardner, M. J. (1996). More informative abstracts revisited. *Cleft Palate Craniofacial Journal, 33*(1), 1–9.

Haynes, W. O. & Johnson, C. E. (2009). *Understanding research and evidence-based practice in communication disorders.* Boston, MA: Pearson.

Hegde, M. N. (2003). *Clinical research in communicative disorders.* Austin, TX: Pro-Ed.

Hegde, M. N. (2010). *Coursebook on scientific and professional writing for speech-language pathology.* San Diego, CA: Singular.

Henson, K. T. (1993, June). Writing for successful publication. *Phi Delta Kappan*, pp. 799–802.

Hirschor, R. F. (2011). A piece of my mind. *Journal of the American Medical Association, 395*, 230.

Holcomb, J., & Roush, R. (1988). A study if the scholarly activities of allied health facilities in southern academic health science center. *Journal of Allied Health, 17*(11), 227–293.

Holmes, T. (2006). *How to write and publish papers in the medical sciences.* Baltimore, MD: Williams & Wilkins.

Huth, E. J. (1999). *Writing and publishing in medicine.* Baltimore, MD: Williams & Wilkins.

Irwin, D. L., Pannbacker, M. D., & Kallail, K. (1992). Writing for communication disorders and related journals. *Journal of the National Student Speech-Language-Hearing Association, 19,* 119–122.

Iverson, C., Flanagin, A., Fontanarosa, P. B., Glass, R. M., Glitman, P., & Lantz, J. C., et al. (1993). *American Medical Association manual of style.* Philadelphia, PA: Lippincott, Williams, & Wilkins.

Jewell, D. V. (2011). *Guidelines to evidence-based physical therapist practice.* Sudbury, MA: Jones and Bartlett.

Kraemer, G., & Lyons, K. (1989). Research productivity of allied health in academic health centers. *Journal Allied Health, 18,* 349–359.

Lackey, K. C., & Ogleetree, R. T. (2012). EBCAI structured abstracts. *Evidence-Based Communication Intervention and Treatment, 10,* 177–165.

Law, M., & Philip, I. (2002). Evaluating the evidence. In M. Law (Ed.), *Evidence-based rehabilitation* (pp. 997–107). Thorofare, NJ: Slack Incorporated.

Leedy, P. D., & Ormrod, J. E. (2010). *Practical research.* Upper Saddle River, NJ: Pearson.

Luey, B. (1987). *Handbook for academic authors.* New York, NY: Cambridge University Press.

Maxwell, D. L., & Satake, E. (2006). *Research and statistical methods in communication sciences and disorders.* Clifton Park, NY: Thomson-Delmar Learning.

McMillan, J. H. (2004). *Educational research.* Boston, MA: Pearson.

Meline, T. (2006). *Research in communication science and disorders.* Upper Saddle River, NJ: Pearson.

Miller, C., & Swift, K. (1988). *The handbook of nonsexist language.* New York, NY: Harper and Row.

Modern Language Association of America. (2003)). *MLA handbook for writers of research papers.* New York, NY: Author.

Mullen, R. (2007, March 6). The state of the evidence. ASHA develops levels of evidence. *ASHA Leader.*

Nichol, A. A., & Pexman, P. M. (2003). *Displaying your findings.* Washington, DC: American Psychological Association.

Novak, J. D. (1998). *Learning, creating, and using knowledge.* Mahwah, NJ: Lawrence Erlbaum Associates.

Paden, E. P. (1970). *A history of the American Speech and Hearing Association, 1925–1958.* Washington DC: American Speech-Language-Hearing Association.

Pierson, D. J. (2004). The top ten reasons why manuscripts are not accepted for publication. *Respiratory Care, 49,* 1246–1252.

Polit, P. F., & Beck, C. T. (2010). *Nursing research: Principles and methods.* Philadelphia, PA: J. B. Lippincott Williams & Wilkins.

Reilly, S. (2004). What constitutes evidence? In S. Rilley, J. Douglas, & J. Oakes (Eds.), *Evidence-based practice in speech pathology* (pp. 18–34). London, UK: Whurr.

Robertson, S. (2004, September 24). I used to have a handle on life, but it broke! *ASHA Leader, 9,* 13, 37.

Roth, A. J. (1989). *The research paper.* Belmont, CA: Wadsworth.

Rudestan, K. E., & Newman, R. R. (2001). *Surviving your dissertation.* Thousand Oaks: CA: Sage.

Sackett, D. L., Strauss, S. E., Richardson, W. S., Rosenberg, W., & Haynes, R. B. (2001). *Evidence-based medicine.* London, UK: Churchill Livingstone.

Schiavetti, N., Metz, D. E., & Orlikoff, R. F. (2010). *Evaluating research in communicative disorders.* Boston, MA: Allyn & Bacon.

Schilling, L. S. (2005). Publish or perish: Writing under pressure. *Pediatric Nursing, 31*(3), 234–236.

Schneider, S., & Soto, A. M. (1989). Sexist language: Should we be concerned? *Journal of the American Women's Medical Association, 44*(3), 79–83.

Schutte, H. K. & Svec, J. G. (2007). Reaction of Folia Phoniatrica et Logopaedica on the current trend of impact factor measures. *Folia Phoniatrica, 59*, 281–285.

Silverman, F. H. (1998). *Research design and evaluation in speech-language pathology and audiology.* Boston, MA: Allyn & Bacon.

Simmonds, D. (1984). How to produce good posters. *Medical Teacher, 6*(1), 10–13.

Sininger, T., March, R., Walden, B., & Wilber, L. A. (2003). Guidelines for ethical practice in research for audiologists. *Audiology Today, 15*(6), 14–17.

Sorrels, B. D. (1983). *How to complete and survive a doctoral dissertation.* New York, NY: St. Martin's Press.

Sternberg, R. J. (1993). *The psychologist's companion: A guide to scientific writing for students and researchers.* New York, NY: Cambridge University Press.

Strunk, W., & White, E. B. (1979). *The elements of style.* New York, NY: MacMillan.

Turabian, K. L. (1995). *A manual for writers of term papers, theses, dissertations.* Chicago, IL: University of Chicago Press.

Yau, N. (2001). *Visualize this.* Indianapolis, IN: Wiley.

12

Evaluating Tests and Treatments

CHAPTER OUTLINE	
Evaluation Issues	Summary
Tests	Discussion Questions
Treatment	References

LEARNING OBJECTIVES

Upon completion of this chapter the reader will be able to:

- Understand reasons for evaluating tests and treatments
- Distinguish between decisions based on evidence and opinions
- Apply specific criteria to evaluation of tests and treatments
- Define terms related to testing: true/false negative, true/false positive, specificity, and sensitivity
- Distinguish between the types of treatment outcome research.

The evaluation of tests and treatments involves both qualitative and quantitative research, that is, multimethod research. In speech-language pathology and audiology, data are collected about individuals for diagnosis and treatment. Options for data collection include tests, checklists, quality of life measuring, observation, and various documents (case history, medical charts, educational records). Evaluating diagnostic tests and treatment outcomes is a type of research relevant to the clinical practice of speech-language pathology and audiology. This type of research involves:

- being skeptical
- considering the source of the information
- distinguishing between cause and effect
- differentiating observation from inference
- ensuring that describing a product is not only to sell it
- recognizing that an example is not evidence for what is claimed (Lum, 2002).

Evidence-based practice and ethics are important in evaluating tests and treatments. It is a method of using the highest available level of evidence to make clinical decisions.

Evidence-based tests and treatments are an ethical responsibility. The present Code of Ethics of the American Speech-Language-Hearing Association (ASHA, 2010) contains several related references to ethical research. Moreover, selection of tests and treatments is significant in terms of cost and benefit.

Speech-language pathologists and audiologists should be discerning con-sumers of diagnostic and treatment resources. A test or treatment should be selected on the best available evidence. Obsolete and outdated evaluation and treatment methods should be discarded. New diagnostic and treatment products constitute a growing market that may be heavily promoted because of high profit margins (Lum, 2002).

Evaluation Issues

Speech-language pathologists and audiologists should assume responsibility for critical review of diagnostic tests and treatment materials to avoid sham products being used because there is great variability in the quality of tests and treatments. With any test or treatment, speech-language pathologists and audiologists should always ask, "What is the evidence?"

An evaluation of diagnostic tests and treatment methods based on opinion is incompatible with evidence-based practice. All sources of evidence are not equal, that is, bad to poor evidence, that is, low (weak) to high (strong) level. Opinion is considered to be weak evidence (Reilly, 2004). Unfortunately, many speech-language pathologists more frequently use clinical experience and opinion than research or clinical practice guidelines to make clinical decisions (Zipoli & Kennedy, 2005). Several trends have decreased the emphasis on general psychometric checklists for evidence about sensitivity and specificity of tests (Pena, Spaulding, & Plante, 2006). Opinion and blind acceptance should not be the basis for making clinical decisions.

Speech-language pathologists and audiologists should be skeptical and admit to not knowing unless there is sound evidence (Lum, 2002).

Tests

Tests are used by speech-language pathologists and audiologists for a variety of different reasons. They may be used to establish whether or not someone has a speech-language-hearing problem, to monitor response to treatment, to make informed treatment decisions, to assess progress, or to assess the risk of developing a speech-language-hearing problem (Mart, 1999).

The primary purpose of any test is to determine whether or not someone has a speech-language-hearing problem. A good test is one that can correctly detect that a problem is really present (true positive) or that someone does not have a problem (true negative). Test results can be misleading if there is a high false negative or false positive result (Mart, 1999). In other words, low false positive and false negative results are more accurate.

Haynes and Pindzola (1998) believe uncritical acceptance of tests "are probably the rule rather than the exception" (p. 83). Test accuracy is based on sensitivity and specificity. The *sensitivity* of a test is the proportion of people who actually have the problem who had a true positive test, that is, accuracy of the test in identifying people with the problem. It is further defined as the probability of a diagnostic test finding a problem among those who have the problem or the proportion of people with the problem who have a positive test result (true

positive) (Melynk & Fineout-Overholt, 2005).The *specificity* of a test is the equal and opposite result of sensitivity. It is the proportion without the problem, that is, a true negative test result (Lum, 2002; Maxwell & Satake, 2006). Specificity is further defined as the probability of a diagnostic test finding no problem among those who do not have the problem or the proportion of people free of a problem who have a negative test (true negative) (Melynk & Fineout-Overholt, 2005). An accurate test will have high positive likelihood ratio and a low negative likelihood ratio indicating that the test correctly identified people who have the problem and those people who do not (Dollaghan, 2004). Sensitivity and specificity can be calculated as follows (Portney & Watkins, 2001):

$$\text{sensitivity} = \frac{\text{true positives}}{\text{true positives} + \text{false negatives}}$$

$$\text{specificity} = \frac{\text{true negatives}}{\text{false negatives} + \text{true negatives}}$$

The composition of normative groups should be considered in interpreting test scores and making diagnostic decisions. Pena, Spaulding, and Plante (2006) reviewed descriptions of the normative groups for 32 child language tests. If the normative group includes a mixed sample of normal and language-impaired children, measurement precision decreases for absolute score interpretation but may increase for relative interpretations.

Thus, clinicians should be aware of two principles: (1) determine if test characteristics are appropriate for interpretation; (2) a single test may not support multiple diagnostic purposes.

Another consideration in evaluating tests is the *predictive value*. It is the predictive value of a test that has practical implications for predicting actual clinical outcome based on test results (Maxwell & Satake, 2006). There are two major components or predictive value of a diagnostic test: (1) predictive value positive; and (2) predictive value negative. Predictive value positive (PV+) is the probability that a person has a problem given the test result is positive. Predictive value negative (PV−) is the probability that a person does not have a problem given that the test result is negative. These values are calculated as (Portney & Watkins, 2000):

$$PV+ = \frac{\text{true positives}}{\text{true positives} + \text{false negatives}}$$

$$PV- = \frac{\text{true negatives}}{\text{true positives} + \text{false negatives}}$$

Many tests have tables for converting raw scores into age and/or grade equivalent scores. These scores according to Haynes and Pindzola (1998) "are the least useful and most dangerous scores to be obtained from standardized tests because they lead to gross misinterpretation of a client's performance" (p. 72). Age and grade equivalent scores are the least useful types of scores because they tend to distort performance and lead to misinterpretations by both consumers and professionals. Nonetheless, these scores are often used to interpret test performance and make diagnostic decisions. Furthermore, many state departments of education mandate the use of age-equivalent scores for making decisions about eligibility for services (Haynes & Pindzola, 2012).

There are two basic types of review for evaluating diagnostic tests and treatment methods: traditional and evidence-based. There are major differences between traditional and evidence-based reviews. The former tend to be subjective and have vague criteria. The latter involve application of specific criteria for evaluating, diagnosis, and treatment. This reduces the risk for bias. ASHA (2005) has provided examples of levels of evidence hierarchies for both diagnosis and treatment as presented in Tables 12–1 and 12–2.

Some evaluation strategies have multiple purposes. For example, ASHA (2006) has a series of questions for evaluation, treatment procedures, purchasing a product, or attending an educational program. These questions can also be used for evaluating tests. Table 12–3 lists ASHA's questions.

Another method of evaluation is to differentiate between science and pseudoscience characteristics of a test or treatment. These criteria are shown in Table 12–4. Several authors have described criteria for evaluating tests (Haynes & Pindzola, 2012; Hutchinson, 1996; Lum, 2002; Mertens, 2005; Shipley & McAfee, 2009; Stein & Cutler, 1996). Basically, these criteria are related to the test manual, descriptive statistics, and the normative sample. Hutchinson presented a series of 20 questions to consider in reviewing a test manual.

Haynes and Pindzola (1998) suggested obtaining a test for evaluation because test brochures and catalogs may not provide adequate information. Furthermore, "if possible, order a test for appraisal, and pay for it only if you are satisfied with its psychometric adequacy and what it will actually tell you about a client" (p. 77). Therefore, psychometric adequacy should be evaluated on the basis of identifiable criteria.

Table 12–1. Examples of Levels-of-Evidence Hierarchies for Diagnostic Studies

Level	Type of Diagnostic Study
1a	Systematic review or meta-analysis of 1c studies (high-quality trials)
1b	Independent replication of a 1c study
1c	A diagnostic study having a representative and consecutive sample and appropriate reference standard (e.g., gold-standard test) in an independent blind comparison demonstrating validated specificity and sensitivity that are almost absolute
2a	Systematic review or meta-analysis 2b diagnostic studies
2b	A cohort study with a good reference standard
3a	Systematic review or meta-analysis 3b studies
3b	A diagnostic study having a nonconsecutive sample or a consistently applied reference standard
4	One or more case-control study Expert opinion without explicit critical appraisal

Note: Levels 1 through 3b could be further fractioned by experimental precision. For example, level 2a could become 2a(+) and 2a(−) for grouping high- and low-precision experiments respectively.

Source: From "Examples of Levels-of-Evidence Hierarchy," by American Speech-Language-Hearing Association, 2005. Retrieved from http://www.asha.org/About/publications/leader-on line/archives/2005/f050524a3.htm

Table 12–2. Examples of Levels-of-Evidence Hierarchies for Treatment Studies

Level	Type of Treatment Study
1a	Systematic reviews or meta-analyses of high-quality randomized controlled trials
1b	High-quality randomized controlled trials
2a	Systematic reviews or meta-analyses of high-quality nonrandomized controlled trials
2b	High-quality nonrandomized controlled trials
3a	Systematic reviews of cohort studies
3b	Individual cohort study or low quality randomized controlled trials
4	Clinical outcome studies
5a	Systematic review of case-control studies
5b	Individual case-control studies
6	Case-series
7a	Expert opinion without explicit critical appraisal

Source: From "Examples of Levels-of-Evidence Hierarchies," by American Speech-Language-Hearing Association, 2005. Retrieved from http://www.asha.org/about/Publications/leader-on line/archives/2005/f05024a3.htm

Table 12–3. ASHA's Questions for Evaluating Treatments, Procedures, Products, or Programs

Stated uses:	What are the stated uses of the procedure, product, or program?
Population:	To which client/patient population does it apply? Is there documented evidence that it is valid for use with a specific population?
Generalization:	To which other populations does it claim to generalize?
Outcomes:	Are outcomes clearly stated?
Publications:	Are there publications about this procedure, product, or program? Is the information published in a peer-reviewed journal? Is promotional material the only published source of information?
Peer-reviewed:	Is there peer-reviewed research that supports or contradicts research: the stated outcomes or benefits?
Developers:	What is the professional background of the developers of the procedure/product/program?
Availability:	Are there similar procedures, products, or programs currently and cost: available? How do they compare in performance and cost?
Experience:	Have you talked with others who have experience with this product, procedure, or program? What was their expertise? Have you considered posting a query on ASHA's interactive member forum on its Web site?
Scope of Practice:	Is it within my profession's Scope of Practice? Is it within my personal scope of practice (i.e., personal training, competence, experience) to use this procedure, product, or program?
Information/ Policies:	Have you checked to see if there are any ASHA statements or guidelines on this topic?
Cost:	Based on the factors above, is the cost reasonable and justifiable?

Source: From "When Evaluating Any Treatment, Procedure, Product, or Program Ask Yourself the Following Questions," by American Speech-Language-Hearing Association, n.d. Retrieved from http://www.asha.org/members/evaluate.htm

Table 12–4. Ten Criteria for Distinguishing Between Science and Pseudoscience

Yes	No	
☐	☐	1. Untestable: Is the treatment unable to be tested or disproved?
☐	☐	2. Unchanged: Does the treatment approach remain unchanged even in the face of contradictory evidence?
☐	☐	3. Confirming evidence: Is the rationale for the treatment approach based only on confirming evidence with disconfirming evidence ignored or minimized?
☐	☐	4. Anecdotal evidence: Does the evidence in support of the treatment rely on personal experience and anecdotal accounts?
☐	☐	5. Inadequate evidence: Are the treatment claims incommensurate with the level of evidence needed to support those claims?
☐	☐	6. Avoiding peer-review: Are treatment claims unsupported by evidence that has undergone critical scrutiny?
☐	☐	7. Disconnected: Is the treatment approach disconnected from well-established scientific models or paradigms?
☐	☐	8. New terms: Is the treatment described by terms that appear to be scientific but upon further examination are found not to be scientific at all?
☐	☐	9. Grandiose outcome: Is the treatment approach based on grandiose claims or poorly specified outcomes?
☐	☐	10. Holistic: Is the treatment claimed to make sense only within a vaguely described holistic framework?

Source: From "Science and Pseudoscience in Communication Disorders: Criteria and Applications," by P. Finn, A. K. Bothe, and R. E. Bramlett, 2005, *American Journal of Speech-Language Pathology, 14*(3), pp. 172–186.

Dollaghan (2004) described criteria from the evidence-based practice literature to use in evaluating diagnostic tests, which are presented in Table 12–5. Three evidence-based propositions were considered:

■ The opinions of expert authorities, singly or in groups such as consensus panels, should be viewed with skepticism and discounted entirely when they contradict evidence from rigorous scientific studies.

■ Not all research is relevant to decisions about clinical practice.

■ Being judgmental about evidence is a goal, not a character flaw.

Another consideration is reporting diagnostic findings which involve both

Table 12–5. Checklist of Questions for Evaluating Evidence of a
Diagnostic Measure

Yes	No	
☐	☐	Was the measure compared to a gold standard (GS)?
☐	☐	Was the gold standard valid, reliable, and reasonable?
☐	☐	Were both measures administered to all participants?
☐	☐	Were both measures administered to all participants?
☐	☐	Were participants identified prospectively?
☐	☐	Were participants described clearly?
☐	☐	Did participants include individuals with and without the disorder of interest?
☐	☐	Did participants exhibit a range of severity levels?
☐	☐	Did participants include some with confusable symptoms?
☐	☐	Were the two measures administered independently, by different examiners?
☐	☐	Were examiners blinded to performance on the other test?
☐	☐	Were examiners blinded to other patient information?
☐	☐	Was the positive likelihood ratio in at least the intermediate range (≥ 4.0)?
☐	☐	Was the negative likelihood ratio in at least the intermediate range (≥ 0.4)?
☐	☐	Was the confidence interval reasonable narrow?
☐	☐	Is the new measure feasible in usual clinical practice?
☐	☐	Does the new measure offer a significant advantage over the gold stand?

Source: From "Evidence-Based Practice in Communication Disorders: What Do We Know and When Do We Know It?" by C. A. Dollaghan, 2004, *Journal of Communication Disorders*, 37(5), pp. 391–400.

quantitative and qualitative data, namely, multimethod research. A worksheet for organizing and interpreting diagnostic findings is shown in Figure 12–1. The worksheet can be used as the final report or as the prerequisite to a narrative report. The worksheet serves as a reminder that diagnosis of communication disorders is a type of research that combines both quantitative and qualitative data.

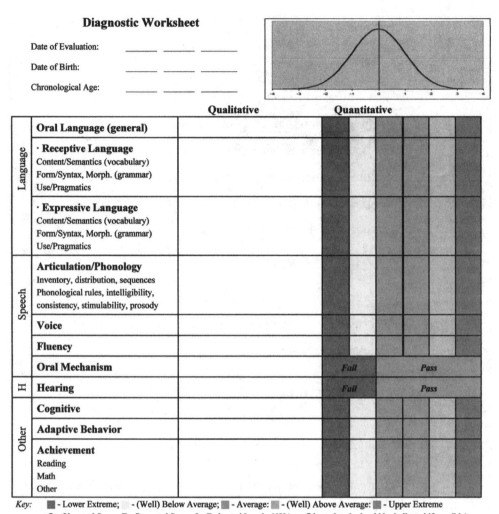

Figure 12–1. Diagnostic worksheet. (From unpublished data, by T. W. Powell, 2006.)

Another consideration is reporting diagnostic findings which involve both quantitative and qualitative data, namely, multimethod research. A worksheet for organizing and interpreting diagnostic findings is shown in Figure 12–1. The worksheet can be used as the final report or as the prerequisite to a narrative report. The worksheet serves as a reminder that diagnosis of communication disorders is a type of research that combines both quantitative and qualitative data.

Treatment

Treatment outcome is a broadly defined term that refers to change, or the lack of it, that may occur as a result of time, treatment, or both (Golper et al., 2001). Moreover, treatment outcomes are generalized, maintained, indirect, and clinically valid results of treatment (Hegde, 2003). A distinction is frequently made between efficacy, effectiveness, and efficiency of treatment. The following questions can be used to make this distinction:

- Has the treatment been shown to be beneficial in controlled research, that is, ideal conditions (efficacy)?
- Is treatment useful in applied clinical settings (average conditions) and if so, with what patients and under what circumstances (effectiveness)?
- Is treatment efficient (minimal waste, expense, unnecessary effort) in the sense of being cost effective relative to other alternative interventions (efficiency) (Golper et al., 2001; Maxwell & Satake, 2006).

There are major differences between various types of treatment research. Uncontrolled or nonexperimental research is designed to document improvement such as case studies (Hegde, 2003). Controlled treatment research, or experimentation, is designed to establish a cause-effect relationship between treatment (independent variable) and positive changes (dependent variable). Controlled treatment research is used to determine effectiveness. It requires either a single subject or group experimental design. Directly replicated research or experimentation is designed to determine if results (improvement or effects) in an uncontrolled or controlled study can be replicated when there is no change in treatment, setting, or clinicians; the only change is new clients.

Two other variations of treatment studies warrant consideration: retrospective (past) and prospective (current) (Lum, 2002). *Retrospective studies* involve examination of existing case records, which has limitations if the records are incorrect or inaccurate. On the other hand, retrospective studies can be completed quickly and economically because they are based on existing data (Maxwell & Satake, 2006). *Prospective* means the data needed for study are determined before they are collected. In prospective studies current information is used to predict future status.

Silverman (1998) provided a series of questions for evaluating treatment that focused on space and time. These questions are listed in Table 12–6. To assess treatment outcomes with a single client, Lum (2002) described a number of factors to consider in evaluating treatments, as presented in Table 12–7. These factors utilize elements related to single-subject research design. Robey and Schulz (1998) and Robey (1998, 2004) described a five-phase outcome model for clinical outcome research that involves: developing a treatment; testing its efficacy; testing its effectiveness; examining its efficacy; and determining its cost effectiveness, cost benefit, and cost utility. The model is presented in Figure 12–2.

Additional measures of treatment outcome include traditional instrumental and behavioral data, cost-benefit analysis, and quality of life scales. Integrated data systems linking these data produce comprehensive reports which provide better information about treatment outcomes. Further information related to treatment outcome research is available in books edited by Frattali (1998), Law (2002), and Schlosser (2003).

Table 12–6. Questions for Evaluating Treatment

— What are the impacts of the treatment on specific behaviors that contribute to a client's speech-language problem at given points in time?
— What are the effects of the treatment on other aspects of a client's speech-language at given points in space-time?
— What are the effects of the treatment on a client other than those directly related to speech-language at given points in space-time?
— What are the client's attitudes about the treatment and its impact on his or her speech-language and other behaviors at given points in space-time?
— What are the attitudes of a client's clinician, family, friends, and others toward the treatment and toward its effect on the client's speech-language and other attributes of behavior in space-time?
— What investment is required of client and clinician at given points in space-time?
— What is the probability of relapse following termination of treatment?

Source: From *Research Design and Evaluation in Speech-Language Pathology and Audiology*, by F. H. Silverman, 1998, Boston, MA: Allyn & Bacon.

Table 12–7. Factors to Consider in Evaluating Treatment

— Specify the nature of the client's problem
— Deciding on the time frame for evaluation
— Selecting the behaviors to be changed
— Deciding on control and treatment behaviors and tasks
— Deciding on the format of the treatment tasks
— Deciding on the content of the treatment task items
— Deciding on the staging of treatment
— Deciding on the strategy for changing behavior
— Deciding which tasks to use to measure performance
— Deciding on the length of the baseline phase
— Deciding on the number of data measurements
— Deciding whether to use probes or continuous measurement
— Defining time intervals for reassessment and maintenance
— Stating predictions about generalization effects
— Developing treatment tasks
— Documenting decisions in treatment and obtaining the client's response

Source: From *Scientific Thinking in Speech and Language Therapy*, by C. Lum, 2002, Mahwah, NJ: Lawrence Erlbaum Associates.

Phase V
- study of efficiency, cost-effectiveness, cost-benefit; cost utility
- patient and family satisfaction; quality of life
- large samples

Phase IV
- test treatment effectiveness
- average conditions
- day to day practice
- typical conditions (patients, clinicians, intensity, and duration)
- large samples
- external control (no-treatment) not required
- a analysis of efficacy studies
- single subject studies with multiple replication; large single group designs
- examine variations in populations, intensity, and duration of treatment, level of clinician training

Phase III
- efficacy of treatment under ideal conditions (ideal patients, ideal clinicians, ideal treatment, ideal intensity and duration, ideal outcome measures)
- typically randomized control trial; (random assigned treatment or no treatment)
- large samples
- multiple sites
- parallel group designs; single subject studies

Phase II
- refine primary research hypothesis
- develop explanation for efficaciously and effectiveness
- specify treatment protocol
- determine discharge criteria
- demonstrate validity and reliability of outcome measures
- case studies, single-subject studies, small, single group studies

Phase I
- develop hypothesis to be tested in later phases
- establish safety of treatment
- demonstrate if treatment active (patients improve)
- brief, small sample size
- does not require external controls
- case studies, single subject studies
- small group pre-post studies, retrospective studies

Figure 12–2. Five-Phase Model for Communication Sciences and Disorders from Highest to Lowest Level (From "A Five-Phase Model for Clinical-Outcome Research," by R. R. Robey, 2004, *Journal of Communication Disorders*, *37*(5), pp. 401–411; and "A Model for Conducting Clinical Outcome Research: An Adaptation of the Standard Protocol for Use in Aphasiology," by R. R. Roby and M. C. Schultz, 1998, *Aphasiology, 12*, pp. 787–810.)

Summary

Careful evaluation of tests and treatments is a fundamental responsibility for justifying clinical services. There are a variety of methods for evaluating tests and treatments, either individually or collectively. Clinical decisions are too often made on the basis of opinion rather than critical review and the best available research evidence. Clinical services are enhanced by evidence-based decisions as opposed to beliefs and opinions.

DISCUSSION QUESTIONS

1. What type(s) of research is involved in evaluating tests and treatments?
2. Why should speech-language pathologists and audiologists be discerning consumers of tests and treatments?
3. Why are clinical decisions based on opinion(s) incompatible with evidence-based practice?
4. How can false negative and false positive results affect clinical decisions?
5. Explain the importance of specificity and sensitivity to test accuracy.
6. What is the difference between positive and negative predictive values?
7. Differentiate between traditional and evidence-based review for evaluating tests and treatments.
8. How do science and pseudoscience differ?
9. What are the criteria for pseudoscience?
10. What are the primary criteria for evaluating tests?
11. What are the evidence-based criteria for evaluating tests?
12. Differentiate between efficiency, effectiveness, and efficacy of treatment.
13. Describe the major differences between various types of treatment research.
14. What is the difference between retrospective and prospective studies?
15. What factors should be considered in evaluating treatment with a single client?
16. Describe a five-phase model for clinical outcome research.

References

American Speech-Language-Hearing Association. (2010). *Code of ethics.* Available from http://www.asha.org /policy

American Speech-Language-Hearing Association. (2005). *Examples of levels of evidence hierarchy.* Retrieved June 4, 2005 from http://www.asha.oralabout/publications/leader-online/archives/2005/f050524q3.htm

American Speech-Language-Hearing Association. (2006). *When evaluating any treatment procedure, product, or program ask yourself the following questions.* Retrieved from http://www.asha.org/members/evaluate

Dollaghan, C. (2004). Evidence-based practice in communication disorders: What do we know, and when do we know it? *Journal of Communication Disorders, 37*(5), 391–400.

Finn, P., Bothe, A. K., & Bramlett, R. E. (2005). Science and pseudoscience in communication disorders: Criteria and application. *American Journal of Speech Language Pathology, 14*(3), 172–186.

Frattali, C. M. (1998). *Measuring outcomes in speech-language pathology.* New York, NY: Thieme.

Golper L., Wertz, R. T., Frattali, C., Yorkston, K., Myers, P., Katz, R., Beeson, P., Kennedy, M. T., Bayles, K., & Wambaugh, J. (2001). Evidence-based practice guidelines for the management of communication disorders in neurologically impaired individuals. *ANCDS, Practice Guidelines Project,* 1–12.

Haynes,W.O., & Pindzola, R. H. (1998). *Diagnosis and evaluation in speech pathology.* Boston, MA: Allyn & Bacon.

Haynes, W. O., & Pindzola, R. H. (2012). *Diagnosis and evaluation in speech-language pathology.* Boston, MA: Pearson.

Hegde, M.N. (2003). *Clinical research in communication disorders.* Austin, TX: Pro-Ed.

Hutchinson, T. A. (1996). What to look for in the technical manual: Twenty questions for test users. *Language Speech and Hearing Services in Schools, 27,* 109–121.

Law, M. (2002). *Evidence-based rehabilitation.* Thorofare, NJ: Slack Incorporated.

Lum, C. (2002). *Scientific thinking in speech and language therapy.*Mahwah, NJ: Lawrence Erlbaum Associates.

Mart, J. (1999). Is this test effective? In M. Dawes, P. Davies, A. Gray, J. Marx, K. Seers, & R. Snowball (Eds.), *Evidence-based practice.* London, UK: Churchill Livingstone.

Maxwell, D. L., & Satake, E. (2006). *Research and statistical methods in communication sciences and disorders.* Clifton Park, NY: Thomson-Delmar Learning.

Melnyk, B. M., & Fineout-Overholt, E. (2005). *Evidence-based practice in nursing and healthcare.* Philadelphia, PA: Lippincott Williams & Wilkins.

Mertens, D. M. (2005). *Research and evaluation in education and psychology.* Thousand Oaks, CA: Sage.

Pena, E. D., Spaulding, T. J., & Plante, E. (2006). The composition of normatic groups and diagnostic decision-making: Shooting ourselves in the foot. *American Journal of Speech, Language Pathologists, 15,* 247–254.

Portney, L. G., & Watkins, M. P. (2000). *Foundations of clinical research: Applications to practice.* Upper Saddle River, NJ: Prentice-Hall Health.

Powell, T. W. (2006). *Diagnostic worksheet.* (Unpublished data).

Reilly, S. (2004). What constitutes evidence? In S. Reilly, J. Douglas, & J. Oates (Eds.), *Evidence-based practice in speech pathology* (pp. 18–34). Philadelphia, PA: Whurr.

Robey, R. R. (1998). A meta-analysis of clinical outcomes in the treatment of aphasia. *Journal of Speech-Language-Hearing Research, 41,* 172–187.

Robey, R. R. (2004). A five-phase model for clinical-outcome research. *Journal of Communication Disorders, 37*(5), 401–411.

Robey, R. R., & Schultz, M. C. (1998). A model for conducting clinical-outcome research. An adaptation of the standard protocol for use in aphasiology. *Aphasiology, 12*, 782–810.

Schlosser, R.W. (2003). *The efficacy of augmentative and alternative communication.* New York, NY: Academic Press.

Shipley, K. G., & McAfee, J. G. (2009). *Assessment in speech-language pathology.* San Diego, CA: Singular.

Silverman, F. H. (1998). *Research design and evaluation in speech-language pathol-ogy and audiology.* Boston, MA: Allyn & Bacon.

Stein, F., & Cutler, S. K. (1996). *Clinical research.* San Diego, CA: Singular.

Zipoli, R. P., & Kennedy, M. (2005). Evidence based practice among speech-language pathologists: Attitudes, utilization, and barriers. *American Journal of Speech Language Pathology, 14*(3), 208–220.

13

Evidence-Based Practice: Application of Research to Clinical Practice

LEARNING OBJECTIVES

Upon completion of this chapter the reader will be able to:

- Define evidence-based practice, research utilization, information literacy
- Recognize myths surrounding evidence-based practice
- Evaluate quality and credibility of ethic communicative evidence to patients and other professionals
- Describe the clinical issues related to evidence-based practice
- Describe clinical traits
- Identify barriers to evidence-based practice
- Locate resources for evidence-based practice
- Recognize the knowledge and skills needed for evidence-based practice.

Evidence-based practice (EBP) is the application of research data to clinical decisions. Speech-language pathologists and audiologists, who base their practice on the best available evidence, use a systematic approach to selecting assessment and treatment procedures (Cornett, 2001). The most compelling reason for speech-language pathologists and audiologist to be evidence-based practitioners is to ensure that clients receive the best possible services (Johnson, 2006).

Speech-language pathologists and audiologist in all work settings should be aware of the advantages of evidence-based practice or research-based practice. Meline (2006) believes evaluating research for its application to clinical practice is one of the most important resources available for ensuring best clinical practice in speech-language and audiology. There is growing interest in developing an evidence-based practice through research that is used in making clinical decisions.

During the past 10 years, changes in education and research have led to an awareness of the need for a better evidence base for the clinical practice of speech-language pathology and audiology. Most training programs have modified their curricula to include evidence-based practice and critical analysis of the research literature. Moreover, standards for the Certificate of Clinical Competence (CCC) in Speech-Language Pathology (ASHA, 2009), require "knowledge of processes used in research and integration of research principles into evidence-based clinical practice" (p. 7). Standards for the CCC-Audiology (ASHA, 2011) also required research and its association to make clinical decisions. There has also been an increased focus on research related to clinical practice. Both students

and practicing professionals need hands-on, interactive, practical experience in translating research into clinical practice (Gallagher, 2001). In 2005, ASHA issued a positive statement about evidence-based practice in communication science and disorders. Additional information about this statement is in the section, Knowledge and Skills Needed for Evidence-Based Practice.

There are other factors that may account for the increasing use of evidence-based practice. Among these factors are: the development of strategies for efficiently finding evidence; systematic clinical practice guidelines; electronic databases, and continuing education (Sackett, Strass, Richardson, Rosenberg, & Haynes, 2001). In spite of these developments, there have not been major changes in research utilization among clinicians; underutilization of research continues to be a problem. Research evidence is not routinely used in making clinical decision about assessment and treatment. Unfortunately, too many clinicians continue to make clinical decisions in the absence of evidence, and on the basis of opinion, testimony, and/or advertisements. Opinions, singly or in groups, even from respected authorities should be viewed with skepticism (Dollaghan, 2004a). In this chapter, various aspects of evidence-based practice are discussed.

Defining Evidence-Based Practice

Evidence-based practice utilizes the best available research to make clinical decisions about patient care. It is based on critical appraisal of research findings and applying what is known to clinical practice

(Frattali & Worrall, 2001). Research utilization is the application of some aspect of research to clinical practice. Polit and Beck (2004) described research utilization as a continuum ranging from direct application of research findings to clinical practice (instrumental utilization) through situations in which research findings are ignored or not used. Research utilization is a matter of degree; clinicians even with limited effort can accomplish some degree of evidence-based practice (Schlosser, 2004). In essence, evidence-based practice is the utilization of research findings to make decisions about patient care.

The major steps in using evidence-based practice are:

■ Selecting a topic or problem (Schlosser & O'Neil-Pirozzi, 2006)
■ Assembling and evaluating evidence; (Law & Plunkett, 2000; Meline, 2006).
■ Assessing for potential implementation (Nye & Harvey, 2006)
■ Developing or identifying evidence-based practice guidelines or protocols (Law & Plunkett, 2006)
■ Implementing the treatment
■ Evaluating outcomes (Bernstein-Ratner, 2006; Herder, Howard, Nye, & Vanryckeghem, 2006).
■ Deciding to adopt or modify the treatment or revert to prior practice (Konnerup & Schwartz, 2006).

Evidence-Based Practice: Terms and Definitions

Evidence-based practice is utilization of the best available research to make clinical decisions about patient care. It is based on critical appraisal of research findings an applying what is known to clinical practice (Frattali & Worrall, 2001).

Other terms related to evidence-based practice are:

■ Clinical expertise-proficiency of clinical skills and abilities, informed by continually expanding knowledge that individual clinicians develop through experience learning and reflection about their professional practice.
■ Cost-effectiveness, Cost benefit, Cost utility-terms that compare cost of service to outcome.
■ Effectiveness-extent to which an intervention or service produces a desired outcome under usual conditions.
■ Efficacy-extent to which intervention an intervention or services produces desired outcome under ideal conditions.
■ Efficiency-extent to which an intervention produces an outcome with a minimum of waste, expense, or unnecessary effort.
■ Evidence-any empirical observation about apparent relations between events constitutes potential evidence.
■ Evidence-based designs-emphasizes importance of using credible evidence.
■ Evidence-based management-evaluation of best evidence for making decisions.
■ Fidelity-truthfulness; degree to which administration of a test or treatment corresponds to the prototype.
■ Intent to treat-analysis based on initial treatment intent.
■ Outcome-result
■ Randomized controlled trail (RCT)-experimental study in which

patients meeting specific criteria are randomly assigned to treatment and no-treatment groups. (Golper et al., 2001: Jewel, 2011; Kaderauck & Justice, 2010)

Research Utilization

Research utilization is the application of research to clinical practice. Polit and Beck (2010) described research utilization as a continuum ranging from direct application of research to clinical practice (instrumental utilization) through situations in which research is ignored or not used. Therefore, research utilization is a matter of degree; clinicians even with minimal effort can use research to some degree to make clinical decisions that is based clinical decisions on evidence or evidence-based practice.

Audiologists and speech-language pathologists use of research to make clinical decision is limited (Gero, Bain & Miller, 2008; Kloda & Barlett, 2009). Zipoli and Kennedy (2006) reported that speech-language pathologists most often consult colleagues and do not use scholarly journals for clinical information.

Information Literacy

Information literacy is the ability to recognize when information is needed and the ability to locate, critically review and effectively use information (Cobus 2008). Many audiologists and speech-language pathologist have inadequate information seeking abilities (Geo, Bain, & Miller 2008; McCurtin & Roddam, 2012; Moodle, Kothan, Seewald, & Soollie, 2011; Nail-Chiwetalu & Rattner, 2006). There is a need for information literacy instruc-

tion in the university curriculum and continuing education for practicing audiologists and speech-language pathologists (Nail-Chiwetalu & Rattner, 2007). It was suggested that librarians work with audiology and speech-pathology training programs to integrate a high level of information into the curriculum and that librarians provide continuing education activities focusing on information literacy for practicing professionals.

Information literacy is essential for evidence-based practice (Nail-Chiwetalu & Rattner, 2006). Five standards for information literacy have been identified (Nail-Chiwetalu & Rattner, 2006). These standards are:

1. Determine the nature and extent of information needed
2. Access needed information effectively and efficiently
3. Evaluate information and is sources critically and incorporate selected information into knowledge based and values system
4. Individually or as a member of a group, use information effectively to accomplish a specific purpose
5. Understand the economic, legal, and social issues about the use of information, and access and use ethically and legally.

Clinical Trials

Clinical trials are typically associated with evidence-based practice. Sometimes referred to as clinical research trials or outcome measures, clinical trials are research designed to study the safety, efficacy, effectiveness, efficiency, and cost-benefit of an assessment or treatment (DePoy & Giltin, 2011; Polit & Beck, 2010).

Clinical trials are classified according to purpose (Portney & Watkins, 2009). The six purposes are: (1) prevention; (2) screening; (3) diagnostic; (4) treatment; (5) quality of life, and (6) compassionate use.

There are six hierarchical phases of clinical trials ranging from preclinical phase to the lowest or highest phase that involves cost-effectiveness, and cost benefit. These phases are listed and described in Table 13–1. Each phase provides information about assessment or treatment.

A major limitation of phase III is related to randomize controlled trials (RCTs). According to Polit and Beck (2009) RCTx are not relevant to real life situations. Moreover, there is the ethical dilemma of having a treatment and no treatment group and blinding or masking which are typically needed to use as a control group, that is, withholding treatment. Therefore, the focus is on practical information which can be used in routine clinical practice. Another problem related to audiology and speech-language pathology is that most studies in audiol-

ogy and speech-language pathology do not adequately address assessment and treatment relative to setting or condition. Other problems are related to extremely limited information from Phase IV treatment in audiology and speech-language pathology.

Advantages and Disadvantages of Evidence-Based Practice

Evidence-based practice has the potential to improve assessment and treatment of children and adults with communication disorders, increase resources for clinical services, and enhance the perception of the professionals of speech-language pathology and audiology (Mullen, 2007).

Disadvantages have been identified. These disadvantages include limited or no evidence about some clinical practices, unrelated to routine clinical practice, conflicting evidenced, increased cost bias, conflict of interest erroneous con-

Table 13–1. Phases of Clinical Trials

Phase	Description
Pre-clinical	Exploratory to determine safety under laboratory conditions.
I	Develop questions to be considered in later phases.
II	Refine primary hypothesis and develop plan for evaluating efficacy and effectiveness of assessment or treatment.
III	Efficacy under ideal conditions: typically a randomized controlled trial.
IV	Efficacy under average conditions
V	Study of efficiency, cost effectiveness, cost benefit, or cost utility.

Source: From "Evidence-Based Practice Guidelines for the Management of Communication Disorders in Neurologically Impaired Individuals," by L. A. Golper et al., 2001, *ANCDS Practice Guidelines.*

cepts, and overemphasis on randomized controlled trials.

There is also the possibility the evidence is wrong (Dodd, 2007). There are other issues; one is the limited discussion of settings and conditions in many research reports. Another is the limited information about the rule of instituting in evidence-based practice (Dodd, 2007).

Myths About Evidence-Based Practice

Several myths surrounding evidence-based practice should be considered. Table 13–2 lists those myths which contribute to misunderstanding evidence-based practice and may make it difficult

Table 13–2. Evidence-Based Practice: Myths and Facts

Myth:	Evidence-based already exists.
Fact:	Many clinicians use opinions not evidence to make clinical decisions.
Myth:	Evidence-based practice is impossible to initiate.
Fact:	It impossible to initiate with minimal time.
Myth:	Clinical experience is not relevant to evidence-based practice.
Fact:	Clinical experience is relevant to evidence-based practice.
Myth:	Cost is not an important consideration.
Fact:	Cost-benefit is an important consideration.
Myth:	Expert opinion is the highest level of evidence.
Fact:	Expert opinion is not considered credible evidence.
Myth:	All research is related to clinical decisions.
Fact:	Basic research is not related to clinical decisions, but applied research is related to clinical decisions.
Myth:	Evidence based on opinion is best.
Fact:	Evidence based empirical research is best.
Myth:	Textbooks contain high levels of evidence.
Fact:	Textbooks contain low levels of evidence copying.
Myth:	Clinical practice guidelines are not detailed
Fact:	Some clinical practice guidelines are detailed.

Source: From "Introduction to Evidence-Based Practice," by M. Law, 2002. In M. Law (Ed.), *Evidence-Based Rehabilitation* (pp. 2–12), Thorofare, NJ: Slack; "Evidence-Based Medicine: What It Is and What It Isn't," by D. L. Sackett, E. M Rosenberg, J. Gray, R. B. Haynes, and W. S. Richardson, 1996, *British Medical Journal, 312*(7023), pp.71–72; and "Evidence-Based Practice: Myths and Misconceptions," by C. Dollagham, 2004, *ASHA Leader.*

if not impossible to implement evidence-based practice. Eliminating or reducing these misconceptions increase the likelihood of using evidence-based practice to support clinical decision-making.

Barriers to Evidence-Based Practice

A major disadvantage of evidence-based practice is related to barriers that prohibit or impede its implementation. These barriers should be considered so that strategies can be developed to reduce or eliminate these barriers, thereby facilitating research use and evidence-based practice. A major barrier to evidence-based practice is failure to integrate research and clinical activities. There have also been delays between the completion of a research study and the time the results were reported, which might make the results no longer applicable to clinical practice.

The evidence base itself is frequently cited as a barrier (Mullen, 2005a, 2005b). Barriers to evidence-based practice were also identified by Woraell and Bennett (2001). These barriers were:

- access and ability to use databases
- all related literature is not listed
- frequently a lack of evidence about the topic
- level of evidence is not high
- evidence does not match the reality of clinical services
- no database of published CATs.

Nonexistent, conflicting, or irrelevant evidence is considered to be a formidable problem. Overreliance on RCTs is also a source of controversy (Elman, 2007). Sackett, Rosenberg, Gray, Haynes, and Richardson (1996) believe that evidence-based practice is not restricted to RCTs and meta-analysis, and it should involve finding the best available evidence to answer clinical questions.

Other barriers to EBP are related to bias about funding, publication, consumer-research mismatch, and reduced clinical applicability (Elman, 2006). There are limited research funds and a trend to allocate funds on the basis of evidence. There is a tendency for positive trials to be published more than once and the possibility of subjective publication decisions. Also, there may be a mismatch between the treatments that are researched and those that are desired or prioritized by consumers. Reduced clinical applicability results from a tradeoff between subject selection criteria and clinical applicability. Clients with severe problems or comorbidities may be underrepresented in clinical trials that have a homogeneous subject selection.

The type of evidence also warrants consideration. The randomized controlled trial (RCT) is considered the gold standard or highest level of evidence, although the information needed to understand human problems is not necessarily amenable to RCT (DePoy & Gitlin, 2011). A related limitation is that RCTs are not the only valid design. RCTs may not be appropriate for evaluating treatment provided to heterogeneous populations that have a wide range of differences, such as, aphasia, dysphagia, and developmental language disorders. For many types of speech-language disorders RCTs cannot be used at this time (Dodd, 2007).

There are other barriers to evidence-based practice research utilization and information literacy, negative attitudes about research, resistance to change, and limited collaboration and communication between researchers and clinicians. Some speech-language pathologists and audiologist do not read research journals or do not critically review published research findings. Lack of knowledge about how to access and critically review research evidence has also been identified as a barrier to using research evidence in clinical practice. On the other hand, research is sometimes reported in a way that makes findings inaccessible for clinicians' complex statistical information and dense research jargon may pose barriers to acquiring knowledge about evidence-based practice (Polit & Beck, 2011). Some speech-language pathologists and audiologists do not attend professional conferences where research is reported. Another consideration is that researchers sometimes ignore the research needs of clinicians.

Other barriers are related to time and change. Sometimes, clinicians are overwhelmed or overstretched because they believe they do not have enough professional time for evidence-based practice (Frattali & Worrell, 2001; Meline & Paradiso, 2003; Mullen, 2005a, 2005b; Zipoli & Kennedy, 2005). Sometimes, clinicians are resistant to change because it requires retraining and reorganization. Other clinicians may lack administrative support to implement evidence-based practice (Rose & Baldac, 2004). Both time and cost are reported as barriers to EBP by some speech-language pathologists (Mullen, 2005; Upton & Upton, 2005). Critical appraisal of research is fundamental to evidence-based practice, yet it may be difficult for some speech-language pathologists and audiologist.

Other barriers to evidence-based practice are related to the shortage of Ph.D. level researchers in speech-language pathology and audiology (ASHA, 2002; Justice & Fey, 2004). In addition, there are associated problems: (1) almost half of new Ph.Ds. choose nonacademic positions, which are probably non-research positions, and (2) an aging faculty and imminent retirement (Meline & Paradiso, 2005).

Last, there are barriers related to organization and the professions. Professional organizations may be reluctant to expend resources for teaching and/or using evidence-based practice. The professionals may also have barriers related to a shortage of role models for evidence-based practice or historical baggage that clinicians perceive themselves as not being capable of doing research or recommending changes based on research results (Polit & Beck, 2010).

Quality of Evidence: Levels and Grades of Evidence

Assessment of the quality of evidence is essential to evidence-based practice. Levels of evidence refer to a hierarchy for evaluating the quality and credibility of evidence. There are several methods for determining levels of evidence.

ASHA (2004) modified the levels of evidence from the Scottish Intercollegiate Guidance Network (Table 13–3). The levels of evidence hierarchical model are based on research design and ranges from highest/most credible or strongest to lowest/least credible or weakest. Randomizing and controlling are considered within research design. Tickle-Degnen

Table 13–3. ASHA's (2005a) Levels of Evidence

Level	Creditability Description
Ia	Well-designed meta-analysis of >1 randomized controlled trial
Ib	Well-designed randomized controlled study
IIa	Well-designed controlled study without randomization
IIb	Well-designed *quasi-experimental* study survey
III	Well-designed nonexperimental studies, i.e., correlational and case studies
IV	Expert committee report, consensus conference, clinical experience of respected authorities

Source: From *Evidence-based practice in communication disorders: An introduction* by ASHA, 2004. Available at http://www.asha.org

and Bedell (2003) criticized this model because "it is wrong when applied in a manner that excludes the use of all relevant valid, and available research evidence for clinical decision making" (p. 234). Other limitations noted were lack of information about patients and causality.

ASHA's Advisory Committee on Evidence-Base Practice and the National Center for Evidence-Based Practice developed a system for levels of evidence (Mullen, 2007). This system is shown in Table 13–4. The system involves four processes: (1) appraising the quality of studies; (2) identifying the research stage of each study; (3) assessing the quality relative to the stage of the research; and (4) synthesizing the information into a single table. Eight factors were identified for evaluation.

The type of clinical study, diagnostic or treatment can be used to determine the level of evidence. ASHA (2005) described hierarchies of evidence for diagnosis and treatment. In addition to these levels of evidence, studies are graded with recommendations about use for making clinical decisions (Figure 13–1). The grades range from A (highly recommended) to D (not recommended.

Regardless of the criteria used for evaluation of the quality of evidence, five common themes were identified by ASHA (2004). These themes are: (1) independent confirmation and converging evidence; (2) experimental control; (3) avoidance of subjectivity and bias; (4) effect sizes and confidence intervals, and (5) relevance and feasibility.

Knowledge and Skills Needed for Evidence-Based Practice

Audiologists and speech-language pathologists should understand that evidence-based practice utilizes the best available evidence in research and clinical practice.

Table 13–4. ASHA's (2007) Levels of Evidence

Study Design
- Controlled Trial
- Cohort Study
- Single-Subject Design or Case Control Study
- Cross-Sectional Study or Case Series
- Case Study

Blinding
- Assessors blinded
- Assessors not blinded or not stated

Sampling
- Random sample adequately described
- Random sample inadequately described
- Convenience sample/hand-picked sample or not stated

Subjects
- Groups comparable at baseline on important factors (between subject design) or subject(s) adequately described (within subject design)
- Groups/subjects not comparable at baseline or comparability not reported or subject(s) not adequately described

Outcomes
- At least one primary outcome measure is valid and reliable
- Validity unknown, but appears reasonable; reliable
- Invalid and/or unreliable

Significance
- p value reported or calculable
- p value neither reported nor calculable

Precision
- Effect size and confidence interval reported or calculable
- Effect size or confidence interval, but not both reported or calculable
- Neither effect size nor confidence interval reported or calculable

Intention to Treat (controlled trials only)
- Analyzed by intention to treat
- Not analyzed by intention to treat or not stated

Source: From "The State of the Evidence," by R. Mullen, 2007, *ASHA Leader.*

A

Good evidence for inclusion
Peer-review evidence
Supporting use for treatment

B

Fair evidence for inclusion
Peer-review evidence supports
Consideration of use for treatment

C

Insufficient evidence
Lack of peer-review evidence: however
recommendation(s) for use possible
on other grounds

D

Fair evidence for exclusion
Peer-review evidence supports treatment
should be excluded

E

Good evidence for exclusion
Peer-review supports treatment
should be excluded

Figure 13–1. Outcomes from systematic review. Reprinted with permission from "Evidence-Based Practice in Schools: Integrating Craft and Theory with Science and Data," by L. M. Justice and M. E. Fey, 2004, *ASHA Leader, 9*(4–5), pp. 30–32. Copyright by American Speech-Language-Hearing Association. All rights reserved.

Research utilization and information literacy are basic perquisites to evidence-based practice. ASHA's (2005) position statement about evidence-based practice outline the skills needed for evidence-based practice. Audiologists and speech-language pathologists should:

■ Recognize the needs, abilities, values, preferences and interests of patients and families and combine this information with best current research evidence and clinical expertise.

■ Acquire and maintain knowledge and skills necessary to provide high quality professional service including knowledge about evidence-based practice.

■ Evaluate clinical services and procedures for cost-effectiveness using recognized appraisal criteria described in the evidence-based literature.

■ Evaluate efficacy, effectiveness, and efficiency of clinical and research protocols using criteria described in the evidence-based literature.

■ Evaluate the quality of evidence in journal reports, textbooks, continuing education newsletters, advertisements, web-based products.

■ Monitor and apply new and high quality evidence.

Haynes and Johnson (2009) provided a detailed discussion for each of these skills. The discussion was related to skills both for students and practicing professionals.

In addition, audiologists and speech-language pathologists should:

■ Use scientific criteria for making decisions about research and clinical practice (Finn, Bothe, & Bramlett, 2005)

- Effectively communicate about evidence to patients, families and other professions
- Determine level of evidence for clinical and research studies (ASHA, 2004; Mullen 2007)
- Educate students and other professionals about the use and application of evidence-based practice
- Evaluate effectiveness and outcomes of education and training about evidence-based practice
- Develop and implement strategies to reduce barriers to evidence-based practice
- Dispel the myths and misconceptions about evidence-based practice
- Create an evidence-based environment
- Document fidelity.

Developing and Implementing Evidence-Based Practice

To utilize EBP, speech-language pathologists and audiologist must: (1) discount the opinions of authorities when there is counterevidence; (2) focus on research relevant to clinical practice, and (3) use rigorous criteria to evaluate the quality of evidence including validity, importance, and precision (Dollaghan, 2004a).

Education and training are the foundation for developing and implementing evidence-based practice. The December 2009 issues of Evidence-Based Communication Assessment and Intervention focused on teaching evidence-based practice to speech-language pathologists. Table 13–5 is a list of the authors and titles of these reports.

The decision-making process can be used to implement and develop evidence-based practice. Boswell (2005) and Kully and Langeven (2005) described similar procedures for evidence-based decision making. The steps were: (1) asking a clear, focused question; (2) finding the best evidence; (3) critically appraising the evidence; (4) integrating the evidence with clinical judgment and clinical values; and (5) evaluating the decision-making process. According to Schlosser,

Table 13–5. Teaching Evidence-Based practice from December 2009 Evidence-Based Communication Assessment and Intervention

Author	Title
Klee and Stringer	Teaching evidence-based practice to speech and language therapy students in the United Kingdom
McCabe, Purcell, Baker, Madill, and Trembath	Case-based learning: One route to evidence-based practice
Proxy and Murza	Building speech-language pathologists capacity for evidence-based practice: A unique graduate course approach
Raghavendra	Teaching evidence-based practice in a problem-based course in speech-language pathology
Schlosser and Sigafoos	Teaching evidence-based practice: An impetus for further curricular innovation and research

Koul, and Costello (2006) the first step in EBP is asking well-built questions but this often difficult for clinicians. To facilitate well-built questions, the PESICO template was proposed. PESICO stands for person (problem), environments, stakes holders, intervention, comparison, and outcome. Johnson, (2006) provided specific examples for making evidence-based decisions about childhood speech-language disorders.

Threats (2002) suggested the World Health Organization's International Classification of Disorders for developing evidence-based practice that could bridge the gap between research and clinical practice by providing a common framework and language. The purpose were to: (1) collect statistical data about functioning and disability, such as in population studies; (2) conduct clinical research, such as measurement of outcomes, quality of life, or impact of environmental factor on disability; (3) use clinically needs assessment, matching treatments with specific conditions, programs outcome evaluation and rehabilitation documentation; and (4) use for social policy, such as social security planning, governmental oversight of disability programs, and policy decision making.

There are several strategies for implementing and developing evidence-based practice. Some of these strategies are:

- Create a culture for evidence-based practice (Fingout-Overholt & Melnyk,2005)
- Provide evidence-based practice training and experience for both students and practicing professions
- Develop critical thinking skills (Finn, 2011)
- Integrate evidence-based practice into speech-language pathology and audiology curriculum (Forrest & Miller, 2001)
- Eliminate dichotomy between research and clinical practice
- Awareness of misconceptions about evidence-based practice
- Provide high levels of research evidence
- Collaboration of researchers and clinicians
- Use of systematic reviews to introduce evidence-based practice (McCauley & Hargrove, 2004; Mullen, 2005b)
- Communicate research results widely and clearly
- Specify clinical implications of research
- Expect evidence that a diagnosis or treatment procedure is effective
- Practice in a journal group
- Collaborative work groups (Johnson, 2006)
- Use ASHA's registry of evidence-based practice guidelines and systematic reviews (Evidence-Based Practice Tool Available, 2006; Mullen, 2006)
- Indicate level of evidence in professional presentations and publications, and continue education
- Seek professional environment that supports evidence-based practice
- Identify and eliminate sources of bias about EBP (Elman, 2005)
- Volunteer to participate in clinical research trials (Logemann & Gardner, 2005)
- Audit the degree and extent of research utilization
- On-site or online journal clubs (Betz, Smith, Melnyk, & Rickey, 2005)
- Multidisciplinary evidence-based practice courses
- Use formats for case presentations and critical reviews such as those

suggested by Dollaghan (2004a, 2004b)(2002), Frattali and Worrall (2001), Threats (2002), and Worrall and Bennett (2001).

Evidence-based practice is a process by which the current best evidence is critically appraised, clinical expertise considered, and a course of action selected. Several decisions may be made. For example, what is the best and most current research evidence? How can the evidence be integrated with clinical expertise and client preferences?

Because of the relative newness of evidence-based practice in speech-language pathology and audiology, little evidence exists to guide identification of the best strategies for implementing evidence-based practice. Some strategies are successful in some settings and with some professional groups but not with other settings or groups (Ciliska, DeCenso, Melynk, & Stetler, 2005).

Organizational Support for Evidence-Based Practice

Professional organizations have supported evidence-based practice. Among these organizations are the Academy of Neurological Communication Disorders and Sciences, American Academy of Audiology, American Speech Language Hearing Association, Australian Speech and Hearing Association, and the Canadian Speech and Hearing Association.

ASHA has devoted considerable effort to increase research utilization through evidence-based practice. The major activities include a Web site for evidence-based practice (ASHA, 2004b), a position statement (ASHA, 2005a), levels of evidence (2005b), a technical report (ASHA,

2005b), and evidence maps for ALS, aphasia, autism, cerebral palsy, cleft lip and palate, dementia, head and neck cancer, Parkinson's disease, TBI-adult, and TBI-children (National Center for Evidence-Based Practice, 2012). In addition to ACEBP, ASHA has established the National Center for Evidence-Based Practice in Communication Disorders. The center has a registry of clinical practice guidelines and systematic reviews (Mullen, 2006). Only guidelines and reviews with an overall rating of highly recommended or recommended with provisions are included in the registry. ASHA also has several practice guidelines, which provide information to assist clinicians in making decisions based on available research evidence and prevailing expert opinion. The purpose of such guidelines is to improve the quality of service, identify the most cost-effective treatment, prevent unfounded practices, and stimulate research (Golper et al., 2001).

ASHA also established the Communication Sciences and Disorders Clinical Trials Research Group (CSDRG), which is devoted solely to the development and conduct of clinical trials by audiologist, speech-language pathologist, and speech, language, and hearing scientists (Baum, Logemann, & Lilenfield, 1998; Logemann, 2004; Logemann & Gardner, 2005). Currently, CSDRG's clinical trials involve dysarthria, dysphagia, and language stimulation.

ASHA's Research and Scientific Affairs Committee had a series of reports about research concept and their application to speech-language pathology and audiology (Feeney, 2006). Topics to date are "Back to the Basics: Reading Research Literature" (Golper, Wertz, & Brown, 2006), "Developing a Research Question" (Nelson & Goffman, 2006), "Bias and Blinding"

(Finn, 2006), and "Interpretation of Correlation" (Oller, 2006).

In addition, two ASHA journals have had issues focusing on EBP. *Communication Issues in Communication Services and Disorders* (CICSD) (2006) described the specific task(s) needed to conduct a systematic review and meta-analysis that would facilitate EBP. The other journal, *Language, Speech, and Hearing in Schools* (LSHSS), discuss making evidence-based decisions for speech sound disorders, reading problems, and child language intervention.

The American Academy of Audiology emphasized EBP in a special 2005 issue of the Academy's Journal, the *Journal of the American Academy of Audiology.* These papers focused on the effectiveness of hearing rehabilitation.

ANCDS applied the principles of evidence-based practice to the development of practice guidelines with support of ASHA's Special Interest Division, Neurophysiologic and Neurogenic Speech and Language Disorders (Golper et al., 2001). "The purpose of such guidelines is to improve and assure the quality of care by reducing unacceptable variation in its provisions" (p. 2). The practice guidelines were completed when research evidence was available in the literature.

There are three types of clinical practice guidelines based on evidence: traditional or narrative (TPG), systematic reviews (SR), and evidence-based practice (Hargrove & Gruffer, 2008. Differences between these clinical practice guidelines were described in Chapter 5.

There is hierarchy of clinical practice guidelines with tradition-narrative reviews lowest (meeting the fewest criteria) and evidence based reviews highest (meeting the most criteria). Specifically,

traditional reviews met only two of seven criteria, systematic reviews met five of seven criteria, and evidence based review met all seven criteria. This information is useful in making decisions about using and recommending clinical practice guidelines.

The National Evidence-Based Center of ASHA (2011) uses the Appraisal of Guidelines for Research and Evaluation (AGREE) for evaluating and recommending systematic reviews. These reviews are highly recommended, recommended with reservations, or not recommended,

The Academy of Neurologic Communication Disorders and Sciences (ANCDS) has developed evidence-based practice guidelines (EBPG). These EBPGs focus on five areas: aphasia, acquires apraxia, cognitive dysarthria, and communication disorders related to traumatic brain injury and dementia.

Obviously, there is a variation in reporting clinical practice guidelines. Shiffner and associates (2003) developed and standardized format for reporting clinical practice guidelines which is based on 15 factors and is followed by systematic reviews by writing committees within ANCDS (Golper et al., 2001; Yorkston et al., 2001a). These guidelines reflected a moderate degree of clinical certainty and are usually based on Class II evidence or strong consensus from Class III evidence (Golper et al., 2001).

The Canadian Association of Speech-Language Pathologist and Audiologists (CASLPA) have promoted evidence-based practice in classrooms, clinics, and research (Orange, 2004). In 1996, CASLPA affiliated with the Canadian Cochrane Network and Center. Evidence-based practice has been incorporated into the academic coursework, clinical practice, and thesis research at the University of Western Ontario.

The Australian Speech Pathology Association published a service of reports about clinical practice (Baker, 2005). The first in this series of articles was, "What Is the Evidence for Oral Motor Therapy" by Bowen (2005). Reports about evidence-based practice have continued to be published in the Association's journal.

Resources for Evidence-Based Practice

Finding evidence is a fundamental aspect of evidence-based practice. Electronic searches can be an efficient way to locate evidence (Dollinghan, 2007). There are several electronic databases related to evidence-based practice: PubMed, Cumulative Index of Nursing and Allied Health (CINHAL), and the Cochrane Collection.

The American Speech Language Hearing Association (n.d.) developed evidence-based maps related to clinical expertise/expert opinion, external scientific evidence, and client/patient/caregiver perspectives. There are evidenced-based maps for amyotrophic lateral sclerosis, autism, spectrum disorders. Parkinson disease, and traumatic brain injury in children and adults.

Several books are available that focus on evidence-based practice in communication disorders. These books are:

- *Evidence-Based Practice in Speech Pathology* (Reilly, Douglas, & Oates (2004)
- *The Efficacy of Augmentative and Alternative Communication: Toward Evidence-Based Practice* (Schlosser, 2000)
- *The Handbook for Evidence-Based Practice in Communication Disorders* (Dollaghan, 2007)
- *Understanding Research and Evidence-Based Practice in Communication Disorders* (Haynes & Johnson, 2009)
- *Introduction to Communication Disorders: A Lifespan Evidence-Based Perspective* (Owens, 2010).

In addition, there are two journals exclusive to evidence-based practice:

- *Evidence-Based Communication: Assessment and Intervention* is published four times per year by Psychology Press. This journal brings together professionals from several different disciplines to facilitate evidence-based services for children and adults with communication disorders. These professionals include speech-language pathologists, special educators, regular educators, applied behavior analysts, clinical psychologists, physical therapists, and occupational therapists.
- *Evidence-Based Practice Briefs in Speech-Language* is a combination electronic and print peer-review journal. It began publication in 2006 by Pearson.

Evidence-based practice guidelines integrate evidence about a single topic (Polit & Beck, 2010). The evidence is summarized and evaluated from previous studies for use in clinical practice. Systematic reviews, meta-analysis, and clinical practice guidelines are useful resources for evidence-based practice.

Communicating Evidence

Communication is important for implementing and developing evidence-based practice. Communicating evidence to clients and others improves understanding, involvement in decisions, and outcomes (Epstein, Alper, & Quill, 2004). Speech-language pathologists and audiologists should discuss possible options, including relevant research evidence, and risks and benefits. The goal is to provide sufficient information to the client and/or family can make an informed decision (Johnson, 2006).

Tickle-Degnen (2002), described four steps for effectively communicating information. These steps are: (1) identify the relative role or the decision maker relative to the clinician; (2) identify the decision that the decision maker will make with the clinician, (3) locate and interpret which evidence is related to the information need of the decision maker and the clinician, and (4) translate the evidence in a comprehensive communication which facilitates informed delegating with the decision maker so that decisions can be made and action taken.

Methods for communicating evidence include visual supplements, tables and groups, decision aids, graphic representation, and quantitative translation of clinical evidence. Systematic reviews and clinical practice guidelines can be used to communicate evidence for clinical decision-making among professionals, third-party payees, and policy makers.

Another approach for communicating evidence among professionals is the peer-reviewed journal *Evidence-Based Communication Assessment and Intervention* (EBCAI) (Taylor & Francis Group,

2006). The primary aims of EBCAI are: (1) promoting EBP in communication assessment and treatment; (2) appraising the latest evidence in communication evaluation and treatment; (3) providing a forum for discussions that advance EBP; and (4) disseminating EBP research.

Critically appraised topics (CAT) have also been used to communicate information among professionals (Worrall & Bennett, 2001). CATs were described in Chapter 11.

Ethical Consideration

There are several ethical principles and practices especially pertinent to evidence-based practice: beneficence, non-maleficence, justice, autonomy, control groups, risk-benefits, and fidelity (Chabon, Morris, & Lemoncello, 2011). Beneficence is doing good or kindness, seeking to maximize benefits for study participants and prevent harm (Polit & Beck, 2010). Non-maleficence means do no harm, in other words avoiding harm to subjects or patients (Aiken 2002). Justice is fairness to equitable distribution of risk and benefits (Portney & Watkins 2009). Autonomy is independence or freedom to make decisions.

Control Groups

The use of control groups (randomized controlled trials, RCTs) has been criticized because withholding treatment is wrong; therefore, many studies have only experimental groups and not control groups. These studies are considered to be weak. RCTs that are considered to be the gold standard for evidence (Golper & Brown, 2001; Brown & Golper, 2012).

Double Blinding

Double blinding is possible in audiology and speech-language pathology research, but is rarely used because of ethical issues related to withholding treatment from a control group (Dodd, 2007).

Risks and Benefits

Risks and benefits are an ethical principle with an element of informed consent in which risks and benefit are compared and relates to outcomes. Studies are compared to the benefits of the study outcome (Portney & Watkins, 2009). Essentially, the question is do the benefits outweigh the risks?

Fidelity

Fidelity is the extent to which a clinical procedure is administered according to the author's instructions. It is an important but neglected concept which can affect clinical research findings. Fidelity can be enhanced by using a detailed unified protocol so that the procedure can be delivered consistently, is producible, and is independent of style; provide training and monitoring through observation or review of audio or video recordings; and training compliance (DePoy & Gitlin, 2011).

Summary

There has been progress in implementing evidence-based practice in speech-language pathology and audiology, although this process has been slow, it does not seem that clinicians have increased their recognition of the need for evidence-based practice, nor research utilization.

Several organizations have undertaken efforts to facilitate implementation and development of evidence-based practice. Among these organizations are ASHA, ANCDS, CASLPA, and ASPA.

There are barriers to evidence-based practice. The primary barriers are related to the evidence based practice. The primary barriers are related to the evidence base itself, time, and resistance to change. On the other hand, there are a number of strategies to implement evidence-based practice that may improve the extent to which research is used for making clinical decisions. Information about evidence in audiology and speech-language pathology must be communicated to decisions makers, that is, patients, third-party payees, and other professionals. Several ethical issues are especially related to evidence-based practice; use of control groups, risks-benefits, and blinding.

DISCUSSION QUESTIONS

1. What is evidence-based practice, research utilization, and information literacy?
2. What factors may account for the increased interest in evidence-based practice?
3. How do speech-language pathologists and audiologist make decisions about assessment and treatment?
4. Why is the research under-utilized? Why is the poorest evidence over utilized?
5. How can research utilization be improved?
6. What is meant by the statement that "research utilization is on a continuum"?
7. How do speech-language pathologists and audiologists make clinical decisions?
8. Why should levels of evidence be considered in making clinical decisions?
9. What are the myths about evidence-based practice? How do these myths affect clinical decisions?
10. What activities has ASHA undertaken to facilitate implementation of evidence-based practice?
11. What is CSDRG?
12. Define clinical trials. What are the phases?
13. What is blinding or masking?
14. What are the indications and contradictions for blinding?
15. What are the steps in making evidence-based decisions?
16. What are the barriers to evidence-based practice? How can these barriers be reduced or eliminated?
17. What can be done to develop and implement evidence-based practice?
18. How can evidence be communicated to patients? Other professionals?
19. How have professional organizations supported evidence-based practice?
20. What resources are available for evidence-based practice?
21. What are the major ethical issues related to evidence-based practices?

References

Aiken, T. D. (2002). *Legal and ethical issues in health occupations.* Philadelphia, PA: W. B. Saunders.

American Academy of Audiology (2010). *The green book.* Washington, DC: Author.

American Speech-Language-Hearing Association, (2002). *PUD program survey results.* Retrieved from http://www.asha.org/mem bers/pudfacilityresearch/reports/pud_survey_sum.htm

American Speech-Language-Hearing Association. (2005a). *Evidence-based practice in communication disorders: Position statement.* Rockville, MD: Author.

American Speech-Language-Hearing Association. (2005b). *Evidence-based practice in communication disorders: An introduction.* Retrieved from http://www.asha.org/about

American Speech-Language-Hearing Association. (2005c). *Examples of levels-of-evidence hierarchies.* Retrieved from http://www.asha.org/about/publication/levels-online/2005/htm

American Speech-Language-Hearing Association. (2009). Background *information and standards and implementation for the Certificate of Clinical Competence in speech-language pathology.* Retrieved from http://www.asha.org/about/membership-certification/handbook/s/slp_standards_new.htm

American Speech-Language-Hearing Association. (2011). *New audiology standards.* Retrieved from http://www.asha.org/about/membershipcertification

Baker, E. (2005). What's the evidence from? *Acquiring Knowledge in Speech, Language, and Hearing,* (3), 144–147.

Baum, H. M., Logemann, J., & Lilenfeld, D. (1998). Clinical trials and their application to communication sciences and disorders. *Journal of Medical Speech-Language Pathology, 6,* 55–64.

Bernstein-Ratner, N. (2006). Evidence-based practice: An examination of its ramifications for the practice of speech-language pathology. *Language, Speech, and Hearing Services in Schools, 37*(4), 257–267.

Betz, C. L., Smith, A., Melnyk, B. M., & Rickey, T. (2005). Disseminating evidence. In B. M. Melynk & E. Fingout-Overholt (Eds.), *Evidence-based practice in nursing and healthcare* (pp. 351–403). Philadelphia, PA: Lippincott Williams & Wilkins.

Boswell, S. (2005, September 27). Finding the evidence for school-based clinical decision-making. *ASHA Leader,* pp. 26–27, 39.

Bowen, C. (2005). What is the evidence for oral motor therapy? *Acquiring Knowledge in Speech, Language, and Hearing, 7*(3), 144–147.

Brown, K. E., & Golper, L.. A. (2012). Applying evidence to clinical practice. In R. Lubinski & M. W. Hudson (Eds.), *Professional issues in speech-language pathology and audiology* (pp. 582–601). Clifton Park, NY: Delmar.

Byiers, B. J. (2012). Single-subject experimental design for evidence-based practice.

American Journal of Speech-Language Pathology, 39, 397–414.

Chabon, S., Morris, J., & Lemoncello, S. (2011). Ethical deliberations: A foundation for evidence-based practice. *Seminar in Speech Language, 31,* 298–308.

Cilisla, D., DeCenso, A., Melynk, B. M., & Stelter, C. (2005). Using models and strategies for evidence-based practice. In B. M. Melynk & E. Fingout-Overholt (Eds.), *Evidence-based practice in nursing and healthcare* (pp. 185–219). Philadelphia, PA: Lippincott Williams & Wilkins.

Cobus, L. (2005). Integrating information literacy into the education of public professional: Roles or librarians and the library. *Journal of the Medical Library Association, 96*(1), 28–33.

Cook, D., & Giacomini, M. (1999). The trials and tribulations of clinical practice guidelines. *Journal of the American Medical Association, 281,* 1900–1905.

Cornett, B. S. (2001). Service delivery issues in health care settings. In R. Lubinski & C. Frattali (Eds.), *Professional issues in speech-language pathology and audiology* (pp. 229–250). Clifton Park, NY: Delmar.

Dennis, J., & Abvorr, J. (2006). Information retrieval: Where's your evidence? *Contemporary Issues in Communication Sciences and Disorders, 33,* 11–20.

DePoy, E., & Gitlin, L. N. (2011). *Introduction to research.* St. Louis, MO: C. V. Mosby.

Dodd, B. (2007). Evidence-based practice and speech-language pathology: Strengths, weaknesses, opportunities, and threats. *Folia Phoniatrica, 9,* 118–119.

Dollaghan, C. A. (2004a). Evidence-based practice in communications disorders: What do we know, and when do we know it? *Journal of Communication Disorders, 3*(5), 391–400.

Dollaghan, C. (2004b). Evidence-based practice myths and realities. *ASHA Leader, 12,* 4–5, 12.

Elkins, M. Y. (2010). Using PICO and the brief report to answer clinical questions. *Nursing,* pp. 59–60.

Elman, R. J. (2005). Evidence-based practice: What evidence is missing? *Aphasiology, 20*, 103–109.

Epstein, R. M., Alper, B. S., & Quill, T. E. (2004). Communicating evidence for participatory decision-making. *Journal of the American Medical Association, 219*(19), 2359–2386.

Evidence-based practice tool available. (2006, June 13). *ASHA Leader, 11*(8), 19.

Feeney, P. (2006, May 2). Primer on research: An introduction. *ASHA Leader, 11*(6), 14, 26.

Fingout-Overholt, E., Cox, T., Robbins, B., & Gray, T. L. (2009). Teaching evidence-based practice. In B. M. Malynk & E. Fingout-Overholt (Eds.), *Evidence-based practice: Nursing and healthcare* (p. 407–441). Philadelphia, PA: Lippincott Williams & Wilkins.

Finn, P. (2006, June 13). Bias and blinding. *ASHA Leader, 11*(8), 16–17, 22.

Finn, P. (2011). Critical thinking: Knowledge and skills for evidence-based practice. *Language, Speech, and Hearing Services in Schools, 42*, 69–72.

Finn, P., Bothe, A. K., & Bramlet, R. F. (2005). Science and pseudoscience in communication disorders: Criteria and application. *American Journal of Speech Language Pathology, 14*, 172–185.

Forrest, J. L., & Miller, S. (2001). A. Integrating evidence-based decision-making into Allied Health curricula. *Journal of Allied Health, 30*(4), 215–222.

Frattali, C., & Worrall, L. E. (2001) Evidence-based practice: Applying science to the art of clinical care. *Journal of Medical Speech-Language Pathology, 9*(1), iv–xiv.

Gallagher, T. M. (2001). Implementation of evidence-based practice in communication disorders coursework and practice. *Proceedings of Academic Programs in Communication Sciences and Disorders* (pp. 29–45).

Golper, L. A., & Brown, K. (2007). Applying evidence to clinical practice. In R. Lubarski, L. A. Golper, & C. M. Fratalli (Eds.), *Professional issues in speech-language pathology and audiology* (pp. 560–576). Clifton Park, NY: Delmar.

Golper, L. C., Wertz, R. T., & Brown, K. E. (2006). Back to basics. Reading research literature. *ASHA Leader, 11*(5), 10–11, 28, 34–35.

Golper L., Wertz, R. T., Frattali, C., Yorkston, K., Myers, P., Katz, R., Beeson, P., Kennedy, M. T., Bayles, K., & Wambaugh, J. (2001). Evidence-based practice guidelines for the management of communication disorders in neurologically impaired adults. *Academy of Neurological Communication Disorders and Science Report Practice Guidelines*, pp. 1–12.

Gueo, R., Bain, B. A., & Miller, J. (2008). Results of an assessment of information needs among speech-language pathologists and audiologist in Idaho. *Journal of the Medical Library Association, 95*(2), 182–188.

Hamre, C. E. (1972). Research and clinical practice: A unifying model. *ASHA, 14*, 542–545.

Hargrove, P., & Gruffer, M. (2008). Procedures for using clinical practice guidelines. *Language, Speech, and Hearing Services in Schools, 39*, 289–302.

Haynes, W. O., & Johnson, C. E., (2009). *Understanding research and evidence-based practice*. Boston, MA: Pearson.

Herder, C., Howard, C, Nye, C., & Vanryckeghem, M. (2006). Effectiveness of behavioral stuttering treatment: A systematic review and meta-analysis. *Contemporary Issues in Communication Sciences and Disorders, 33*, 61–73.

Hooper, T., Mahendra, N., Kim, E., Azuma, T., Bayles, K. A., & Cleary, S. J. (2005). Evidence-based practice recommendations for working with individuals with dementia: Space retrieval training. *Journal of Medical Speech-Language Pathology, 13*(4), xxvii–xxxiv.

Huang, X., Lin, J., & Demner-Fushmann, D. (2006). Evaluation of PICO as a knowledge representation for clinical questions. *Annual Symposium Proceedings*, pp. 359–363.

Jewell, D. V. (2011). *Guide to evidence-based physical therapy*. Sudbury, MA: Jones and Bartlett.

Johnson, C. E. (2006). Getting started in evidence-based practice for childhood speech-language disorders. *American Journal of Speech-Language Pathology, 15*, 20–35.

Johnson, C. E., & Danhalier, J. L. (2006). Evidence-based practice in audiology: A tutorial. *Audiology Today*, pp. 16–20.

Justice, L. M., & Fey, M. E. (2004, September 21). Evidence-based practice in schools: Integrating craft and theory with science and data. *ASHA Leader*, pp. 30–32, 45.

Kaderavk, J. N., & Justice, L. M. (2010). Fidelity: An essential component of evidence-based practice in speech-language pathology. *American Journal of Speech-Language Pathology, 19*, 269–279.

Klee, T., Stringer, H., & Howard, D. (2009). Teaching evidence-based practice to speech and language therapy students in the United Kingdom. *Evidence-Based Communication Assessment and Intervention, 3*, 195–207.

Kloda, L., & Bartlett, J. C. (2009). Clinical information behavior of rehabilitation therapists: A review of the research or occupational therapists, physical therapists, and speech-language pathologists. *Journal of the Medical Library Association, 97*, 194–202.

Konnerup, M., & Schwartz. J. (2006). Translating systematic reviews into policy and practice. *Contemporary Issues in Commumnication Sciences and Disorders, 33*, 79–82.

Kully, D., & Langeven, M. (2005, October 18). Evidence-based practice in fluency disorders. *ASHA Leader*, pp. 10–11, 23.

LaRue, E. M., Draus, P., & Klem, M. L. (2009). A description of a web-based educational tool for understanding the PICO framework in evidence-based practice with a citation ranking system. *Computer information Nursing, 27*, 44–49.

Law, J., & Plunkett, C. (2000). Grading study quality in systematic reviews. *Contemporary Issues in Communication Disorders and Sciences, 33*, 28–36.

Law, M. (2002). Introduction to evidence-based practice. In M. Law (Ed.), *Evidence-based rehabilitation* (pp. 2–12). Thorofare, NJ: Slack Incorporated.

Logemann, J. A. (1998). *Evaluation and treatment of swallowing disorders*. Austin, TX: Pro-Ed.

Logemann, J. A. (2004). Clinical trials: CSDRGG overview. *Journal of Communication Disorders, 37*(5), 419–423.

Logemann, J. A., & Gardner, P. M. (2005, August 16). Help find the evidence clinicians need. *ASHA Leader*, pp. 8–9.

Lum, C. (2002). *Scientific thinking in speech and language therapy*. Mahwah, NJ: Lawrence Erlbaum Associates.

McCabe, P., Purcell, A., Baker, E., Mago, C., & Trembath, D. (2009). Case-based learning: One route to evidence-based practice. *Evidence-Based Communication Assessment and Intervention, 3*, 20.

McCauley, R. J., & Hargrove, P. (2004). A clinician's introduction to systematic reviews in communication disorders: The course review paper with muscle. *Issues in Communication Sciences and Disorders, 31*, 173–181.

McCurtin, A., & Roddam, H. (2012). Evidence-based practice: SLT's under siege opportunity for growth: The use and nature of research evidence in the profession. *International Journal of Language and Communication Disorders, 17*, 22–26.

Meline, T. (2006). *Research in communication science and disorders*. Columbus, OH. Pearson.

Meline, T., & Paradiso, T. (2003). Evidence-based practice in schools. *Language, Speech, and Hearing Services in Schools, 34*, 273–283.

Melnyk, B. M., & Fineout-Overholt, E, (2005). *Evidence-based practice in nursing and healthcare*. Philadelpjhia, PA: Lippincott, Williams and Wilkins.

Moodle, S. T., Kotuari, A., Kothan, A., Bagatto, M. P., Seewald, R., & Miller, L. T. (2011).

Knowledge translation in audiology: Promotion the clinical application of best evidence. *Trends in Amplification 15*, 5–22.

Mullen, R. (2005a, August 16). Evidence-based practice planning addresses member needs skills. *ASHA Leader, 1*, 21.

Mullen, R. (2005b, November 8). Survey test members' understanding of evidence-based practice. *ASHA Leader, 4*, 14.

Mullen, R. (2006). *The N-CED registry of clinical practice guidelines and systematic reviews.* Retrieved from http://www.asha.org/members/ebp/registry/NCEP-registry

Mullen, R. (2007 March 6). The state of the evidence. ASHA develops levels of evidence for communication sciences and disorders. *ASHA Leader*, pp. 8-9, 24–25.

Nail-Chiwetalu, B. (2005). Information literacy: Essential for evidence-based practice. *ASHA Administration and Supervisors*, pp. 14–17.

Nail-Chiwetalu, B., & Ratner, N. (2006). Information literacy for speech-language pathologists: A key to evidence-based practice. *Language, Speech, and Hearing Services in Schools, 17*(2), 151–167.

Nail-Chiwetalu, B., & Ratner, N. (2007). Assessment of the information seeking abilities and needs among speech-language pathologists. *Journal of the Medical Library Association, 95*(2), 182–188.

National Center for Evidence-Based Practice in Communication Disorders. (2012). Retrieved from http://www.ncepmap.org

Nelson, P., & Goffman, L. (2006, May 2). Primer on research: Developing research questions. *ASHA Leader, 11*(6), 15, 26.

Nicholson, D. (2002). Practice guidelines algorithms and clinical pathways. In M. Law (Ed.), *Evidence-based rehabilitation* (pp. 195–220). Thorofare, NJ: Slack Incorporated.

Nollan, R., Fingout-Overholt, E., & Stephenson, P. (2005). Asking compelling clinical questions. In B. M. Melnyk & S. E. Fingout-Overholt (Eds.), *Evidence-based practice* (pp. 25–37). Philadelphia, PA: Lippincott Williams & Wilkins.

Nye, C., & Harvey, J. (2006). Interpreting and maintaining the evidence. *Contemporary Issues in Communication Sciences and Disorders, 33*, 56–60.

Oller, D. K. (2006, November 7). Interpretation and correlation. *ASHA Leader*, pp. 24–26.

Orange, J. B. (2004). Evidence-based clinical practice: A Canadian perspective. *American Journal of Speech-Language Pathology, 13*(3), 1264–1265.

Owens, R. E. (2012). *Introduction to communication disorders: A lifespan evidence-based perspective.* Boston, MA: Allyn & Bacon.

Pain, K., Magill-Evans, J., Darrah, J., Hagler, P., & Warren, S. (2004). Effects of processing and facilitating type of research utilization by rehabilitation professionals. *Journal of Allied Health, 33*(7), 3–9.

Polit, P. F., & Beck, C. T. (2010). *Nursing research.* Philadelphia, PA: Lippincott.

Portney, L. G., & Watkins, M. P. (2009). *Foundations of clinical research: Applications to practice.* Upper Saddle River, NJ: Pearson.

Pring, T. (2004). Ask a silly question: Two decades of troublesome tricks. *International Journal of Language Communication Disorders, 39*(3), 285–302.

Proxy, J., & Mural, K. A. (2009). Building speech-language pathology capacity for evidence-based practice: A unique graduate course approach. *Evidence-Based Communication Assessment and Intervention, 3*, 220–231.

Raghavendra, P. (2009). Teaching evidence-based practice in a problem-based learning course in speech-language pathology. *Evidence-Based Communication Assessment and Intervention, 3*, 232–237.

Reilly, S., Oates, J., & Douglas, J. (204). Evidence-based practice in speech-language pathology: Future directions. In S. Reilly, J. Douglas, & J. Oates (Eds.), *Evidence-based practice in speech-language pathology*, (pp. 330–352). London, UK: Whurr.

Richardson, W., Wilson, N., Nishisawa, J., & Haywsdt. (1995). The well-built question: A key to evidence-based design. *ACP Journal Club, 123*, A12-A13.

Ringel, R. (1972). The clinician and the researcher: An artificial dichotomy. *ASHA, 14*, 351–353.

Robey, R. R. (2004). A five-phase model for clinical outcome research. *Journal of Communication Disorders, 37*(5), 401–411.

Robey, R. R. (2005, May 24). An introduction to clinical trials. *ASHA Leader*, pp. 6-7, 22–23.

Robey, R. R. (2008). A model for conducting clinical outcome research: An adaptation of the standard protocol for use in aphasiology. *Aphasiology, 12*, 787–810.

Rose, M. I., & Baldac, S. (2004). Translating evidence into practice. In S. Reilly, J. Douglas, & J. Oates (Eds.), *Evidence-based practice in speech pathology* (pp. 317–329). London, UK: Whurr.

Sackett, D. L., Rosenberg, W. M., Gray, J., Haynes, R. B., & Richardson, W. S. (1996). Evidence-based medicine: What it is and what it isn't. *British Medical Journal, 312*(7023), 71–72.

Sackett, D. L., Strauss, S. E., Richardson, W. S., Rosenberg, W. M., & Haynes, R. B. (2001). *Evidence-based medicine.* London, UK: Churchill Livingstone.

Schlosser, R. W. (2000). *The efficacy of augmentative and alternate communication: Evidence-based practice.* St Louis, MO: Elsevier.

Schlosser, R. W. (2004). Evidence-based practice in ACC: 10 points to consider. *ASHA Leader*, pp. 6–7, 10–11.

Schlosser, R. W. (2009). Referring to clinical expertise and to client perspectives as evidence: Methods and perils. *Evidence-Based Communication Assessment and Intervention, 3*, 131–135.

Schlosser, R. W., Koul, K., & Costello, J. (2007). Asking well-built questions for evidence-based practice in augmentative and alternative communication. *Journal of Communication Disorders, 40*, 225–238.

Schlosser, R. W., & O'Neil-Pirozz, T. M. (2006). Problem formulation in evidence-based practice and systematic reviews. *Contemporary Issues in Communication Sciences and Disorders, 33*, 5–10.

Schlosser, R. W., & Sigafoos, J. (2008). Identifying evidence-based practice versus empirically supported treatment. *Evidence-Based Communication Assessment and Intervention, 2*, 61–62.

Schlosser, R. W., & Sigafoos, J. (2009). Teaching evidence-based practice: An imperative for further innovation and research. *Evidence-Based Communication Assessment and Intervention, 3*, 191–194.

Sheneyfelt, T. M., Mayo-Smith, M. F., & Rothwangl, J. (1999). Are guidelines following Guidelines? *Journal of the American Medical Association, 281*(20), 1900–1905.

Shiffner, R. M., Shekelle, P., Overcharge, M., Slutsky, K., & Grimshaw, J. (2002). Standardizing reports of clinical practice guidelines. *Annals of Internal Medicine, 139*, 493–498.

Silverman, F. H. (1998). *Research design and evaluation in speech-language pathology and audiology.* Boston, MA: Allyn & Bacon.

Snowball, R. (2000). Critical appraisal of clinical guidelines. In M. Dawes, P. T. Davies, A. M. Grey, J. Mant, K Seers, & R. Snowball (Eds.), *Evidence-based practice.* (pp. 122–132). New York, NY: Churchill Livingstone.

Taylor & Francis Group. (2006). *Evidence-based communication and intervention.* Retrieved from http://www.tandfico/journals/titles/17489539.asp

Threats, T. T. (2002). Evidence-based practice research using a WHO framework. *Journal of Medical Speech-Language Pathology, 10*(3), xvii–xxiv.

Tickle-Degnen, L., & Bedell, G. (2005). Hierarchy and hierarchy: A critical appraisal on the "level of evidence" as a tool for clinical decision-making. *American Journal of Occupational Therapy, 57*, 234–237.

Tickle-Degnen, N. (2002). Communicative evidence to clients, managers, and funders. In M. Law (Ed.), *Evidence-based rehabilitation* (pp. 221–254) Thorofare, NJ: Slack Incorporated.

U.S. Preventive Services Task Force. (1989). *Examples of outcomes from systematic review.* Retrieved from http://www.asha

.org/about/publicaitons/leader-online/archives/2004/fo4092/al.htm

Upton, D., & Upton, P. (2006). Knowledge and use of evidence-based practice by allied health and health science professional in the United Kingdom. *Journal of Allied Health Professionals, 35*(3), 127–133.

Wertz, R. T. (2002). Evidence-based practice guidelines: Not all evidence is created equal. *Journal of Medical Speech-Language Pathology, 103*(3), x–xv.

Worral, L. E., & Bennett, S. (2001). Evidence-based practice: Barriers and facilitators for speech-language pathologists. *Journal of Medical Speech-Language Pathology, 9*(2), xi–xvi.

Yorkston, K. M., Spencer. K. A., & Duffy, J. R. (2003). Behavioral management of respiratory/phonatory dysfunction from dysarthria: A systematic review of evidence. *Journal of Medical Speech-Language Pathology, 11*, xiii–xxxviii.

Yorkston, K. M., Spencer. K. A., Duffy, J., Beukelman, D., Golper, L. A., & Miller, R. (2001a). Evidence-based medicine and practice guidelines: Application to the field of speech-language pathology. *Journal of Medical Speech-Language Pathology, 9*(4), 243–256.

Yorkston, K. M., Spencer. K. A., Duffy, J., Beukelman, D., Golper, L. A., & Sullivan, M., (2001b). Evidence-based practice guidelines for dysarthria: Management of velopharyngeal function. *Journal of Medical Speech-Language Pathology, 8*(4), 257–274.

Zipoli, R. P., & Kennedy, M. (2005). Evidence-based practice among speech-language pathologist: Attitudes, utilization, and barriers. *American Journal of Speech-Language Pathology, 14*, 208–220.

14

Research Grants

LEARNING OBJECTIVES

Upon completion of this chapter the reader will be able to:

- Identify the three phases of the grants acquisition process

- Identify reference sources available for the seeking of grants from federal and private agencies

- List general principles of the grant seeking process

- Discuss preliminary considerations in grant proposal writing

- Identify the major sections of a research grant proposal

- List and define the major categories in the budget section of a research grant proposal

- Differentiate direct costs and indirect costs associated with a research grant proposal

- Discuss the sources of ideas/problems for research projects

- Identify basic principles of grant proposal writing

- List some suggestions for grant proposal writing

- Identify the characteristics of a fundable research grant proposal

- Describe the grant proposal review process.

Introduction

There is a strong association between research activities and grants. Without grants from the government and private sector, much of the research in communication disorders (and, for that matter, in many fields) would not be possible. In addition to any available internal funds, for those involved in research, it is essential to locate a specific external source(s) of support for their activities. For example, a university professor or hospital audiologist or school speech-language pathologist who has an interest in a specific communication disorder and wishes to pursue a research project to learn more about the disorder, may find that funds are not available within her/his agency to support the necessary personnel, equipment, materials, travel, and other items that are needed to conduct the research. The only feasible approach for obtaining funds for the research may be through external sources (such as the federal government or private foundations), and the only way to obtain external support is to write a grant proposal to a particular funding agency. Moreover, the importance of grants is further accentuated in academia, where support for research activities is essential for conducting research, and conducting research is essential for publications in scholarly journals which, in turn, are essential for the awarding of tenure, which is essential for maintaining one's position in a university. Therefore, grants may be the mechanism for job stability and may play a major role in the "publish or perish" philosophy in institutions of higher education.

The Grants Acquisition Process

Acquiring grant support may appear to the uninitiated as somewhat "mystical" in nature. However, in reality, there is nothing magical about the grants acquisition process. In fact, it is a systematic process which can be considered in three phases: grant seeking, grant proposal writing, and grant management. First, the investigator seeks sources of support whose mission and interests coincide with the goals and nature of his or her project. Then the investigator writes a grant proposal following the guidelines established by the sponsoring agency. Then, if a grant is awarded, the investigator manages the research project, including the expenditure of awarded funds.

Grant Seeking

Grant seeking involves searching for a source of funding for a specific research project, thus matching the nature of the topic with the objectives of the support source. There are various sources of external support for research projects, the largest being the federal government. In addition, national organizations and private corporations are potential sources for competitive grants.

Foundations are another major source of support in the private sector. A foundation is a nongovernmental, nonprofit organization whose funds and programs are managed by its own trustees or directors and established to maintain or aid educational, charitable, or other activities serving the common welfare, primarily through the awarding of grants. There are different types of foundations, but the type that serves as the primary source of support for research projects is the independent foundation.

In addition to *extramural* (outside the institution) *funding* sources, colleges and universities provide support for research in the form of relatively small grants as "seed money" for starting new research projects. These *intramural* (in-house) *funds*, although relatively small, are essential for collecting preliminary data and providing the foundation for more extensive research projects to be supported by extramural funding. They can be a very important component in the decisions for funding made by outside agencies.

Numerous references are available to locate potential funding sources in both the public and private sector. Much of this information can be found online, some of it free and some fee-based. The following are representative samples of references available for grant seeking purposes.

- *Catalog of Federal Domestic Assistance* (http://www.cfda.gov) is a valuable reference source to learn about relevant federal programs, eligibility requirements, and application deadlines. It provides access to a database of all available federal programs that can be searched in a number of ways, including keywords, agency, applicant eligibility, type of assistance, and several other factors. There is a category specifically for finding grants that would be of most relevance to seekers of support for research grants. There is also a CFDA User Guide that can be downloaded.

- *Foundation Center* (http://www .foundationcenter.org) collects, organizes, and communicates information on U.S. philanthropy; provides education and training on the grant seeking process; allows public access to information and services through its Web site, print, and electronic publications, library/ learning centers, and a national network of Cooperating Collections. Included on its Web site are general and specialized information retrieval tools.

- *Foundation Directory Online* (http://www.fconline.fdncenter.org), developed by the Foundation Center, is part of an online subscription set of databases that provides access to information on grant makers and their giving interests. Searches include text-based foundation searches, grant searches, and IRS 990 searches.(IRS 990 forms are the tax forms completed by foundations that contain information on awarded grants, including recipients and titles of projects funded, which could be very useful information to grant seekers.)

- *Sponsored Programs Information Network (SPIN)* (http://orsp .umich.edu/funding/databases.html) is a computer database containing information on grant opportunities from federal and private sponsoring agencies. The database is targeted primarily to institutions of higher education. InfoEd, the company that maintains the SPIN database, also offers an alert service called SMARTS, which sends E-mail messages whenever there is a match between the grantseeker's choice of keywords and the funding programs in the SPIN funding opportunities database.

- **Grants.Gov** (http://www.grants .gov), a central storehouse for information on grant programs offered by federal grant-making agencies, allows grantseekers to electronically find and apply for competitive grant opportunities from these federal agencies. Those interested in research grants can register for e-mail notification of grant opportunities; access, download, complete, and submit active grant application packages; and check the status of grant applications submitted via Grants.gov.

- **GrantSelect** (http://www.grant select.com) provides an extensive list of funding opportunities from state and federal government agencies (including NIH, NSF, CDC, and others), corporations, foundations, research institutes, and other nonprofit organizations. Grant seekers can subscribe to the entire research grants database or choose from customized segments, including Arts and Humanities, Biomedical and Health Care, Children and Youth, Community Development, International Programs, and others.

- **Guidestar** (http://www.guidestar .org) allows grant seekers to search for information on nonprofit organizations, including foundations. It provides general information as well as specifics, including foundations' current IRS Form 990, income range, contact information, mission, programs, goals, board of directors, grants awarded, and other relevant information.

- **Pivot** (formerly **Community of Science**) (http://pivot.cos.com)

is a resource for hard-to-find information critical to scientific research and other projects across all disciplines. It provides grant seekers the opportunity to search a very comprehensive resource for funding opportunities. It also contains prepopulated scholar profiles worldwide to match a given institution's profiles against funding opportunities and to find potential collaborators from among the scholar profiles.

- **Society of Research Administrators (SRA) International** (http:// www.srainternational.org/sra03/ grantsweb/index.cfm) is a source for finding funds available from local, state, federal, and international governments. It also contains information to locate private funding for projects, including links to foundations, nonprofit centers, charities, and others.

- **NIH RePORTER** (http://project reporter.nih.gov/reporter.cfm) contains a searchable database of NIH-funded intramural and extramural research projects, and provides access to publications and grants resulting from NIH funding.

- **GrantsNet** (http://www.hhs.gov/ grantsnet) is an Internet application tool created by the Department of Health and Human Services (HHS) for finding and exchanging information about HHS and other federal grant programs. In support of its mission, HHS is the largest grant-awarding agency in the federal government.

- **Ed.Gov** (http://www.ed.gov), the Web site of the U.S. Department of Education (ED), contains answers to frequently asked questions about funding opportunities; information on and instructions for completing grant application packages; application packages for ED grant competitions that are currently open; announcements of grant competitions; all programs and competitions under which ED has invited or expects to invite applications for new awards; deadlines for the submission of applications; and the Guide to ED Programs, which describes all programs administered by ED [including the National Institute on Disability and Rehabilitation Research (NIDRR)]. It also provides a search tool to find ED programs relevant to grantseekers' interests.

■ *National Science Foundation* (http://www.nsf.gov/index.jsp) is an independent federal agency created by Congress " . . . to promote the progress of science; to advance the national health, prosperity, and welfare; to secure the national defense . . . " It is the funding source for approximately 20% of all federally supported basic research conducted by U.S. colleges and universities. The Web site includes information about research projects that NSF has funded since 1989 by searching the Award Abstracts database. The information includes abstracts that describe the research as well as names of principal investigators and their institutions. The database includes both completed and current research projects.

■ *National Endowment for the Humanities* (http://www.neh .gov/grants) is an independent grantmaking agency of the U.S. government dedicated to supporting research, education, preserva-

tion, and public programs in the humanities. This Web site contains information on grant programs; application materials and guidelines; lists of NEH-supported projects by division and program; a procedure for matching a project to a specific NEH-sponsored grant program; information on how to apply for a grant; information on eligibility and preparing the grant application; deadline dates for grant applications; and the various grant programs that NEH offers.

■ *American Speech-Language-Hearing Association* (http:// www.asha.org) contains information on research grants offered by the American Speech-Language-Hearing Foundation (http://www .ashfoundation.org) and federal agencies (including the National Institutes of Health, Agency for Healthcare Research and Quality, Department of Education, National Science Foundation, Centers for Disease Control and Prevention, and U.S. Department of Veterans Affairs) as well as private foundations and organizations (http://www .asha.org/research/grants-funding/ Funding-for-Researchers.htm). Also included on this Web site is information and suggestions on the grants acquisition process, including grant seeking and grant proposal writing. A bimonthly subscription to the *ASHA Access Academics and Research E-Newsletter* (http:// www.asha.org/publications/enews/ accessacademics.htm), which serves the specific needs of researchers, including information, resources, services, educational opportunities, as well as funding, research, and grant opportunities, is available at this Web site.

- *American Academy of Audiology* (http://www.audiology.org) contains information on research grants offered by the American Academy of Audiology Foundation (http://www.audiology.org/about/foundation) to support research, education, and public awareness in audiology and hearing science, as well as other sources, including federal agencies, private foundations, and national organizations in hearing and balance. (www.audiology.org/education/research/funding/Pages/default.aspx)

- *American Hearing Research Foundation* (AHRF) (http://american-hearing.org) funds research in hearing and balance disorders. It awards an average of five to ten research projects per year, with an average grant of approximately $20,000. Priority is given to investigators early in their careers who need seed funds to generate results and data that can be used to support later applications for larger grants (e.g., NIH grants) in the future. The AHRF also gives two special grants: the Birtman Grant, and the Wiley H. Harrison, MD Grant. This site has links to a research grant application as well as a list of former recipients and their research topics from 1996 through the present.

- *Capita Foundation* (http://www.capitafoundation.org) is dedicated to the support of cutting-edge innovative auditory research worldwide. The majority of Capita Foundation grants fund early-stage research and projects by early-career research scientists, allowing them to produce the preliminary results needed to secure grants from the National Institutes of Health (NIH) and other major funders. Grant applications are welcomed from scientists conducting research in line with the Foundation's mission statement to "support innovative research that works toward the prevention and cure of hearing disorders."

- *Federal Grants & Contracts* (http://www.federalgrantsandcontracts.com/about.aspx) is a comprehensive biweekly review of the latest funding opportunities across all federal agencies. It covers relevant grant opportunities announced each week, provides information on upcoming grant initiatives, and offers news on standing cyclical grant competitions. It researches many online and print channels of federal information and resources, and provides specific information on scope, deadline, funds, eligibility, and contact needed to start the grant application process.

- *The Grantsmanship Center* (http://www.tgci.com) offers training programs which include information, resources, best approaches, tips, and insights to avoid trial-and-error learning. These training programs provide an overview of the entire proposal development process, highlighting the key elements that make proposals competitive. Also addressed is an understanding of federal application guidelines and designing a proposal development work plan. Other reference sources on research grants include the following directories. Information on their availability can be obtained via online searches (e.g., Google) as well as at other Web sites (e.g., Amazon.com):

- *Annual Register of Grant Support* is a directory of grant and fellowship programs of foundations, governmental agencies, as well as business, professional, and other organizations.
- *Directory of Biomedical and Health Care Grants* includes U.S. and international grant programs of governmental agencies, foundations, corporations, and professional organizations.
- *Directory of Research Grants* contains a listing of grant opportunities from federal agencies as well as U.S. and international foundations, corporations, government agencies, and other organizations. Included are grants for basic research, equipment, building construction/renovation, fellowships, and other program types.
- *Taft Foundation Reporter* provides comprehensive profiles and giving analyses of America's major private foundations in annual grants to nonprofit organizations.
- *Taft Corporate Giving Directory* contains information on corporate foundations and direct giving programs.

General Principles of Grant Seeking

The following are some general principles applicable to the grant seeking process:

- Search databases of existing grants from relevant funding agencies
- Know a funding agency's mission and what it wishes to fund
- Match an agency whose goals fit your research project

- Contact the contact person (program officer) to discuss your proposed project to determine its feasibility for support. Additional information on the grant seeking process is provided by Bauer (2003) and Hollis (2004).

Grant Proposal Writing

Preliminary Considerations

Once the grant seeking phase has been completed and the agency located as a potential funding source for the proposed research project, the next major step is to write the grant proposal. However, before the writing begins, there are some preliminary considerations:

1. Request an application from the sponsoring agency.
2. Carefully review the agency's guidelines (located in the application material) for the relevant grants program, which should contain the following important information:
   - suggested format for the proposal
   - any necessary appendices
   - deadline dates
   - any applicable cost-sharing requirements for the applicant
   - allowable indirect cost rates
   - criteria used to judge each proposal
   - relative weighting of each factor in the criteria.

The guidelines should be followed exactly as specified. If any of the above information is missing from the guidelines, or if there are questions about the guidelines, the sponsoring agency's contact person (whose name, E-mail and postal addresses, and telephone number are listed in the application material) should be contacted for clarifications.

The Grant Proposal

The grant proposal usually contains the following major sections:

Introduction

Problem Statement (Needs Assessment)

Objectives

Methodology

Budget

Writing a research grant proposal is somewhat similar to writing a manuscript for publication in a journal or a masters degree thesis or doctoral dissertation, because all include a review of the pertinent literature, a statement of purpose of the research, and a description of the methodology to study a proposed purpose or problem. However, since a research grant proposal is written before the proposed research is conducted, it includes a budget section requesting funds to conduct the research.

The Budget

The major categories of the budget usually include the following:

- *Personnel*—the people who will be working on the project, including the principal investigator and other personnel, as well as the amount of time they will be working on the project.

- *Fringe Benefits*—usually include social security, workmen's compensation, health insurance, unemployment compensation, and retirement plan. It is a percentage of the base salary of the people working on the project and will vary from institution to institution.
- *Travel*—funds to travel to professional meetings to present the findings of the research project and, depending on the nature of the research, may include funds to travel to collect data and other related research activities.
- *Equipment*—any necessary instrumentation to conduct the research. For most organizations, equipment is defined as any item with a unit acquisition cost of $5000.00 or more and a life span of two or more years.
- *Supplies*—needed supplies and materials.
- *Contractual*—any necessary contractual agreements with other agencies or individuals as part of the research project.
- *Other*—other items not covered in the previous six categories.
- *Total Direct Costs*—the sum of the seven budget categories listed above.
- *Indirect Costs*—expenditures not included directly in any of the budget categories listed above, such as the cost of heating/cooling; electricity; maintenance; security of facilities used for the research project; the processing of paperwork for purchases associated with the project; administrative costs; and other related expenses.
- *Total Project Costs*—the total cost of the research project, including all direct and indirect costs.

It should be noted that grant proposals need not include all seven budget categories listed above. Only budget items that can be justified because they relate directly to the methodology employed should be included in the proposed budget for the research project.

The Idea/Problem

A fundable proposal includes a good idea/problem that is expressed well and with an appropriate plan for implementation. The idea/problem for a research grant proposal should ask an important theoretical or applied question(s) capable of being systematically studied. A few questions to ask and answer about the idea/problem for a research study are:

- Is it important (re: discovery, improvement, or application of knowledge)?
- Is it timely?
- Is it capable of being investigated (re: the availability of personnel, expertise, techniques, instrumentation, facilities, etc.)?

Ideas/problems for a research project come from various sources, including the following:

- the applicant's previous experiences (e.g., teaching, research, clinical practice, administration, etc.);
- the applicant's literature reading and familiarity with the area of investigation;
- unresolved problems in the applicant's field of study;
- potential applications of previous research findings;
- priority areas for funding established by sponsoring agencies.

Unsolicited and Solicited Proposals

An *unsolicited proposal* is one that is written without any specific guidelines provided by a sponsoring agency and is not in response to a particular need or problem expressed by a sponsoring agency. Instead, it originates from a need perceived by the applicant who tries to find a sponsor to support the proposal. Unsolicited proposals have no specific deadline dates for submission and usually are accepted and reviewed by sponsoring agencies at any time rather than at specified dates each year.

Solicited proposals, on the other hand, originate with a sponsoring agency that recognizes a need for something to be done or learned. Solicited proposals usually are announced by a Request for Application (RFA) or Request for Proposal (RFP), which identifies problem areas and may include specific objectives to be met.

Basic Principles of Grant Proposal Writing

- The grant proposal should contain clear, concise writing, with definitions/explanations for all appropriate terms. (Grants will not be awarded for projects that are not understood by a sponsoring agency's reviewers.)
- All factual statements should be documented with cited references to support them.
- An objective and strong case for funding should be provided, with sufficient empirical evidence presented to support the investigator's position.

- The idea/problem for funding should be feasible, important, contemporary, and relevant.
- The methodology proposed should be well-designed for accomplishing the objectives of the project.
- The project personnel should be shown (via their vitae or resume) to be qualified to conduct the research.
- The budget should be realistic, containing only items that are relevant to the proposed project.
- A knowledge of grant application deficiencies is helpful. Some common deficiencies are: inadequate control of relevant variables; deficiency in methodology; research design problems; poor conceptualization of problem(s); and inappropriate statistical analyses.

Suggestions for Grant Proposal Writing

- Read and follow the sponsoring agency's guidelines.
- Begin writing early, well in advance of the submission deadline.
- Set a deadline to complete each section of the grant proposal.
- Define a focused, specific problem.
- Develop procedures to study the problem.
- Draft the body (narrative) of the proposal.
- Develop a realistic budget, with valid justifications for all items in the budget.
- Add any required additional components to the proposal (e.g., relevant assurance forms)
- Submit a draft of the proposal to colleagues for their review and comments.

- Revise the proposal based on colleagues' relevant comments/suggestions before submitting the finalized proposal.

Characteristics of a Fundable Research Grant Proposal

In summary, a fundable research grant proposal, one that should receive serious consideration for funding, should contain the following features:

- A clearly established need for the proposed research, preferably with supporting data.
- Clear objectives of the project.
- A detailed schedule of activities for the project, with realistic timelines.
- If relevant, commitment of all involved agencies/consultants verified with letters of commitment in the appendix.
- Any relevant cost-sharing included in the proposal.
- All budget items are justifiable and consistent with the proposed purpose and procedures of the research project. All budget explanations/justifications provide an adequate basis for the dollar figures used in the budget section.
- All major items included in the funding agency's guidelines are addressed in the proposal.
- All appropriate assurance forms are completed, indicating that all governmental requirements have been fulfilled.
- All sections of the proposal contain sufficient details and address all relevant issues.
- All directions in the funding agency's guidelines have been followed.

■ Appropriate appendixes have been included to provide evidence of careful planning of the research project.

■ The length of the proposal does not exceed the funding agency's guidelines.

■ The qualifications of project personnel are clearly indicated (via resumes, curriculum vitae, etc.) in the proposal.

■ The writing style is clear and concise.

Additional information on the writing of grant proposals (some of which include grantseeking as well as grant proposal writing) is provided by Carlson and O'Neal-McElrath (2008), Clarke and Fox (2006), Coley and Scheinberg (2008), Geever (2007), Gitlin and Lyons (2008), Grayson (2005), Henson (2004), Hollis (2004), Johnson (2011), Karsh and Fox (2009), Kiritz (1980), Miner and Miner (2005), Ogden and Goldberg (2002), Pequegnat, Stover, and Boyce (2011), Reif-Lehrer (2004), Smith and Works (2006), Ward (2012), Wason (2004), and Yang (2005), as well as online at the Web sites of various funding agencies (e.g., http://www.ninds.nih.gov/funding/write_grant_doc.htm).

The Grant Proposal Review Process

Although the specific process of reviewing research grant proposals may vary from one funding agency to another, there are some commonalities applicable to all reviews. Proposals usually are reviewed by the investigator's peers, generally colleagues at other institutions or laboratories who are knowledgeable about the topic of the proposal. Sponsoring agencies base their decisions about the awarding of grants on reviewers' comments. Usually, reviewers are required to follow specific criteria and use some type of rating scale established by the sponsoring agency to judge the merits of each proposal. Moreover, some agencies, like the National Institutes of Health (NIH), have a specific rating system for all proposals and a face-to-face meeting of a panel of peers to arrive at decisions for funding proposals. Additional information on the peer-review process can be found online at the Web sites of various funding agencies (e.g., http://www.drg.nih.gov/Video/Video.asp; http://www.csr.nih.gov; http://www.nsf.gov/pubs/gpg/nsf04_23/3.jsp).

Grant Management

Each grant usually has one principal investigator (project director) who is responsible for all activities and expenditures associated with the grant. Once a grant is awarded, there needs to be competent management of the funds because the grantee is held accountable for all expended funds. In addition, there are reporting requirements, frequently annual reports to the sponsoring agency delineating progress in research activities and fund expenditures. However, some agencies require more than an annual report. The award notification letter or an addendum to the letter should specify all reporting requirements.

Usually, funds awarded in a grant are specified and earmarked for particular budget categories (e.g., personnel, equipment, travel, etc.). However, on occasion, because of unexpected expenses or unexpected increases in approved budget items, there is a need to modify the existing approved budget. Most sponsoring agencies have an established rule of allowing the transfer of no more than a specific percentage of the entire budget from specific line items to other specific line items without the need for prior approval from the sponsoring agency. However, in cases that exceed this maximum percentage, the principal investigator must make a written request to transfer funds from one budget category to another and must receive approval in writing from the person at the sponsoring agency who is authorized to do so. In addition, the same is true for other necessary non-monetary changes in the research project: the principal investigator must make a request in writing and must receive approval in writing from the appropriate authorized representative of the sponsoring agency.

Thus, once a grant is awarded, the grantee's responsibilities begin. In addition to conducting the proposed research, the principal investigator is responsible for the expending of funds approved by the sponsoring agency (and in the amounts approved) as well as for any fiscal and programmatic reporting requirements.

Summary

Grants are essential for conducting research. The process of grants acquisition involves three phases: grant seeking, grant proposal writing, and grant management. Grant seeking is searching for funds from internal as well as external sources, including governmental agencies, private foundations, corporations, and national organizations. Grant proposal writing involves the preparation of a proposal that makes a strong case for financial support and follows the guidelines established by the sponsoring agency. Grant management involves conducting the research project and expending funds associated with the project as delineated in the grant proposal and approved by the sponsoring agency. In addition, it includes the preparation of fiscal and programmatic reports to the sponsoring agency. Detailed information and suggestions concerning each phase of the grants acquisition process are presented in this chapter.

DISCUSSION QUESTIONS

1. What are the three phases associated with the grants acquisition process?
2. What are some available online and hard copy reference sources for locating information on research grant opportunities from federal and private agencies?
3. What are some preliminary considerations in writing a research grant proposal?
4. What are the major sections of a research grant proposal?
5. What are the major categories in the budget section of a research grant proposal?
6. What is the difference between direct costs and indirect costs associated with a research grant?
7. What are some sources of ideas/problems for research projects?
8. List some basic principles of grant proposal writing.

9. List some suggestions for research grant proposal writing.
10. What are the characteristics of a fundable research grant proposal?
11. Who reviews research grant proposals and makes recommendations for funding?
12. What are the responsibilities of the principal investigator in the management of research grants?

STUDY EXERCISES

1. Locate 10 online (and/or hard copy) research grant references and prepare a brief summary of one entry from each reference. Select five sources of federal grants and five sources of foundation grants. Include in the summary the following:
   - title of the entry
   - a brief description of the funding program.

2. Obtain a grant application online or by contacting an appropriate federal agency (or obtain one from the sponsored programs office at your institution or agency). Read it thoroughly and indicate whether or not each of the following items is included in the application:
   - legislation relevant to the federal agency's research grants program
   - eligibility requirements for grantees
   - priorities (topics/areas) for funding for a particular fiscal year
   - restrictions (if any) on topics/areas to be funded
   - amount of funds available for grant awards for a particular fiscal year
   - maximum dollar amount (or range) to be awarded per grant
   - cost-sharing requirements (if any)
   - indirect cost rate restrictions (if any)
   - cover page and instructions for completion
   - budget sheets and instructions for completion
   - assurance forms and instructions for completion
   - instructions for completion of narrative section of grant application
   - page limitations for narrative section of grant application
   - deadline date(s) for submission of grant application
   - criteria to be used to judge each grant proposal for funding, including any relative weighting of each criterion
   - any necessary appendixes
   - name, E-mail address, and telephone number of contact person.

3. Read two funded grant proposals, one by a governmental agency and one by a foundation (these may be obtained from your institution or agency or else contact the sponsoring agency) and prepare a brief abstract of each proposal.

Include in the abstract the following information:
- title of proposal
- agency to which submitted
- purpose/objectives
- methodology
- budget summary.

References

Bauer, D. G. (2003). *The "How To" grants manual: Successful grantseeking techniques for obtaining public and private grants* (5th ed.). Westport, CT: Praeger.

Carlson, M., O'Neal-McElrath, T., & The Alliance for Nonprofit Management (2008). *Winning grants step by step* (3rd ed.). San Francisco, CA: Jossey-Bass Nonprofit Guidebook Series.

Clarke, C. A., & Fox, S. P. (2006). *Grant proposal makeover: Transform your request from no to yes.* San Francisco, CA: Jossey-Bass.

Coley, S. M., & Scheinberg, C. A. (2008). *Proposal writing: Effective grantsmanship* (3rd ed.). Thousand Oaks, CA: Sage.

Geever, J. C. (2007). *The Foundation Center's guide to proposal writing* (5th ed.). New York, NY: The Foundation Center.

Gitlin, L. N., & J. Lyons, K. J. (2008). *Successful grant writing: Strategies for health and human service professionals* (3rd ed.). New York, NY: Springer.

Grayson, H. M. (2005). *Guide to government grants writing: Tools for success.* Lincoln, NE: iUniverse.

Henson, K. (2004). *Grant writing in higher education: A step-by-step guide.* Old Tappan, NJ: Pearson Education.

Hollis, A. (2004). *Everything you need to know about grants: How to write the grant—how to get the grant—where to get the grant.* New York, NY: iUniverse.

Johnson, V. (2011). *Grant writing 101: Everything you need to start raising funds today.* New York, NY: McGraw-Hill.

Karsh, E., & Fox, A. S. (2009). *The only grantwriting book you'll ever need* (3rd ed.). New York, NY: Basic Books.

Kiritz, N. J. (1980). *Program planning and proposal writing* (Reprint). Los Angeles, CA: Grantsmanship Center.

Miner, J. T., & Miner, L. E. (2005). *Models of proposal planning and writing.* Westport, CT: Praeger/Greenwood.

Ogden, T. E., & Goldberg, I. A. (Eds.). (2002). *Research proposals: A guide to success* (3rd ed.). San Diego, CA: Academic Press.

Pequegnat, W., Stover, E., & Boyce, C.A. (Eds.). (2011). *How to write a successful research grant application: A guide for social and behavioral scientists* (2nd ed.). New York, NY: Springer.

Reif-Lehrer, L. (2004). *Grant application writers handbook* (4th ed.). Burlington, MA: Jones & Bartlett.

Smith, N. B., & Works, E. G. (2006). *The complete book of grant writing: Learn to write grants like a professional.* Naperville, IL: Sourcebooks.

Ward, D. (2012). *Writing grant proposals that win* (4th ed.). Burlington, MA: Jones & Bartlett.

Wason, S. D. (2004). *Webster's new world grant writing handbook.* Hoboken, NJ: Wiley.

Yang, O. O. (2005). *Guide to effective grant writing: How to write an effective NIH grant application.* New York, NY: Kluwer Academic/Plenum.

Glossary

A-B design: single-case design with two phases: A represents the baseline phase, and B represents the intervention phase.

A-B-A design: a single-case withdrawal design in which a second baseline phase is introduced.

Abstract: brief description of a paper, usually located at the beginning of an article.

Applied research: research that seeks to answer practical questions such as those pertaining to prevention and management of communication disorders; also known as clinical research.

Assurance forms: standardized forms completed by the applicant agency to assure the funding agency that the applicant agency meets all requirements to qualify for funding.

Baseline measure: measurement of dependent variable before experimental intervention.

Basic research: research that is often theoretical; designed to seek answers that explain and/or predict phenomena.

Between-subject design: design that uses two groups of subjects, each group assigned to a different level of the independent variable.

Bias: any influence that affects results.

Bivariate statistics: test used to analyze significance of the relationship between two variables simultaneously, for example, correlation.

Blinding: process of preventing those involved in a study (subjects, clinicians, data collectors) from having information that could bias. Same as masking.

CADE: critically appraised topic of diagnostic evidence.

CAPE: checklist for appraising patient/practice evidence.

CAPP: checklist for appraising evidence on patient preference.

CASM: critical appraisal of systematic review or meta-analysis.

CATE: critical appraisal of treatment evidence.

Case-control studies: when individuals are selected whether they have a particular disorder or not.

Case study research: intensive study of the background, current status, or environmental interactions of an individual, group, institution, or community.

Charge master: a spreadsheet that is part of the budgetary process and includes all expenses related to the implementation of a research study.

Class I level of evidence: the highest level of evidence provided by at least one well-designed, randomized controlled clinical trial.

Class II level of evidence: evidence provided by at least one or better designed observational, clinical studies with concurrent controls, that is, single case control or cohort control studies.

Class III level of evidence: the lowest level of evidence; provided by expert opinion, case studies, case reports, and studies with historical controls.

Clinical practice guidelines: literature review usually a consensus by a group of experts for use in making clinical decisions. Three types: traditional clinical practice guidelines, systematic reviews, and evidence-based clinical practice guidelines.

Clinical research: research designed to generate knowledge to guide the clinical practice in speech-language pathology and audiology; also known as applied research.

Clinical trial: study designed to investigate outcome.

Cohort study: follows the temporal sequence of factors that may have impacted the development of a disorder.

Complementary design: the result of the dominant research method being enhanced or clarified by results from the findings of the other type of research.

Complex hypothesis: the hypothesis contains more than one independent and dependent variable.

Concept maps: require selecting important relevant concepts to add to the map and identifying salient cross-links; and indicating relationships between concepts in different sections of the map.

Confidence interval: an inferential statistic for estimating range of values within which a population parameter lies.

Confirmability: refers to sharing findings with participants by informant checks or feedback sessions to confirm view of the person being studied.

Conflict of commitment: conflicting demands on professionals who have obligations to their patients and to others including students and other professionals.

Conflict of interest: situations where personal and/or financial considerations compromise judgment in any professional activity.

Consent process: involves meeting with a potential subject, finding out whether he or she is capable of giving consent, and discussing the purpose, risks, and benefits of participation.

Constant variable: variables that describe the population investigated by a study; variables that do not change from individual to individual (such as a diagnosis of stuttering).

Construct validity: the extent to which a test or questionnaire measures what it is supposed to measure.

Content validity: a logical examination of all behaviors that need to be measured in order to adequately answer the question.

Continuous variable: a quantitative variable that can theoretically take on values along a continuum.

Control group: a group that does not receive treatment; equivalent to the experimental group in age, sex, and so on.

Convenience sampling: using the most readily available persons as participants, sometimes called accidental sampling.

Coordinated substudies: qualitative studies that are part of a larger program project or long-term study.

Correlation: tendency for variation in one variable to be related to variation in another variable; an interrelation between two or more variables.

Correlation coefficient: a measure of the direction and strength of the relationship between variables usually ranging from +1.00 (perfect positive) through zero (no relationship) to −1.00 (perfect negative) relationships.

Correlational research: used to determine possible relationships among factors.

Cost-benefit analysis: an evaluation comparing financial costs with financial gains attributed to a program or intervention.

Cost-sharing requirements: expenses associated with a grant that are to be incurred by the applicant agency to share the expense of the research project with the funding agency.

Cover letter: typically includes the purpose, conveys appreciation to the participant, states that the survey has been approved by the appropriate committee or advisor, and offers to provide a summary of the results.

Credibility: the extent to which data are believable and trustworthy, that is, confidence in the truth of the data.

Criterion-related (predictive) validity: the measure of an attribute to predict future performance.

Critical Appraisal Topic/Paper (CAT/CAP): a summary of a critical review of the best evidence on a specific topic; a written outcome of the evidence-based practice (EBP) process.

Cross-sectional research: involves selecting subjects from various age groups and observing differences between the behavior and characteristics of the group.

Database: information accessed by using electronic hardware.

Deception: deliberate withholding of information or misinformation

Dependability: the qualitative equivalent to reliability of quantitative research.

Dependent variable: variable that is the effect of unknown etiology(ies) and must be described in operational terms.

Descriptive research: designed to systemically describe situations or events as they naturally occur, in other words, the status of phenomena of interest as they currently exist.

Descriptive statistics: procedures for describing and analyzing quantitative data.

Design: the structure of a study organized for the purpose of revealing cause-and-effect relationships by controlling variables, comparing groups, or analyzing specific characteristics of individuals or groups.

Direct costs: expenses related to personnel, fringe benefits, travel, equipment, supplies, and contractual matters.

Directional hypothesis: when a researcher states there will be a change or describes a relationship in a certain direction (i.e., high or low; positive or negative; etc.).

Discrete variable: a variable that can only be measured in separate units and that cannot be measured in intervals less than 1.

Dissertation: research project/paper typically associated with a doctoral degree.

Double-blind studies: a study in which the investigator and the subject do not know group assignment.

Editing analysis: involves interpretation of the data on which categorization is used for coding, sorting, and organizing the data.

Effect size: a statistical expression of the magnitude of difference between two treatments or the magnitude of a relationship between two variables.

Effectiveness: in research is defined as the benefits and use of the procedure under "real world" conditions.

Efficacy: in research is the benefit of an intervention plan as compared to a control or standard program.

Evaluation research: the collection and analysis of information related to the effects of a program, policy, or procedure.

Evidence-based practice: such practice increases professionalism, accountability to clients and other professionals, and the social relevance of the health services delivered in an economy with increased costs and decreased resources; utilization of the best available research to make clinical decisions about patient care.

Expansion design: involves using different methods for different components for a multimethod research project.

Experimental research: examines possible cause-and-effect relationships by exposing one or more experimental groups to one or more conditions and comparing the results to one or more control groups.

Experimental treatment: utilizes the principles of experimental research investigating the use of new or novel treatment.

Exploded pie chart: emphasizes the proportion of time devoted to a topic or area that is displayed in a pie chart.

Exploratory research: examines how one event or events relate to other factors.

External validity: degree results of a study can be generalized to persons or settings outside the experimental situation.

Extramural funding: funding for research projects provided by agencies outside the researcher's institution.

Extraneous variable: a variable that confounds the relationship between the independent and dependent variable.

Extrinsic variables: variables associated with the research situation or environment; related to the place and time the research was conducted and adherence (or not) to the research specification or protocols.

Fabrication: making up data or results and recording or reporting data for experiments never conducted.

Factorial designs: manipulating two or more independent variables; one group in the design accounts for each possible combination of the levels of the independent variables.

Feasibility test: a researcher reviews factors that could influence the possibility of a study being conducted.

Fidelity: maintaining integrity in use of test or treatment.

Focus groups: a method of interviewing a group of individuals about a specific topic or issue.

Foundation: a nongovernmental, nonprofit organization whose funds and programs are managed by its own trustees or directors and established to maintain or aid educational, charitable, or other activities serving the common welfare, primarily through the awarding of grants.

Frequency polygon: a graphic display of a frequency distribution; created by drawing a straight line between the success midpoints of class intervals.

Fringe benefits: an item in the budget section of a grant proposal that usually includes social security, workmen's compensation, health insurance, unemployment compensation, and a retirement plan. It is a percentage of the base salary of personnel on a funded research project and will vary from institution to institution.

Ghost authorship: failure to name as an author an individual who has made substantial contribution that merits authorship or an unnamed individual who participated in writing the manuscript; also known as honorary authorship.

Gold standard: An instrument that is considered a valid measure and that can be used as the standard for assessing validity of other instruments.

Grant seeking: the process involved in searching for a source of funding for a specific research project, thus matching the nature of the topic with the objectives of the support source.

Grants acquisition process: the process for securing a funding source that involves three phases: grant seeking, grant proposal writing, and grant management.

Group designs: design involving comparison of average or typical performance of a group to other groups or conditions; includes between-subject designs, within-subject designs, and mixed group designs.

Health Insurance Portability and Accountability Act of 1996 (HIPAA, Title II): required the Department of Health and Human Services (HHS) to establish national standards for electronic health care transactions and national identifiers for providers, health plans, and employers. It also addresses the security and privacy of health data.

Histogram (graph): graphic display of frequency distribution data in which scores (often in group intervals) are plotted on the x-axis and frequency (or percent of cases) is plotted on the y-axis.

Historical research: sometimes referred to as archival or library research, it is a type of research aimed at establishing facts and relationship about past events.

Hyperclarity: suggesting that research is likely to achieve what it is unlikely to achieve.

Hypothesis: statement concerning the relationship between variables; formulated to test theories.

Immersion method: a form of qualitative data analysis that involves total immersion in the problem; considered to be an insider's perspective.

Impact evaluation: to determine whether a program should be discontinued, replaced, modified, continued, or replicated.

Independent variable: variable with known qualities that explains the dependent variable; may be manipulated to determine effect on dependent variable.

Indirect costs: costs such as heating/cooling, electricity, maintenance, security, and administrative costs.

Inferential statistics: statistics used to test hypotheses by drawing inferences or generalizations from small groups to larger groups.

Informed consent: requires obtaining the consent of the individual to participate in a study based on full prior disclosure of risks and benefits.

Institutional Review Board (IRB): a group of diverse individuals who review research proposals to protect human and animal subjects through analysis of risks and benefits.

Interaction effect: combined effect of two or more independent variables on a dependent variable.

Interexaminers reliability: implies agreement among different observers measuring the same phenomenon.

Internal estimation: a statistic that indicates the upper and lower limits of a range of values in which the parameter has a given probability of occurring.

Internal validity: degree of relationship between independent and dependent variables is free from the impact of extraneous/confounding variables.

Interquartile range: difference between the first and third quartiles in a distribution.

Interval scale: level of measurement in which values have equal intervals, but no true zero point.

Interview: a form of data collection in which questions are asked orally and participants' responses are recorded; may be structured, semistructured, or unstructured.

Intraexaminer reliability: implies that in repeated observations of the same subject, the same examiner gets similar results.

Intramural funding: in-house funds used to support research projects.

Intrinsic variables: variables associated with subjects of an investigation such as age, gender, socioeconomic status, and marital status.

Level of significance: significance level selected to reject the null hypothesis established before statistical analysis to reduce the risk of making a Type I or Type II error; also known as limit of confidence.

Longitudinal research: the same group of subjects is followed over time; sometimes known as cohort study, follow-up study, incidence study, or perspective study.

Main effect: separate effect of one independent variable in a multifactor design.

Mañana syndrome: procrastination; frequently results in missing deadlines.

Mean: simple arithmetic average.

Measures of central tendency: measures representing the average or typical score in a distribution (mean, median, mode).

Median: a statistic describing the central tendency of scores in an ordinal scale; the midpoint in a set of values (same number of values as above and below the median).

Meta-analysis: a technique for quantitatively combining results of several studies on a given topic.

Mixed group design: combines within-subjects and between-subjects designs to investigate effects of treatment for which carryover effects would be a problem while repeatedly sampling the behavior.

Mode: the most frequently occurring value in a distribution.

Multifactor baseline designs: include more than one independent variable and require that different combinations of the independent variable be tested across the study.

Multimethod or mixed research: combines both quantitative (outcome) and qualitative (process) features in the design, data collection, and analysis.

Multivariate designs: two or more dependent variables; provides information about the effect of the independent variable on each dependent variable and on a composite dependent variable.

Multivariate statistics: statistical procedures used to study the relationships between three or more variables.

Narrative review: nonsystematic review of the literature that synthesizes particular topics of interest; also known as a "review of the literature" in most research proposals.

Nested design: a variation of the mixed group design that involves more than one task for each level of the independent variable.

Nominal scale: level of measurement for classification variables; values are assigned based on mutually exclusive and exhaustive categories with no inherent rank order.

Nonequivalent groups posttest-only design: a comparison between an experimental and control group both of whom are tested after treatment and not before treatment.

Nonexperimental research: descriptive (nonstatistical) organization of data; or ex post facto research.

Nonparametric statistics: a type of inferential statistics that does not involve vigorous assumptions about the parameters of the population from which the sample was drawn; used for nominal and ordinal measures.

Normal distribution: symmetric graphic display of the numerical values.

Null hypothesis: statement that there is no relationship between variables under study.

Online: data that are accessed by the user who interacts directly with the electronic program to retrieve desired information.

One-group postdesign: a type of preexperimental design; involves study of the presumed effect of an independent variable in one group of subjects by administering a posttest after some treatment.

One-tailed (directional) test: a test of statistical significance in which only values at one extreme (tail) of a distribution are considered in testing significance.

Ordinal scale: level of measurement in which scores are ranked.

Outliers: scores that are outside the range of most scores.

Parallel designs: involve qualitative methods such as case studies, focused ethnographic observation, multiple linked in-depth interviews, or some combination of time in combination with other methods.

Parameter estimation: used to estimate a single parameter such as a mean.

Parametric statistics: a type of inferential statistics that involves making assumptions about the parameters of the population from which the research sample was drawn; used for interval measures.

Participant observer: when the researcher is an active participant in the activity being studied, that is, the researcher participates as a member of the group and is not known as the researcher.

Passive participant: is detached from the group being studied and is known as the researcher.

Peer review: the process by which the quality of research is assessed; involves multiple activities.

PESICO: framework for asking question. P = person or problem, E = environments, S = stakeholder, I = intervention, C = comparison, O = outcome.

PICO: P = patient/population, I = intervention/treatment/exposure, C = comparison, and O = outcome; a method used in evidence-based practice/research.

Pie charts: used to represent the proportion of data falling into certain categories in the form of a circle containing segments that are also called slices, sections, or wedges.

Plagiarism: use of another person's ideas, processes, results, or words without giving appropriate credit.

Predictive value: the degree to which a test or instrument can determine an outcome.

Predictive value negative (PV−): the probability that a person does not have a problem, given that the test result is negative.

Predictive value positive (PV+): the probability that a person has a problem, given the test result is positive.

Pre-experimental designs: sometimes referred to as pseudoexperimental designs because they do not meet at least two of the three criteria for true experiments: randomization; manipulation; or control.

Principal investigator (PI): the project director of a research grant who is responsible for all expenditures and programmatic issues associated with the grant.

Priorities: topics/areas for research support that have been established by a funding agency for a particular fiscal year.

Point estimation: calculated by dividing the observed values from the sample by the size of the sample.

Power: the probability of a statistical test to reject the null hypothesis when in fact it is false.

Primary source: firsthand data that the researcher obtains directly from the source.

Prospective study: researcher contacts the subjects before they develop the disorder, but after exposure to risk factors.

Protected health information: related to HIPAA privacy rule about individual's past, present and future health conditions, treatment for conditions and financial history related to health care.

Qualitative research: research designed to investigate real-life events or situations without reference to hypothesis or theory, allowing researchers' subjective point of view; also known as field research, hermeneutic, naturalistic inquiry, phenomenological research, symbolic interactionism, descriptive research, interpretive research, and ethnographic study.

Quantitative research: research that generates data capable of being organized in graphs and descriptive statistical forms; stresses numbers, measurement, deductive logic, control, and experiments.

Quantitative or statistical analysis: the organization and integration of quantitative data according to systematic mathematical rules and procedures.

Quasiexperimental research: like experimental research, involves manipulation of an independent variable but does not have a comparison group or randomization; also known as preexperimental and pseudoexperimental.

Quasistatistical analysis: involves preconceived ideas about the analysis that has been specified in a code book, and then using these ideas (codes) to sort the data; also known as manifest analysis.

Randomization: a method of selecting subjects that ensures that everyone in the population has an equal chance of being included in the study.

Randomized control trial (RCT): involves the experimental group receiving the variable of interest and the control group not receiving any form of treatment; also known as the "gold standard" for clinical research.

Publish or perish: academic requirement of publishing to obtain or maintain position or be promoted.

Range: distance between the lowest and highest value in a distribution.

Ratio scale: The highest level of measurement, in which there are equal intervals between score units and a true zero point.

Reliability: repeatability, consistency among repeated measures or observations.

Research hypothesis: the question being asked by an investigator; sometimes known as the working hypothesis.

Research utilization: the application of some aspect of research to clinical practice.

Retrospective study: researcher determines subjects have already been exposed to risk factors.

Risk-benefit: comparison of relative cost and benefit.

Scales of measurement: a means of assigning numbers to events or objects according to prescribed rules. Nominal, ordinal interval or ratio.

Scatter plot: a graphic display of the relationship between two variables; also know as scatter diagram or scattergram.

Scientific approach: a systematic, empirical, controlled, and critical examination of hypothetical propositions about the association among natural phenomena.

Scientific method: a method of efficiently or methodically generating knowledge by recognizing a problem capable of objective study, collecting data by observation or experimentation, and drawing conclusions based on analysis of the data.

Secondary analysis: involves research that uses previously gathered data; examining unanalyzed variables, testing unexplored relationships, focusing on a specific subsample, or changing the unit of analysis.

Secondary sources: secondhand documentation based on what is seen or heard by someone else, or a summary of primary information.

Seed money: funds provided by colleges and universities to support research in the form of relatively small grants for starting new research projects in the hope that this intramural support will help secure extramural funding.

Self-plagiarism: involves duplicate submission or publication: duplicate/previous submission means that the manuscript is simultaneously being considered for publication elsewhere.

Self-reports: a method of collecting data that involves a direct report of information by the person being studied.

Semilongitudinal approach: compromise designed to maximize the strengths and minimize the weaknesses of the cross-sectional and longitudinal approaches; selecting subjects at the low end of designated age spans and following them until they reach the upper limits of that age span.

Semistructured observation: a method used in qualitative research that is more concerned with some aspects of the situation for the participants than others.

Sensitivity: a measure of validity based on the probability that someone with a disease or condition will test positive.

Sequential clinical trials (SCTs): does not require a fixed sample size before the study can begin; can be used to compare two treatments such as an "old" or standard treatment to a "new" experimental treatment.

Simple hypothesis: the hypothesis includes one independent variable and one dependent variable.

Single-blind studies: a study in which only the investigator does not know the assignment of a subject to a group.

Single or one group pretest-posttest design: compares pretest and posttest data subsequent to treatment.

Single-subject discrete trial designs: individual subjects receive each treatment condition of the experiment dozens of times.

Single-subject research: focuses on the behavior of one or a few subjects; applied behavioral analysis designs or behavioral analysis; idiographic designs; single-subject experimental designs; single-case designs; intrasubject replication designs; small approach; and within-subjects designs.

Snowball sampling: selection of participants by nomination or referral from earlier participants in a study.

Solicited proposals: grant proposals that originate with a sponsoring (funding) agency that recognizes a need for something to be done or learned; usually are announced by a Request for Application (RFA) or Request for Proposal (RFP), which identifies problem areas and sometimes includes specific objectives to be met.

Specificity: a measure of validity of a procedure based on the probability that a person who does not have a disease will test negative.

Standard deviation: a variability measure of the degree to which each value deviates from the mean.

Statistic: a number derived by counting or measuring sample observations drawn from a population that is used in estimating a population parameter.

Statistical Package for Social Sciences® (SPSS): statistical program used in behavioral and social sciences published by Prentice-Hall, a division of Pearson Education, Inc.; can be used for qualitative and quantitative research analyses.

Structured observation: a method used in qualitative research; what to observe is decided in advance and there is an observational schedule.

Sum of squares: a measure of variability in a set of data, equal to the sum of squared deviations for a distribution; used in analysis of variance as the basis for partitioning between-groups and within-groups variance components.

Survey research: designed to provide a detailed inspection of the prevalence of conditions, practices, or attitudes in a given environment by asking people about them rather than observing them directly.

Synthesis: collecting, analyzing and integrating information.

Systematic review: a summary of the evidence typically conducted by an expert or expert panel that uses a rigorous process for identifying, appraising, and synthesizing studies to answer a particular question or draw a conclusion.

Template analysis: involves the development of a template or analysis guide to sort the data.

Test-retest reliability: how well subjects perform on one set of measurements as compared to their performance on a second evaluation of the same measurements.

Theoretical sampling: selection of participants based on emerging findings as the study progresses so adequate representation of important themes is ensured; also known as purposeful sampling.

Thesis: research project/paper typically associated with a master's degree.

Time series design: involves repeated measures before and after treatment using the same instruments with the same or similar subjects over an extended period of time.

Total project cost: total cost of a research project, including all direct and indirect costs.

Transferability: the extent to which findings from a qualitative study can be transferred to similar circumstances.

Treatment outcome: a broadly defined term that refers to change, or the lack of it, that may occur as a result of time, treatment, or both.

Trend chart: illustrates frequencies or percentages of change in a data set which is organized in a developmental or temporal order.

Triangulated designs: both quantitative and qualitative methods are used to study the same entity or concept with a focus on convergence (similarities) and increased validity.

Triangulation: refers to the use of multiple methods to improve the credibility of findings or the truth and it may involve comparison of data from different sources or analyses to reduce or eliminate bias and errors.

True experimental design: characterized by manipulation (treatment or intervention), randomizations, and use of a control group.

Two-tailed test: test of a hypothesis using both ends of the distribution to determine a range of improbable values.

Type I error: incorrectly rejecting the null hypothesis.

Type II error: incorrectly accepting the null hypothesis.

Unsolicited proposals: grant proposals written without any guidelines provided by a sponsoring (funding) agency and are not in response to a particular need or problem expressed by the agency; originate from a need perceived by the applicant who tries to find a sponsor to support the proposal.

Unstructured observation: a method used in qualitative research when there is no attempt to manipulate the situation.

V diagrams: used to diagram the components of knowledge and clarify their relationships.

Variable: a trait capable of change or modification.

Variance: a measure of variability equal to the square of the standard deviation.

Within-subjects designs: a design in which every subject in the experiment is exposed to all the experimental conditions.

Index

Note: Page numbers in **bold** reference non-text material.